Clinical Clerkship Manual

Edited by
Larry E. Boh
Associate Professor (CHS)
Chair, Pharmacy Practice Division
School of Pharmacy
University of Wisconsin
Madison

Applied Therapeutics, Inc., Vancouver, Washington 98682

Printing and Binding: Delta Lithograph Co., Valencia, CA
Typesetting: Impressions, Madison, WI
Cover Design: Steven B. Naught

Applied Therapeutics, Inc.
P.O. Box 5077
Vancouver, Washington 98668-5077
(206) 253-7123

ISBN: 0-915486- 17- 2

First Printing November 1992

CONTENTS

Contributing Authors

Susan Lynn Bathke, B.S.
Consultant Pharmacist
Pharmacy Plus Dimondale
St. Lawrence Hospital
Lansing, Michigan

Marilyn G. Bufton, Pharm.D.
Assistant Director of Clinical Services
St. Joseph Hospital
Bellingham, Washington

Robert M. Breslow, B. S.
Clinical Instructor/Clinical Pharmacist
Department of Pharmacy
School of Pharmacy
University of Wisconsin
Madison, Wisconsin

Larry E. Boh, M.S.
Associate Professor (CHS)
Chair, Pharmacy Practice Division
School of Pharmacy
University of Wisconsin
Madison, Wisconsin

Linda M. Calkins, B. S.
Pharmacist Arizona Cancer Center
Department of Pharmacy
University Medical Center
Tucson, Arizona

Bill R. Check, B. S.
Senior Clinical Pharmacist and Clinical Instructor
Department of Pharmacy
School of Pharmacy
University of Wisconsin Hospital and Clinics
Madison, Wisconsin

Richard Carl Christopherson, B. S.
Senior Clinical Pharmacist and Clinical Instructor
Department of Pharmacy
School of Pharmacy
University of Wisconsin Hospital and Clinics
Madison, Wisconsin

Steven C. Ebert, Pharm.D.
Clinical Specialist in Infectious Diseases/Pharmacokinetics
Department of Pharmacy
Meriter Hospital
Clinical Assistant Professor
Department of Pharmacy
School of Pharmacy
University of Wisconsin
Madison, Wisconsin

Kathryn L. Grant, Pharm.D.
Director, Drug and Poison Information
Clinical Instructor
Department of Pharmacy
School of Pharmacy
University of Wisconsin Hospital and Clinics
Madison, Wisconsin

Lucy Schneller Hazebrook, M.S.
Assistant Director/Clinical Instructor
Department of Pharmacy
School of Pharmacy
University of Wisconsin Hospital and Clinics
Madison, Wisconsin

Randolf William Hurley, M.D.
Instructor, Introduction to Clinical Medicine
Department of Medicine
University of Wisconsin Medical School
Madison, Wisconsin

Kristin Krumbiegel Hanson, M.S.
Assistant Director
Clinical Pharmacy Services
Froedtert Memorial Lutheran Hospital
Milwaukee, Wisconsin

Michael Madalon, B. S.
Senior Clinical Pharmacist and Clinical Instructor
Department of Pharmacy
School of Pharmacy
University of Wisconsin Hospital and Clinics
Madison, Wisconsin

Cheryl A. Ray, B. S.
Clinical Pharmacist/Clinical Instructor
Department of Pharmacy
School of Pharmacy
University of Wisconsin Hospital and Clinics
Madison, Wisconsin

Mary E. Swandby, B. S.
Senior Clinical Pharmacist/Clinical Instructor
Department of Pharmacy
School of Pharmacy
University of Wisconsin Hospital and Clinics
Madison, Wisconsin

Karen E. Vick, M.S.
Investigational Drug Pharmacist
Department of Pharmacy
Milwaukee County Medical Complex
Milwaukee, Wisconsin

David A. Wegner, B. S.
Senior Clinical Pharmacist and Clinical Instructor
Department of Pharmacy
School of Pharmacy
University of Wisconsin Hospital and Clinics
Madison, Wisconsin

Timothy D. Wolf, Pharm.D.
Clinical Pharmacist and Clinical Instructor
Department of Pharmacy
School of Pharmacy
University of Wisconsin Hospital and Clinics
Madison, Wisconsin

Acknowledgments

My sincere appreciation to the contributing authors for their outstanding contributions, dedication and commitment to Clinical Clerkship Manual and to their families and friends who sacrificed evenings and weekends to meet the numerous deadlines over the past several years. A special thanks to the Section Coordinators for their extraordinary effort in reviewing and coordinating the works of the individual contributors; the Contributors/Reviewers for sharing their experience and knowledge helping to make this a unique and practical resource. I am gratefully indebted to the decentral clinical pharmacists/clinical instructors at the University of Wisconsin Hospital and Clinics (UWHC) for their constructive input and feedback to the individual authors. To Tom Thielke, Pam Ploetz, and the assistant directors at UWHC, a special thank you for your never-ending encouragement and support of a project in which we all so strongly believe.

Special recognition to Ms. Audrey Fish for her countless hours of formatting and typing the original manuscripts and endless patience when changes were required.

To Linda Young, Nannette Naught, Lloyd Y. Young, Mary Anne Koda-Kimble, and other members of the Applied Therapeutics staff, my deepest gratitude for your continued interest and encouragement. Your support, good humor, smoked salmon, and countless days, nights, and weekends toward making this publication a reality are truly appreciated.

To our students, thank you for your constant quest for knowledge and reminding us that we can learn from each other and that there is a student in all of us.

Finally, to my wife Dawn and daughters Kimberly and Andrea, thank you for your love and endless patience but mostly for your understanding and support.

Notice to Reader

Drug therapy information is constantly evolving. Our ever-changing knowledge and experience with drugs and the continual development of new drugs necessitates changes in treatment and drug therapy. The editors, authors, and the publisher of this work have made every effort to ensure the information provided herein was accurate at the time of publication. *It remains the responsibility of every practitioner to evaluate the appropriateness of a particular opinion or therapy in the context of the actual clinical situation and with due consideration of any new developments in the field.* Although the authors have been careful to recommend dosages that are in agreement with current standards and responsible literature, we recommend the student or practitioner consult several appropriate information sources when dealing with new and unfamiliar drugs.

Preface

The traditional practice of pharmacy has evolved over the past three decades from a practice primarily focusing on the preparation of medications to a practice primarily emphasizing rational pharmacotherapeutics. The selection of the most appropriate medication, regimen, and dose while minimizing problems such as drug interactions, adverse drug reactions, and IV incompatibilities become central to this new patient focused approach. This transition was assisted by the initiation of introductory clinical clerkships which place pharmacy students in patient care areas alongside medical students, physicians, residents, and other health care providers. Unfortunately, these students often were immediately overwhelmed by the volume of medical information, terminology, jargon and procedures that were perhaps minimally understood.

In each university, busy clinical faculty developed various educational tools to assist their students during this mentoring process. A course workbook, supplemented by various reading assignments, was usually made available on the first day of instruction and students were instructed to review these materials. Although the clerkship syllabus at each university was created specifically to meet the needs of its own students, a review of syllabi from various programs noted considerable common similarities. Introductions to laboratory tests, medical procedures, medical abbreviations, and pharmacokinetics all seemed to be covered despite marked differences in these introductory clinical clerkships.

This **Clinical Clerkship Manual (CCM)** was developed by the University of Wisconsin clinical preceptors and faculty over several years to provide the novice clinical practitioner with a reference source during the first few weeks of an introductory clerkship. This clerkship manual was well received by our students because it helped alleviate some of their anxiety and uncertainty during this challenging and exciting time. It also served to establish a clear code of conduct for our students and clearly stated expectations for their responsibilities to their patients.

This **Clinical Clerkship Manual** should meet many of the core needs of most introductory clinical clerkships. Although clinical faculty may need to supplement this manual with additional materials for specialized clerkship rotations, this CCM should serve the needs of students from other universities as well as it has the University of Wisconsin.

Since this is the first edition of the **Clinical Clerkship Manual,** comments concerning its usefulness and suggestions for revisions would be gratefully appreciated.

Larry E. Boh
October 1992

Clinical Clerkship Manual

Goals, Objectives, and Activities

Larry E. Boh

Kristin Krumbiegal Hanson

As the pharmacy profession has moved from the traditional product orientation to a patient orientation, curricula within the schools and colleges of pharmacy have evolved to include more experiential coursework to foster this patient orientation. This change has been supported by the philosophy of pharmaceutical care which encourages pharmacists to assume a patient advocacy role in optimizing a patient's drug therapy while minimizing the adverse effects of the medication. The role of experiential education, and especially the clerkship experience, is to hasten and enhance the development of this concept and philosophy for pharmacy students.

Before we describe the contents and components of clerkships, a brief explanation of the various types of experiential education is warranted as considerable confusion exists among students, preceptors, and colleges of pharmacy.

There are currently three types of experiential programs for pharmacy students: externships, clerkships, and internships. *Externships* and *clerkships* are school sponsored programs for which students receive academic credit. *Internships*, however, are not school sponsored and students do not receive academic credit. Rather, students in internship programs are paid for their work and must complete a set number of hours, as determined by the respective state, prior to licensure. Some states require that at least a portion of the internship experience be completed after graduation from pharmacy school. Other states allow all internship hours to be completed before graduation. In addition, several states allow clerkship or externship hours to count toward the total number of internship hours required for licensure.

The difference between clerkships and externships is more subtle. The primary focus of an externship is to give students experience with the technical and distributive aspects of providing medication to patients. This includes experiences such as filling and dispensing a prescription, preparing an intravenous solution, and filling a unit dose medication cart. As with an internship, externships can be completed in a community, chain, clinic, or hospital pharmacy setting.

Clerkships, whether in a hospital, ambulatory clinic, community, or nursing home setting, use patient care experiences to integrate and apply information from prior didactic coursework. Their goal is to develop and enhance a student's therapeutic problem-solving skills and knowledge of the appropriate use of medications. This experience is often thought of as the laboratory component to a therapeutics course, because information on appropriate medication selection, use, dosing, and monitoring is applied in a patient care environment. Traditionally, clerkships take place in an inpatient hospital setting which provides a wealth of experience in understanding terminology, abbreviations, laboratory tests, physical examination parameters, diagnostic tests, and use of medications in a controlled setting over a relatively short period of time. This is in contrast to an ambulatory clerkship setting, where patients are often not acutely ill. The response of ambulatory patients to therapy may be more gradual; thus, students need to be present at that particular setting for a longer period of time to observe responses to therapy. For example, a patient with rheumatoid arthritis started on gold therapy usually requires at least three months of continued therapy before a response is observed. There is, however, an increased interest in providing more clerkship experiences in ambulatory and community settings as these settings more closely reflect the evolution and status of health care delivery in the United States.

Traditionally, the school sponsored programs of clerkships and externships described above are separate entities. However, as pharmacy has evolved, the line between distributive and clinical functions has begun to fade and both activities are often handled by the same individual. Furthermore, technicians and technology are increasingly relied upon to attend to many of the distributive aspects of pharmacy practice. Therefore, while pharmacists must understand and participate in distributive aspects of pharmacy, their major emphasis and concentration has shifted to the clinical aspects of pharmaceutical care. School sponsored experiential programs are reflecting this change. The remainder of this chapter will discuss the common goals, objectives, and activities typically found in today's clerkship programs.

CLERKSHIP GOALS

Within a clerkship experience, several general goals are aimed at developing and enhancing students' skills in implementing this philosophy of pharmaceutical care. Through participation in an institutional clerkship, students should:

>> **Gain** an appreciation and understanding of the concept of pharmaceutical care and its importance in the delivery of health care to an institutionalized patient.

>> **Develop** the skills necessary to effectively and efficiently apply and integrate information from the basic pharmaceutical and medical sciences to direct patient care.

>> **Gain** experience in prospectively solving medication related problems.

>> **Develop** the skills necessary to communicate effectively with patients and health care professionals.

Course Competencies and Objectives

More specifically, upon completion of a clerkship rotation, students should be able to:

>> **Understand** symptoms, pathophysiology, laboratory tests, physical examination, diagnosis, and prognosis of acute and chronic disease.

>> **Formulate,** on a prospective basis, a therapeutic management plan for drug and non-drug treatments for a particular disease state.

>> **Demonstrate** competency and efficiency in monitoring therapy using subjective and objective parameters for efficacy and toxicity.

>> **Formulate** patient specific medication dosing adjustments.

- ›› **Utilize** the problem-solving approach effectively and efficiently in the patient care setting.

- ›› **Provide** basic life support (i.e., CPR).

- ›› **Discuss** the chemical properties such as stability, compatibility, and storage requirements of drugs and drug products.

- ›› **Understand** the mechanisms of action of drugs and drug products.

- ›› **Identify** the pharmacokinetic properties and administration methods of drugs and drug products.

- ›› **Describe** adverse reactions, side effects, or contraindications of drugs and drug products.

- ›› **List** potential drug-drug, drug-food, and drug-laboratory interactions for drugs and drug products.

- ›› **Describe** available product formulations for drugs and drug products.

- ›› **Provide** drug information to patients and health care professionals in an effective and efficient manner using both written and verbal communication skills.

- ›› **Communicate** therapeutic recommendations to the prescriber.

- ›› **Conduct** a patient medication history to identify medication use and allergies.

- ›› **Provide** discharge medication instructions to patients.

- ›› **Prepare and Present** educational information to classmates and preceptors.

- ›› **Use** primary literature and reference sources to effectively answer questions and provide information.

- ›› **Demonstrate** a technical knowledge of drugs and drug products.

- ›› **Communicate** effectively with patients and other health care professionals.

In general, the above objectives are focused on the student's ability to demonstrate an appreciation and understanding of diseases, principles of therapeutics, and the role of drug therapy for disease states commonly observed on the assigned rotation.

CLERKSHIP ACTIVITIES

To accomplish these objectives, a variety of structured patient oriented activities and experiences are incorporated into typical institutionally based clerkship programs. These activities normally include, participation in patient care rounds; application of therapeutic drug monitoring principles; provision of pharmacokinetic consultations, patient counseling, and answers to day to day drug-related questions; presentation of cases to peers, faculty, and other health care providers; and obtainment of admission drug histories.

Patient Care Rounds

In a teaching hospital, patient care rounds or "work rounds" typically occur early in the morning (7 a.m. to 9 a.m.) for medical services and even earlier for surgical services. Rounds are used by physicians to systematically evaluate each patient's response to therapeutic intervention, review the results of diagnostic or therapeutic procedure(s), and establish and communicate future treatment plans to the patient and the team. During work rounds, the physician gathers subjective data from patient communications and objective data from routine physical examination, laboratory tests, and nursing notes. He then analyzes the data and further formulates therapeutic and diagnostic plans.

A variety of health care professionals take part in rounds and the types of practitioners on rounds at any one time depends upon the hospital and the specific types of patients receiving care. Participants in work rounds at a teaching hospital generally include an attending physician, a medical resident, a medical intern, a nurse, a pharmacist, and perhaps one or two students from each health care discipline.

Work rounds provide excellent opportunities for learning. For many students this often is their first face-to-face contact with hospitalized patients and health care professionals. In this environment, students have the opportunity to review a variety of clinical patient data (e.g., laboratory tests, blood pressure and other measurements of vital signs, fluid and electrolyte balance, and physical examinations) for a variety of medical problems. Most importantly, students see patients on a daily basis and can evaluate these patients' responses to drug therapy both in terms of efficacy and toxicity. In addition, with so many students and other health care professionals participating in rounds, this is an excellent atmosphere for discussion of disease states, drug therapy, prognosis, and other patient care issues in a multi-disciplinary setting.

As pharmacists, attendance at work rounds allows direct patient observation and information gathering that can be used to monitor a patient's medication therapy; to plan admissions and discharge counseling; and to anticipate daily workloads. Work rounds also provide a means for communication between health care professionals and serve as a continuing source of educational experiences. However, because of their design, work rounds cannot serve as a forum for extensive discussion of any given topic.

Objectives. By attending work rounds, students should be able to:

›› **Identify and Gather** subjective and objective data necessary to monitor medication therapy for efficacy and toxicity.

›› **Establish** a prospective therapeutic management plan that includes therapeutic endpoints, monitoring parameters, individualization of dosages, and patient counseling.

›› **Communicate** effectively with other members of the health care team on topics such as therapeutics, drug information, policies and procedures, and patient planning needs.

›› **Assess** patient medication teaching needs and communicate medication information to the patient, including why drug changes are made, and when the patient should expect to notice results from therapy changes.

>> **Resolve** questionable or unclear medication orders and explain any medication errors such as missed doses or incorrect drug or dose.

>> **Prioritize** daily workload based on information obtained during rounds.

>> **Develop** a formal working relationship with the health care team.

>> **Assess** patient medication needs upon discharge, solving problems such as drug and dosage discrepancies, where prescriptions should be filled, and when drugs are needed.

Activities. When attending work rounds, students should:

>> **Orient** new medical house staff and nursing staff to pharmacy policies and procedures unique to the particular unit.

Hints for Rounds

1 Introduce yourself to the medical team if you are not already acquainted.

2 Be prepared to answer and ask questions. Support any information with the necessary literature references.

3 If you are unable to answer a question, do not hesitate to say so. However, add that you will attempt to locate the answer. Do this in a timely fashion, or if you are unable to do so, communicate the question to the person who receives your report. Be sure to follow through.

4 Obtain the necessary monitoring parameters (e.g., vital signs, laboratory test results) **before** rounds.

5 Review the medication administration record (patient profile) **before** rounds. Check for the administration of all PRN medications and any missed scheduled doses.

6 Be assertive and discuss therapeutic management concerns.

7 Voice concerns in a calm, courteous manner with rationale for disagreement.

8 Be consistent. Attend rounds daily and for the entire duration if possible.

9 Anticipate medication orders, especially discharge prescriptions.

10 A clipboard or a pocket full of 3 x 5 index cards is handy for recording information while on rounds.

Activities (Continued)

>> **Review** patient medication therapy on a daily basis *before* rounds to ensure their understanding of the indications, dosages, routes of administration, efficacy, and toxicity of their patient's medications.

>> **Obtain** information to update and correct the medication profile.

>> **Formulate and Document** a problem list for new or existing patients seen by the service. This list should focus on disease, drug, and socioeconomic factors.

>> **Attend** work rounds on a consistent basis.

>> **Communicate** the following information to others on rounds:

> Patients' current medication use.

> Deviances in patient's therapy (e.g., incorrect dosage, missed or refused doses, intravenous infiltration, late doses).

> Observed subjective or objective signs of efficacy or toxicity.

> Drug distribution problems (e.g., non-formulary status).

> Prospective therapeutic management plans for patient problems (e.g., change of therapy, discontinuation of a drug, change in pain medication, use of prophylactic antibiotics, identification of therapeutic alternatives).

>> **Gather** the following information:

> Subjective and objective data for monitoring a patient's medication therapy.

> Changes in *patient status* including: improved or worsened condition, discharge date, surgery, planned diagnostic procedures, and the results of those procedures.

> Changes in nondrug therapy (e.g., dietary, socioeconomic, physical therapy, respiratory therapy, occupational therapy).

> Changes in medication therapy (e.g., new drug orders, discontinued orders, or changes in dose, route of administration, or duration).

> When chemotherapy, pre-ops (preoperative medications), or intravenous solutions are needed.

> Patients' understanding of medication, name, strength, and expected benefits and toxicities.

> Projected discharge date, including any special teaching needs (e.g., home antibiotics or total parenteral nutrition).

>> **Communicate** to the unit pharmacist any information gleaned from rounds if she is unable to attend.

Therapeutic Drug Monitoring

Clerkship students are generally required to monitor drug therapy on a daily basis for patients on their assigned service. This activity is aimed at optimizing the benefits while minimizing risks associated with a patient's medication therapy. Institutions have different formats in which this activity is performed, but typically it is a variation of the traditional "SOAP Note." SOAP stands for the terms Subjective, Objective, Assessment, and Plan, each of which describe a portion of the progress note. (See Chapter 13: Clinical Drug Monitoring for a more detailed discussion.)

Pharmacokinetic Consults

The blood concentration of drugs with narrow therapeutic ranges (i.e., aminoglycosides, digoxin, phenytoin, theophylline) must be monitored closely to enhance the probability of therapeutic efficacy and to minimize toxicity. Pharmacists today are active participants in pharmacokinetic programs in most teaching hospitals; however, the extent of their involvement varies greatly among institutions. Some pharmacists operate solely as a consultant when the medical team faces a difficult case. Others take responsibility for prescribing and administering the dose and drawing blood for drug concentration analysis.

Participation in pharmacokinetic monitoring allows clerkship students to practice calculations learned in school and to combine these skills with their clinical patient assessment abilities. Patient parameters such as changing renal or liver function or volume of distribution, require insights and interpretations when recommending doses and establishing plans for subsequent monitoring.

Pharmacokinetics are performed as a formal consult in some hospitals. With this type of program, pharmacists are responsible for evaluating the patient, recommending the dosing regimen, and documenting their actions as a formal note in the patient chart. This documentation must be complete and accurate as this note is usually included in the patient's permanent record.

The format for written pharmacokinetic consultative notes varies considerably among institutions, but the underlying concept remains the same. The drug, dose, dosing interval, day of therapy, infusion time for the anticipated dose, and times and results of previous blood concentrations should be included. Calculated values such as extrapolated peak, half-life, and volume of distribution, should follow the demographic data. Fluctuating laboratory values may also be included (e.g., serum creatinine, WBC counts, and differentials) in support of the recommendations. The note should end with a recommendation, the statement "will continue to follow" if therapy is to continue, and the pharmacist's signature and title.

Self Assessment For Work Rounds

Directions: Answer each of the following questions. If you answer "no" to any of the questions, you have identified an area of possible improvement.

1 Do you know the names of the members on the service?

2 Do the members on the service know your name?

3 Do you actively participate on rounds and not just tag along?

4 Do members of the service ask you therapeutic questions?

5 Do you return information accurately and in a timely manner?

6 Do you communicate in a courteous manner with members of the service?

7 Do you know the patients' medical problems?

8 Do you know the rationale for the patients' medications?

9 Do you ask questions concerning therapeutic rationale that you do not understand?

10 Do you ask questions about diagnostic or physical examination information as related to drug therapy?

11 Do you attend all the rounds or see just a few patients?

12 Do you remind the service to write discharge medications and pre-ops and to okay chemotherapy on rounds?

13 What percent of the time are you asked therapeutic questions prospectively (asked before the medication is ordered)? (circle one)

| 0% | 10% | 30% | 60% | 90% | 100% |

Admission Histories and Discharge Medication Counseling

In order to obtain an accurate record of a patient's medication history, pharmacists in many hospitals obtain admission interviews for some or all hospitalized patients. This experience is often included in clerkship rotations. During an admission interview it is important to collect information such as:

>> The patient's height and weight.

>> A history of drug allergies or adverse reactions. (If present, type of reaction, how long ago the reaction occurred, and whether or not the patient was rechallenged with the offending agent).

>> All current prescription medications including dose, route, frequency, indication, duration, and number of doses already taken for the day.

>> Any significant past medications the patient has received (and, if pertinent, why they were discontinued).

(Continued on page 1–10)

Pharmacokinetic Results

EXAMPLE 1

Initial Work-up

9/26/92 Pharmacokinetic Consult
        Day #1 of tobramycin therapy

One time bolus of 140 mg infused over 60 minutes (0855–0955), followed by three post-infusion levels.

Time	Post-Infusion	Level
1109	1 hr, 14 min	3.0 µg/mL
1303	3 hr, 8 min	1.2 µg/mL
1427	5 hr, 32 min	0.6 µg/mL
Extrapolated peak	4.4 µg/mL	
Half-life	1.52 hr	
Volume of distribution	0.25 L/kg	

To achieve a peak of 7.0 and a trough of 0.2 µg/mL, recommended regimen: tobramycin 220 mg Q 12 hr

Will continue to follow.   *Larry Boh, MS RPH*

EXAMPLE 2

Peak and Trough Work-up

9/27/92 Pharmacokinetic Consult
        Day #8 of gentamicin therapy

Current regimen: 180 mg Q 12 hr. Patient afebrile x 3 days   WBC = 9000
180 mg gentamicin infused over 60 minutes (0910–1010).

Time	Time Post-Infusion	Level
0908	11 hr, 8 min (trough)	0.4 µg/mL
1109	59 min (peak)	6.9 µg/mL
Extrapolated peak	9.1 µg/mL	
Half-life	2 hr, 28 min	
Volume of distribution	0.33 L/kg	

Recommend discontinuing gentamicin therapy.

                            Kristin–Krumbiegal Hanson, MS RPH

>> Over-the-counter (OTC) medications the patient takes and approximately how often.

>> Any history of social drug use, such as consumption of alcohol, smoking, or illicit drug use.

During the interview, the reliability of the patient or caregiver and the patient's compliance with the prescribed regimen should be assessed and any specific requirements which may affect the patient's compliance should be noted. For example, an elderly frail patient with arthritis may be incapable of opening prescription vials with child-proof caps. The pharmacist should use this information to counsel the patient at time of discharge and ensure that medications are dispensed in easy-to-open containers.

In many institutions, pharmacists are responsible for first dose teaching and/or medication counseling at the time of a patient's discharge from the facility. This activity may also be incorporated into the clerkship experience. When counseling patients on use of their medications, it is important to use words that patients will understand and to provide them with the following information:

>> Drug name.

>> The drug's purpose and expected benefits the patient should watch for (e.g., clearing of a rash, decreased pain).

>> Dose, frequency, and route of administration.

>> Special dosing instructions.

>> Duration the patient is to remain on the medication.

>> Frequent minor side effects.

>> Significant adverse effects that warrant notification of the physician if encountered by the patient.

>> Information on refills and storage.

Drug Information Questions

Drug information questions, whether formal or informal, are a common activity of clerkships. Other health care professionals frequently ask questions regarding specific drugs, potential side effects, doses, or a recommended therapy. Often the answers to these inquiries are not be obvious. It is important **NEVER** to guess if you are unsure of the correct answer. The best response is to say, "I'm really not sure. Let me check some references and get back to you." Health care professionals will respond to you better if you take the time to research an answer rather than guess, especially if you guess incorrectly! You must, however, ask when the information is needed and provide it in a timely manner.

In addition to drug information questions, formal written answers to drug-related questions that may arise while monitoring a patient's medication therapy are often a component of clerkships. These formal written responses may be provided to a preceptor, physician, nurse, or other health care professional. The prepared answer should restate the question, establish an answer, and support the answer with appropriate references.

Researching an answer will help students understand the issue and familiarize them with the various available references. (See Chapter 3: Providing Drug Information for a more detailed discussion on how to answer drug information questions.)

Case Presentations

Most clerkships require students to prepare and present patient cases. In general, the cases are 20 to 30 minutes in length and may be presented to pharmacists at the clerkship site, classmates, or perhaps both. These case presentations give students an opportunity to strengthen their communication skills and should consist of a handout, a discussion of disease states, a discussion of drug therapy, and a summation which critiques therapy and draws conclusions from the presentation.

The Handout. Students should begin their presentations with a handout no longer than two pages. (See example on page 1–13.) Additional visual aids that assist in clarifying confusing issues are encouraged. References must be cited in the correct (ASHP) format.

›› **Components.** The handout should include:

> *Demographic data (Dem data)* such as age, sex, race, weight, and service the patient is on.

> *Chief complaint (CC)* or reason for the patient's admission.

> *History of present illness (HPI).*

> *Past medical history (PMH)* consisting of a brief list of all illnesses, surgical procedures, and previous hospitalizations that have a direct effect on the present illness.

> *Social history (SH).*

> *Family history (FH).*

> *Medications (Meds) and allergies or adverse drug reactions (ADRs).* This list of information is obtained during the medication history and should include the length of treatment and any allergic or adverse drug reactions. Be sure to list how reactions were treated and if the patient was rechallenged.

> *Pertinent physical examination (PE) data.* For example an abnormal examination in a patient with congestive heart failure (CHF) may include the presence of 3+ ankle edema, + hepato-jugular reflex (HJR), + jugular venous distention (JVD), and the presence of rales in both lung fields. Pertinent negatives such as a normal rate and rhythm in a patient admitted to rule out myocardial infarction (R/O MI) should also be included.

> *Pertinent laboratory values (Labs).* For example in a patient with anemia, the data may include hemoglobin (Hgb), hematocrit (Hct), mean cell volume (MCV), hemoglobin concentration (MCHC), serum iron, total iron binding capacity (TIBC). Again, pertinent negatives should also be included. Be sure to include normal value ranges and the creatinine clearance (Cl_{Cr}) and liver function test (LFT) assessments.

> *Problem list.*

>> **Duration:** Approximately 5 minutes.

Discussion of Disease States

>> **Purpose:** This is a general discussion of the disease process and should cover underlying pathologic and physiologic changes. *Remember:* The discussion of the disease state is important. It will be the foundation for discussing drug therapy and monitoring parameters for both efficacy and toxicity. Be brief (about 5 minutes).

>> **Components:** State the cause of the disease, symptoms, physical, and laboratory findings of a *typical* case.

> *Discuss* the diagnosis and prognosis of the disease state.

> *Compare* these items to your particular patient case.

> *State* the possible complications of the disease.

>> **Duration:** Approximately 5 minutes.

Discussion of Drug Therapy

>> **Purpose:** This is a discussion of the therapeutic approaches to the disease.

>> **Components:** State the objective of drug therapy for the disease, including selection of drug, mechanism of action, dosage, route of administration, and duration of therapy.

> *Discuss* common and serious side effects for each medication. The *relative importance* and frequency of these reactions should be stressed. Be sure to include limits and management of reactions.

> *Describe and Outline* the monitoring parameters to evaluate response to therapy, including therapeutic endpoints.

Case Presentation Example

GASTROINTESTINAL BLEED
PEPTIC ULCER DISEASE (PUD)

Dem. Data   G.Z. is a 48-year-old female who was admitted to the intensive care unit on November 25th. She was transferred to a regular medical floor two days later. G.Z. weighs 61 kg and is 167.6 cm tall.

CC   Coughing up blood.

HPI   G.Z. presented to the emergency room on November 25th 30 minutes following an episode of hematemesis. She stated she had experienced mid-epigastric pain with nausea on 11/24, which was relieved by antacids. This morning following breakfast she had one melanotic stool. She is feeling increasingly fatigued and complains of dizziness when standing. She denies abdominal pain, shortness of breath (SOB), dysuria, hematuria, or chest pain.

PMH   The patient has no history of liver disease, PUD, GI bleed, hypertension, or DM. She denies previous hematemesis, hematochezia, and melena. She does report several weeks of vague abdominal discomfort. She is s/p (status post) appendectomy.

SH   Negative alcohol and tobacco use.

FH   One brother with PUD.

Meds   Patient denies use of any medications including ASA and other NSAIDs.

Allergies   G.Z. has no known allergies.

PE   General appearance: Well nourished female.

Vital signs:
Lying: p = 91 (60–80 BPM); BP = 110/80 (120–140/<90 mm Hg)
Sitting: 128; BP = 80/0.
T = 37.2 (35.8–37.3 °C)
Abdomen: Soft, negative distention/tenderness, hypoactive bowel sounds

Rectal	Melanotic, guaiac positive stool in vault

Labs

Heme		
RBCs	3.4 (3.8–5.0 m/uL)*
Hgb	10.6 (11.8–15.4 gm/dL)*
Hct	31 (35–45 mL/dL)*
MCV	92 (82–98 fL/RBC)
MCHC	34 (32–36 gm/dL)
Platelets	249 (170–380 K/uL)

Continued

Case Presentation Example (Continued)

Labs

Chem	Lytes		
		Na	141 (135–144 mmol/L)
		K	3.5 (3.6–4.8 mmol/L)*
		Cl	103 (9—106 mmol/L)
		CO_2	25 (22–32 mmol/L)
		Glu	124 (70–110 mg/dL)*

LFTs: WNL

BUN	24 (7–20 mg/dL)*	Creatinine	0.6 (0.6–1.3 mg/dL)
PT	13.6 (11–13 sec)*	aPTT	25.4 (20–30 sec)

Problem List   Painless UGI bleed

REFERENCES

1. Grossman MI et al. Gastrointestinal diseases: peptic ulcer. In: Wyngaarden JB, Smith LH, eds. Cecil Textbook of Medicine. Philadelphia: WB Saunders; 19th ed. 1992:635–54.

2. Mitros FA. Atlas of Gastrointestinal Pathology. Philadelphia: JB Lippincott; 1988.

3. Garnett WR. Antacid products. In: American Pharmaceutical Association. Handbook of Nonprescription Drugs. 8th ed. Washington, DC: APhA; 1986:19–51.

4. Berardi RR. Peptic ulcer disease and Zollinger-Ellison syndrome. In: Pharmacotherapy: A Pathophysiologic Approach. DePiro JT et al (eds). New York: Elsevier;1989:418–43.

5. Dammann HG et al. The 24-hour acid suppression profile of nizatidine. Scand J Gastroenterol. 1987:22(Suppl.136):56–60.

6. Emas S. Medical principles for treatment of peptic ulcer. Scand J Gastroenterol. 1987;22(Suppl.137):28–32.

7. Freston JW. H2-receptor antagonists and duodenal ulcer recurrence: analysis of efficacy and commentary on safety, costs and patient selection. Am J Gastroenterol. 1987;82:1242–249.

8. Lewis JH. Hepatic effects of drugs used in the treatment of peptic ulcer disease. Am J Gastroenterol. 1987;82:987–1003.

9. Ostro MJ. Pharmacodynamics and pharmacokinetics of parenteral histamine (H2)-receptor antagonists. Am J Med. 1987;83(Suppl.6A):15–21.

10. Wolfe MM. Considerations for selection of parenteral histamine (H2)-receptor antagonists. Am J Med. 1987;83 (Suppl.6A):82–88.

11. Hollander D. Peptic disease therapy. Am J Med. 1989;86(Suppl.6A):152–53.

12. Knodell RG et al. Newer agents available for treatment of stress-related upper gastrointestinal tract mucosa damage. Am J Med. 1987;83(Suppl.6A):36–40.

13. Kastrup EK, Olin BR, Connell SI et al. Drug Facts and Comparisons. St. Louis: JB Lippincott; 1988.

14. Lanza FL, Sibley CM. Role of antacids in the management of disorders of the upper gastrointestinal tract. Review of clinical experience 1975–1985. Am J Gastroenterol. 1987;82:1223–241.

Discussion of Drug Therapy (Continued)

> *Define* the potentially clinically significant drug-drug, drug-laboratory, or drug-nutrient test interactions.

> *Describe* factors that would modify choice of drug, dose, or route of administration (e.g., a comatose patient would receive no oral medication). Be sure to include methods for modifying a dosage when necessary for patients with compromised renal or hepatic function.

> *Define* problems likely to be encountered during the administration of medications including compliance problems.

> *Describe* nondrug treatment modalities (e.g., diet instruction, physical therapy, occupational therapy, respiratory therapy).

> *Field* any questions related to your rational for discussed drug therapy.

>> **Duration:** Approximately 10 minutes.

Conclusions and Critique of Therapy

>> **Purpose:** This is a summary of the entire case presentation that focuses on the following questions:

> How closely does the specific patient fit the "classic" case? What were the differences or similarities?

> Did any adverse reactions occur? Could they have been avoided?

> Do you agree with the therapy used? If not, what would you do differently and why?

> What medications were given at the time of discharge? What would or did you tell the patient? Is compliance a potential problem?

> What were the most important therapeutic principles you learned?

>> **Duration:** Approximately 5 minutes.

Helpful Hints for Case Presentation

■ Think ahead! Be able to answer the question: "What if . . . . ?" Or if this happens, what should I do?

■ Remember to be brief; you do not have a lot of time.

■ Vocabulary may be understood by you but to your fellow students, it may be Greek. Define any unusual terminology. Upon questioning, you should be able to define any medical vocabulary you have used.

■ Pronunciation and articulation are important parts of effective communication. If you do not know how to pronounce a term, or drug, find out before you present the case. Stumbling over words decreases your credibility.

■ Remember you are playing the role of a teacher. Be sure to bring out the important teaching points illustrated by this patient.

■ If all questions were answered during the course of your presentation, it would stretch into a two-hour presentation. Use the outline on page 1–11 as a guideline and extract only the most important information under each section for presentation. If you have answered all questions in this outline before the case presentation you should be able to field any question posed by your fellow students or the instructor.

■ When presenting your case, you should be able to answer the following questions if asked:

• What was the probability for success with this patient's therapeutic regimen, and how long will it take before success is achieved? How long before a lack of sufficient response during any segment of therapy could be interpreted as therapeutic failure?

• What clinically significant interactions or adverse effects of drug therapy might occur?

■ What is the nature of this possible interaction or side effect? What would be its significance in this particular patient?

■ What is the probability that an interaction or side effect may occur and with what frequency is it encountered in the general population?

■ What parameters will you inspect during treatment as an indication of drug interaction or side effect?

• What is the overall benefit versus risk assessment of therapy? Would long-term treatment modify the overall benefit?

• What routine alterations in drug therapy can be expected to occur as a matter of course and when should they occur? *Hint:* This might be an alteration of dose, route of administration, or nature of drug. Are there any special procedures to be considered in making these changes (i.e., patients on anticoagulants are unsuitable for intramuscular injection)?

• What drugs were discontinued during the course of the patient's illness? Why? Was this considered a therapeutic failure?

Continued

- What drugs were added to the therapeutic regimen and why? Was adequate time allowed to determine whether the previous regimen was inadequate?

- Include intravenous therapy as it affects the overall treatment of the patient.

- What laboratory tests, symptoms, or other clinical signs were used as criteria to determine the degree of response to therapy?

- Did any drug-drug or drug-laboratory interactions occur? If so, how were they handled? Be sure to include synergism and additive and antagonistic effects.

- Did any adverse reactions occur? If so, how were they managed?

- If complications arose, how were they treated?

- If the patient was discharged, were the discharge medications correct? Would you expect any problems with patient compliance or the medications themselves? What directions (by the pharmacist) should be or were given to the patient at the time of discharge regarding their medications?

HINTS ON CLERKSHIP SURVIVAL

To help you adjust to the hospital setting and maximize your clerkship rotation, the authors have compiled the following list of suggestions. Remember that although each clerkship program is unique, these ideas should apply to all.

>> Ask questions of pharmacists, technicians, nurses, physicians, and other health care students. This is a learning experience for you, teaching is the responsibility of all health care professionals and usually a part of their job description.

>> If you are unsure of the answer to a question, do not guess or make one up. Look up the answer and return promptly with the requested information.

>> Be prepared. Review old class notes or portions of textbooks (especially therapeutics) if necessary.

>> Prepare for work rounds. Depending on the number and complexity of patients on your service, this normally requires about 30 minutes. This is the time to review what has happened with each patient since you left the unit and catch up on new admissions.

>> Participate during rounds. Avoid standing at the back of the group. This is an excellent time to view disease manifestations and the effects of drug therapy on patients.

>> Eat a good breakfast. The sights, sounds, and smells in a hospital are not all pleasant, especially to someone not accustomed to them.

>> Take advantage of any additional opportunities (e.g., special lectures or conferences). Some hospitals will allow you to observe a variety of tests and procedures or even a surgery. These types of observations are even more beneficial if someone is available to explain the procedure.

>> Remember to dress and act in a professional manner. This will reflect positively on your profession, your school, and most importantly, you.

>> Patient confidentiality is extremely important. Do not discuss patients in public places or in a loud voice, regardless of whether or not you are using names or initials. You never know who may be listening. *Remember:* The patient is an individual, not just a case.

>> Do not fall behind. This is an extremely busy time and if you are stressed to complete work, you will not learn as much from this experience as you would if you had kept up. In addition, much of what you learn in a clerkship builds on what you learned the previous week.

>> Remember to work "smart." This translates to working on assignments effectively and efficiently. The clerkship experience does not necessarily require you to work long hours, though this may be necessary if your background is weak in a particular area. A daily calendar can help you organize your days to increase efficiency.

EVALUATION OF STUDENT PERFORMANCE

An important aspect of experiential education is the evaluation of the student's performance. Often, the chosen approach varies considerably by site and institution, as well as by college. Attempts to remove the subjectiveness associated with evaluating a student and improve the evaluation process in experiential education are currently ongoing.

Despite an apparent deficiency, there are several important concepts which can aid preceptors in the difficult area of student performance evaluation. The following general principles are intended to help preceptors eliminate the subjectiveness often associated with performance evaluations.

>> **Establish** specific clerkship goals and expectations before beginning the clerkship rotation. The object of the clerkship should be documented and measures to determine its completion should be clearly identified.

>> **Provide** students with the opportunity for input into clerkship objectives. This allows students to tailor their rotation to meet specific needs and interests.

>> **Provide** specific feedback to students concerning their progress both at the midpoint (a formative evaluation) and at the end of the rotation (a summative evaluation).

>> **Identify** students' strengths and weaknesses. Suggest ways they can improve or correct deficiencies.

>> **Document** student performance and progress with specific examples.

>> **Evaluate** performance as it is currently being performed. Do not evaluate performance based upon anticipated performance or progress that has occurred since the last evaluation.

>> **Separate** the evaluation process from the assignment of grades.

>> **Encourage** students to self-evaluate their own performance (see page 1–8). This approach is critical for encouraging life-long learning and growth throughout your students' professional careers.

Although some objective measures of student performance evaluation exist and others are being developed, preceptors still need to be appropriately trained in using available evaluation instruments and students need to understand the various objectives and expectations these instruments measure. Much of the frustration and confusion concerning grading in experiential education can be minimized by maintaining and encouraging open communication between student and preceptor. Differences, should be addressed and corrected together, with assistance from the clerkship coordinator when necessary.

ACKNOWLEDGMENTS

We acknowledge the contributions of Sandy Hoel, Paula Ploetz, Teresa Geier, Kathy Skibinshir, and Ruth Bruskiewitz to this chapter.

Standards of Professional Conduct

Lucy Schneller Hazebrook

The first day on a patient care unit can be stressful. You are surrounded by sick or injured patients in various states of undress, as well as by busy, purposeful, and professional health care workers. You must adapt to an environment that is focused on cleanliness and a system guided by numerous policies and procedures structured to minimize errors and to maximize the quality of patient care. You are in unfamiliar surroundings and are expected to quickly become knowledge-able about the disease states, clinical condition, and treatment regimens of specific patients. Furthermore, you must communicate in an unfamiliar "language" often using medical terminology to discuss the clinical response of patients to drug therapy.

As you make the transition from a campus setting to a health care arena, take time to reflect on the image and conduct needed to reassure and to comfort the sick, while maximizing your opportunities to learn. Developing a professional image can facili-tate your interactions with patients and with physicians, nurses, and other health care workers who will participate in your clinical education. Your image affects how patients, their families, and others interpret your comments and contributions to patient care. A non-professional image can undermine your confidence and compe-tence and make your clinical experience unfruitful and unrewarding.

While you may be focused on *what* you are communicating, your listeners are focused on *you*. Your selection of words and your professional image affect how well the listener hears and understands your message. Skill and knowledge are nonvisual attributes, therefore, the components of an image (e.g., dress, grooming, language, and communication techniques) are critical to the successful delivery of your mes-sage. You will meet many patients during your clerkship; consider how your initial impressions and interactions will impact the success of your clerkship. More impor-tantly, consider how your conduct will add to, or minimize, the stress of patients already anxious about their illness.

HOW TO DEMONSTRATE
PROFESSIONALISM AS A PHARMACY STUDENT

Competence, professional integrity, and genuine concern, for the health and well-being of others are essential to your success in a patient-care setting. A professional image supported by good grooming, language, and a congenial personality will encourage the cooperation of both patients and health care professionals.

Competence

Passing the state boards does not assure competency. Competence in pharmaceutical care can only be achieved by developing a significant knowledge base and repeatedly applying that knowledge to various clinical situations to resolve therapeutic dilemmas. You must establish a life-long commitment to learning because clinical knowledge reflects the evolution of ongoing scientific discoveries.

Integrity

Integrity can be defined as a state or quality of being complete, undivided or unbroken. Moral soundness, purity, honesty, and uprightness are frequently used synonyms for "integrity." Integrity also can be manifested by adherence to a code of personal and professional values that embraces honesty and truth. As a pharmacist, you have accepted the responsibility for the pharmaceutical care of your patients and need the cooperation of fellow health care professionals. Without integrity, trust from patients and other health care professionals may never be established, even if you possess a wealth of pharmacotherapeutic data.

Professional Concern

You can express professional concern in many ways: careful listening, going "above and beyond" the call of duty on matters that affect the health and well-being of patients, and participation in decisions being made by fellow health care team members. Therefore, you must be readily available and present in the patient care arena to provide answers to questions concerning drugs.

Being accountable for patients' pharmaceutical care and making a commitment to optimize patients' drug therapy are of utmost importance. You must accept the con-

---

Self-Assessment Checklist: Professional Conduct in a Patient Care Area

Directions: Answer each of the following questions. If you answer "no" to any of the questions, you have identified an area of possible improvement.

1 Do you communicate in a courteous manner with patients and other health care team members?

2 Is your grooming, dress, non-verbal behavior, and language acceptable to all your patients and team members?

3 Do patients or health professionals ask you questions related to providing pharmaceutical care?

4 Can your team members find you when they have a question?

5 Do you actively participate in the care of your patients?

6 Do you know the names of your health care team?

7 Do your fellow team members know your name?

8 Do you practice universal precautions and inform others if they are not adhering to universal precautions?

9 Are you on time for rounds, meetings, and answering questions?

10 Do any of your patients have problems with drug misadventures?

sequences of adverse or negative responses to drug therapy and missed opportunities which would have, had they been taken, improved patient care. When a patient's clinical condition responds favorably to your interventions, welcome your feelings of enhanced self-esteem, and remember that the positive feelings resulted from your professional concern for your patient.

Personality

Personalities of professionals vary as much as students in your class and it is okay to "be yourself." However, remember that approachability is very important. Patient and health care professionals need to be comfortable in soliciting your participation in drug therapy decisions.

Professional Dress/Appearance

Patients often are elderly and conservative in philosophy. As a result, dressing conservatively is always acceptable and in good taste. Men should wear a necktie, women should wear hose. Blue jeans and revealing clothing (e.g., very short skirts, low necklines) are unacceptable for men and women.

A clean, pressed white lab jacket and your name tag help to identify health care professionals. In some practice locations (e.g., pediatric or psychiatric institutions) white jackets may not be appropriate. When in doubt, base your dress decisions on other health care workers in your patient care unit, or make inquiries of your preceptor.

Scrub suits, often worn by health care professionals "on call" during the night, are not proper attire for pharmacy students in the patient care area. Do not dress in a manner others may find distracting: this detracts from your professional image. The way you dress makes a statement and should reflect your respect for patients and coworkers, and good professional judgment.

Athletic shoes and sandals, though comfortable, detract from your professional image. Comfortable, non-flashy shoes are most appropriate. Although high heel shoes appear professional, they are not recommended in patient care areas because they can be noisy and uncomfortable when standing for prolonged periods of time.

Grooming also affects your professional image. Your hairstyle, jewelry, fragrance, breath, and the length and cleanliness of your fingernails affect other people's perception of your professional competence. Many people are repulsed by, or even allergic to, heavy fragrances, and exotic hair fashions may overwhelm elderly patients. Again, being conservative is always safe.

Language

Adapt your language to your audience. When speaking with patients, assess their understanding to optimize the effectiveness of your communications. Watch attentively as you speak to ensure your listeners understand you. Avoid "medicalese" and use plain English whenever possible.

Address the patient with courtesy and respect. Patients are not at their best in the hospital setting; they are often anxious, confused, and uncomfortable. Be sensitive and careful in your selection of words. Although you can speak more directly with other health care professionals, you need to be aware of their feelings, attitudes, and communication styles. Never refer to a specific patient unless you are sure that the patient, the patient's relative, friends, and other non-health care team members are not within hearing range. Avoid patient specific conversations in elevators, hallways, cafeterias, and general public areas. As always, cursing and derogatory language are inappropriate in public and patient care areas. If you have a disagreement or are upset with a preceptor, colleague, or health care professional, discuss the issue in a private location away from the patient care setting.

HOW TO IMPROVE YOUR PROFESSIONAL IMAGE

At the beginning of your clerkship, introduce yourself to other health care professionals with whom you will be working. Strive to become an active part of the team rather than an observer. Adhere to the appropriate institutional policies regarding lab jackets, grooming, dress, and name tags. Most importantly, be on time for patient care discussions, meetings, or specific appointments. If you are unable to fulfill a commitment, contact the appropriate individual in advance. Follow-up after the event to receive an update.

Show respect for others by using their appropriate titles. Address patients by their surname (i.e., Mr., Mrs., Dr., Ms.) unless asked by the individual to address them differently. When talking with patients and health care professionals do not interrupt. Listen carefully and observe their nonverbal behavior. A demeanor of attentiveness, cooperation, and concern is important when communicating with patients, family members, and others. Your communications should reflect a mutual courtesy, respect, openness, and honesty, as well as a commitment to the patient. In meetings with other health care professionals, do not hold personal conversations during patient care discussions. This is distracting and, more importantly, you might miss critical patient care information.

YOUR RESPONSIBILITY FOR
PROVIDING PHARMACEUTICAL CARE TO PATIENTS

As a clerkship student, you have the same responsibility for the pharmaceutical care of your patients as the pharmacist. Your preceptor or pharmacist, however, is *accountable* for the legal and ethical delivery of pharmaceutical care to the patient. While you are not directly accountable, you *are* responsible for all drug therapy a patient receives. This responsibility includes optimization of drug therapy outcomes (e.g., cure or prevention, reduction, and slowing of the disease process) avoidance of drug-induced illnesses, and prevention of inappropriate prescribing (e.g., indication, dose, interval, duration). The inappropriate administration or delivery of a medication and the appropriate assessment of efficacy or toxicity also are your responsibilities to address. Therefore, to effectively practice a pharmaceutical care philosophy, you must place a clear emphasis upon patient welfare. In essence, you must assume a patient advocacy role in order to optimize patients' drug therapy while preventing harmful effects.

YOUR RESPONSIBILITY TO THE HEALTH CARE TEAM

The health care team consists of professionals who provide patient care. This team often includes the attending or staff physician, medical residents, nurses, pharmacists, dietitians, social workers, interns, and students from any of these disciplines. In a hospital setting, daily work rounds are typically the major meeting time for the team. Those team members not attending rounds either use the medical record to document, receive, and communicate pertinent information or verbally follow-up with the physician.

Your responsibilities, as a clerkship student, include: monitoring all aspects of pharmaceutical care for each patient (e.g., identifying and resolving pharmaceutical problems), communicating all pertinent information obtained from the patient and other documents to the health care team, and responding to any requests or educational needs related to pharmaceutical care. This requires your active participation in rounds and collaboration with other team members to ensure quality patient care and the achievement of desired therapeutic outcomes.

WHEN OTHER HEALTH CARE PROFESSIONALS LIMIT YOUR PROFESSIONAL INTERACTIONS

Your response to individuals who do not accept you as an individual or as a member of the health care team reflects on your professionalism. When faced with these situations, you should seek advice from your preceptor. Most professionals have been confronted with difficult people many times during their professional careers. Your preceptor or another professional may be able to help you and hopefully, you can turn the situation into a positive learning experience.

YOUR ROLE IN MAINTAINING PATIENT CONFIDENTIALITY

Patients have the right to complete confidentiality regarding their health status, including admission into the hospital. Patients have entrusted the institution and the health care team with the privilege of, and authority for, their care. Therefore, any use of patients' names by an unauthorized individual away from the patient care unit constitutes a betrayal of this confidence. For classroom presentations to, and discussions with, faculty and other students regarding the clinical management of patients, do not identify patients by their formal names.

The medical record documents every aspect of a patients' health status. Therefore, it too is an important component of confidentiality. These documents should never be manually or mechanically copied or taken away from the patient care environment. These actions increase the risk of unauthorized disclosure of confidential information and jeopardize patient care. Any document produced by the institution that contains confidential patient information should be handled like the medical record (e.g., prescriptions, medicine profiles). Any betrayal of this confidence is a breach of patients' rights to privacy and may result in legal action.

WHY YOU NEED TO TREAT PATIENTS DIFFERENTLY THAN OTHER PEOPLE

Patients have granted the physician and hospital the authority to diagnose and treat their illnesses as needed. The psychological and social implications of hospitalization are complex and involve patients, significant others, and family.

Consider the experience of being a patient in the hospital. Individuals whom you have never seen before come into your "private room" while you are not fully clothed. They perform diagnostic procedures, take blood, and ask questions at various times during the day. Every morning a group of two to six people walks into your room and asks you personal questions about your body and mind. Meanwhile, you may have concerns about your quality of life, the effect of your hospitalization or illness upon your family, financial obligations, and even your own mortality. At the very least you are a bit frightened and feeling vulnerable. It is essential that you treat patients with respect and empathy and make every effort to protect their dignity.

WHEN YOUR ILLNESS IS A HEALTH ISSUE FOR YOUR PATIENTS AND PEERS

If you have any potentially communicable disease, you have a professional responsibility to protect patients and other members of the community. Once your disease is diagnosed, you must obtain guidelines for controlling the spread of the infection from your physician or student health service. Due to variations in institutional policies, you should also contact the employee health service of the institution(s) where you are training, regarding their precautions.

An example of a health policy for students assigned to patient care areas is presented on page XX. It requires all students to receive a tuberculin skin test and provide a record of immunization or susceptibility testing for varicellla (chicken pox), rubella (German measles) and rubeola (measles) before participation in a clerkship. The policy also addresses the issue of persons or students infected with HIV (active and seropositive) and requires that infected students be fully informed by the University Health Service on how to conduct themselves responsibly in public and in the patient care environment to protect others from becoming infected. In addition, an infection control procedure entitled "Universal Precautions" is detailed on page XX. This procedure outlines behaviors which decrease the opportunity for transmission of any type of communicable disease to or from patient and health professionals.

As with patients, your health status is a confidential issue and will be handled as such. You will not be excluded from access to the institution unless the welfare of other members of the institution or patients is at risk.

YOU ARE RESPONSIBLE FOR ENSURING DISCRIMINATION IS NOT INVOLVED WITH THE PROVISION OF HEALTH CARE

Avoid any conduct that could potentially be interpreted as discriminatory and report any observed discriminatory conduct to the appropriate people at your training site. Misconduct includes acts of physical abuse, sexual harassment, intimidation, threats of bodily harm, and any other verbal, visual, or written acts that may be demeaning to others. Any misconduct related to discriminatory issues undermines your professional image and violates the professional code of ethics.

PLAGIARISM

Plagiarism is "submission of others' ideas/works/papers as one's own." Accepting responsibility or credit for the work of another individual is both unprofessional and unethical. Unintentional plagiarism can be avoided by adopting a consistent method of differentiating word-for-word notes from thoughts obtained from readings. Keep a list of all your references to clarify to yourself and others the source of your ideas. This also enables you to double check your references if there is concern about similarities in statements.

Sample Health Policy for Students Assigned to Patient Care Areas

Purpose

To ensure that students rotating through hospitals and clinics as part of their training program have been:

- Properly screened for infectious diseases before reporting for duty.

- Informed that if they are susceptible and are exposed to an infectious disease, they report the exposure to their preceptor/supervisor and are not allowed in the hospital until it has been determined that they do not pose a risk of transmission.

Policy

It is the responsibility of the School of Pharmacy to ensure that students, before beginning their clinical training, have been screened for the infectious diseases listed below:

- **Tuberculosis.** A 5 TU tuberculin skin test is required within the past 12 months unless it is known that the student is already positive. Tuberculin-positive (>10 mm of induration with standardized 5 TU PPD skin test) students should be able to provide documentation that they have been judged not to be infectious.

- **Measles/Mumps/Rubella.** A record of immunization or the results of a serologic (antibody) testing confirming immunity must be on file. If not medically contraindicated, immunization is required for all students found to be susceptible by serologic testing. The most recent recommendations of the Centers for Disease Control (CDC) and the Public Health Service Advisory Committee on Immunization Practice (ACIP) should be used to determine whether additional immunization is necessary.

- **Varicella (Chicken Pox).** If it cannot be confirmed that the student has had chicken pox, an immunofluorescent antibody (IFA) test is strongly recommended. If the history or antibody test indicates that the student is susceptible, the student must be counseled as to the serious implications of exposing vulnerable hospital patients and staff to chicken pox. Assignment to patient care areas where exposure is uncommon is encouraged. If a susceptible student is exposed to varicella or herpes zoster (shingles) during the rotation, they must *immediately* report the exposure to their preceptor, course coordinator, and the Employee Health Service and Infection Control. A determination will then be made on whether or not the student poses a risk of transmission in the current clinical rotation assignment and whether he will be allowed to continue the rotation or assignment, be assigned to another service, or be allowed in the hospital.

- **General Health.** A general health history should be obtained to determine any other conditions that may need to be evaluated medically or for which the student may need counseling to protect themselves or patients before reporting to their clinical rotation.

Adapted from the University of Wisconsin Hospital and Clinics
Policy and Procedure 13.01, December 1989.

Sample Universal Precautions for Pharmacy Students Assigned to Patient Care Areas

Direct Patient Care

1 Wash hands thoroughly with liquid soap or antimicrobial skin cleanser after contact with a patient.

2 Do not recap needles.

3 Dispose of syringes and needles in appropriate containers.

4 Care for patients in isolation areas according to the isolation technique specific to that patient's diagnosis.

5 Use clean latex or vinyl gloves for all nonsterile contacts (i.e., if there is a risk of contacting blood or body fluids) requiring a barrier between the patient and the care giver. Discard gloves between patient contacts.

6 Wash hands routinely after gloves are removed.

7 Wear a gown if there is a risk of splashing blood or other body fluids.

8 Wear masks and protective eye wear or face shields during procedures likely to generate splashes or aerosolization of blood or other body fluids.

9 Contact the Employee or Student Health Service to determine guidelines for patient contact if you have open skin lesions, weeping dermatitis, diarrhea, or rashes of unknown etiology.

Sample Universal Precautions for Pharmacy Students Assigned to Patient Care Areas

Sterile Products Preparation

1 All personnel involved in sterile compounding must wash their hands with an antimicrobial cleanser before engaging in the preparation of sterile products. If sterile compounding is interrupted, repeat the hand washing procedure.

2 All personnel with upper respiratory tract infections who are assigned to compound sterile products, must wear a face mask during the compounding.

3 Dispose of sharp objects in appropriate boxes.

4 Clean both the laminar and vertical flow hoods at least once per shift with 70% isopropyl alcohol and wipe with gauze pads.

5 Dispose of needles in the red needle containers which will be removed by housekeeping.

6 Surgical latex gloves and isolation gowns are required for chemotherapy preparation.

7 Prepare all oncology drugs in the Type II vertical flow hood.

REFERENCES

1. University of Wisconsin School of Pharmacy. Inpatient clerkship-externship clinical instructor manual. Pharmacy Practice 728-662. 1990–1991.

2. University of Wisconsin School of Pharmacy. Student Handbook. 1990–1991.

3. Practice Standards of ASHP. American Society of Hospital Pharmacists. 1990–1991.

4. University of Wisconsin Hospital and Clinics. Department of pharmacy policy and procedure manual. Administrative Standards. 1990 September.

5. University of Wisconsin School of Pharmacy. Policy Regarding Health Issues of Pharmacy Students. 1988 December.

6. Hepler CD, Strand LM. Opportunities and responsibilities in pharmaceutical care. Am J Hosp Pharm. 1990;47:533–43.

7. Penna RP. Pharmaceutical care: pharmacy's mission for the 1990s. Am J Hosp Pharm. 1990;47:543–49.

8. University of Wisconsin System Student Conduct Rules. 1989.

9. Furlow TW. Clinical etiquette: a critical primer. JAMA. 1988;260(17): 2558–559.

ACKNOWLEDGMENT

We acknowledge the University of Wisconsin Hospital & Clinics Infection Control Committee for their assistance with the Student Health Policy and Universal Precaution Guidelines.

Providing Drug Information
Kathryn L. Grant

Learning to provide drug information entails learning a process to help you efficiently, accurately, and quickly answer drug information questions. This chapter contains questions students frequently ask about providing drug information and each question reflects an important step in the process of providing quality drug information. As with other clinical skills, the process will seem slow and cumbersome at first. Practice and experience will help you use this process to successfully provide quality drug information. However, this chapter is not a substitute for a drug literature evaluation course.

WHAT IF I AM ASKED A QUESTION AND I AM UNSURE OF THE ANSWER?

When in doubt look it up! Never be intimidated into providing an answer when you are unsure of your answer's accuracy. A patient's health is not worth the risk.

WHAT TYPES OF QUESTIONS ARE ASKED?

The vast majority of drug information questions fall into one of nine major categories:

>> Adverse drug reactions   >> Indications

>> Doses   >> IV or IM compatibilities

>> Drug administration   >> Pharmacokinetics

>> Drug identification   >> Teratogenicity

>> Drug interactions

Table 3–1 lists examples in each category. Review these examples to prepare for the scope of questions often asked concerning drug therapy or drug delivery. Other drug information categories include requests for information concerning breast feeding, carcinogenicity/mutagenicity, chemistry, contraindications, costs, patient information, pharmacology, poisoning/overdose, preparations, stability, storage, and more.

WHO ASKS DRUG INFORMATION QUESTIONS?

Pharmacists are recognized as drug experts and pharmacy students are considered "drug experts in training." As a result, patients, nurses, physicians, other pharmacists, students, respiratory therapists, and in short, anyone who needs drug knowledge asks drug information questions. Your answer must be tailored to the questioner: a nurse may need a concise, patient-specific answer, while a physician may require a more

TABLE 3–1: Major Drug Information Question Categories

Question Catagories	Sample Questions
Adverse drug reactions	What is the incidence of flushing with niacin? Can ranitidine cause liver toxicity? What are the side effects of nimodipine?
Doses	What is the dose of phenytoin for status epilepticus? What is the dose of gentamicin in a patient with renal failure? What is the dose of acetaminophen in a 6 month old infant?
Drug administration	Can carbamazepine be given rectally? How rapidly can cimetidine be given IV? Should iron dextran be given as a Z-track injection?
Drug identification	What is a new drug called ondansetron? What is the new, approved drug for endometriosis? What is the drug's name which is a round, white tablet imprinted MSD 214?
Drug interactions	Can aspirin and warfarin safely be given concurrently? Can tetracycline be taken with milk? Will cephalexin interfere with a serum glucose determination?
Indications	What is epoetin used for? What is the first line drug therapy for endometriosis? How effective is mesalamine for the treatment of ulcerative colitis?
IV or IM compatibilities	Can heparin and nitroprusside be added to the same IV bag/bottle? Can morphine and diphenhydramine be drawn into the same syringe?
Pharmacokinetics	What is the half-life of streptokinase? How much phenytoin should be given to a patient with a steady-state concentration of 5 µg/mL?
Teratogenicity	What would the risk to the fetus be if a woman took aspirin 650 mg BID for two weeks during her first trimester? Which antibiotics could be used to treat a urinary tract infection in a woman entering her third trimester?

detailed explanation of where you found the information. A patient, however, needs to have information provided in understandable terminology.

HOW CAN I ANSWER DRUG INFORMATION QUESTIONS QUICKLY?

As with any new skill you need to learn a process which, when practiced and used, helps you efficiently and accurately locate the information you need to answer drug information questions.

5 Step-Process For Providing Drug Information

1 Define and understand the question,

2 Search for an answer,

3 Evaluate and compile the facts,

4 Formulate an answer,

5 Follow up.

The key to the whole process is *step 1*. You can waste a considerable amount of time if you do not thoroughly understand the question. An inaccurate or incomplete answer can result when insufficient background or patient-specific data is obtained. Table 3–2 provides background and patient-specific data commonly needed to help you accurately answer a question.

HOW LONG CAN I TAKE TO ANSWER A DRUG INFORMATION QUESTION?

Ask the questioner how soon the answer is needed; remember, a detailed search for a complicated question takes time. The answer to a patient-related question, however, loses its impact the longer the turnaround from question to answer. Therefore, a less thorough search may be acceptable if the answer is timely for the patient in question. If the questioner appears to have an unrealistic expectation, negotiate.

WHERE DO I LOOK FOR INFORMATION?

Hundreds of texts and thousands of journals provide information to answer questions. Knowing which reference to use, along with when and how to use principal references, are the keys to finding pertinent and accurate information quickly. Medical information can be pictured as a pyramid (see Figure 3–1). Medical knowledge relies upon reports of clinical experience and clinical trials published in journal articles; these publications are referred to as *primary literature*. The most efficient way to find current, relevant primary literature is to complete a primary literature search using *secondary sources* (guides to primary literature). Performing literature searches for every question, no matter how minor, would be impractical. Health care educators write *textbooks and reference books* which, depending on their focus, compile, review, or eval-

TABLE 3–2: Defining Drug Information Questions

Category	Background or Patient Specific Information
Adverse drug reactions	Description of reactions Medications/duration of therapy Known allergies Concurrent disease states Age, weight, race, sex
Doses	Indication Route Renal function[a] Liver function Age, weight, race, sex Concurrent medications Known allergies Concurrent diseases

Drug administration	Route
	Concurrent medications
	If IV:
	    peripheral versus central access
	    infusion fluid
	    other IV medications
	If IM:
	    ability to tolerate pain
	    availability of sites
	    platelet levels
	If Oral:
	    bowel sounds present
	    patient absorbing orally
	If Rectal:
	    colon disease present
	    diarrhea

Drug identification	Correct spelling
	Imprint code
	Trade versus generic name
	Marketed, investigational, or foreign
	Indication
	Dosage form
	If Foreign:
	    country of origin
	    container information

Drug interactions
  Drug-drug
	Current medications
	Symptoms of the interaction, if occurring
	Adding a new drug
	Stopping a drug known to be causing an
	  interaction

(Continued)

3–4

TABLE 3–2: Defining Drug Information Questions *(Continued)*

Category	Background or Patient Specific Information
Drug interactions *(Continued)*	
Drug-drug	Age, weight, race, sex Disease state(s)
Drug-food	Current medications Dose/schedule Timing of meals Specific food problem (e.g., milk)
Drug-laboratory	Current medications Laboratory test(s) Specific test method used
Indications	Disease state severity, onset, duration Previous drug therapy Previous nondrug therapy See doses above
Infectious diseases	Microorganism culture and susceptibility results Infection site as above
IV or IM compatibilities	Medications/doses/schedules/routes Infusion fluid IV set-up[b] number and types of access sites available

Pharmacokinetics	Medication/dose/schedule
	Age, weight, race, sex
	Previous serum levels
	Drug pharmacokinetic parameters
	   elimination half-life
	   volume of distribution
	   serum peak concentrations
	   serum trough concentrations
	   time to peak concentration
	   compartment model
	   area-under-the-curve (AUC)

Teratogenicity	Medications/doses/schedules/duration Trimester Medical status Drinking/smoking history Can therapy be postponed until postpartum

[a] Renal function parameters include serum creatinine, creatinine clearance, dialysis method, and dialysis schedule.

[b] IV setups include: Continuous infusions: two drugs added to the same liter bag/bottle; Piggyback or Y site: one drug infused in the IV line of another drug; Injection port: one drug pushed from a syringe into the line of another drug.

FIGURE 3–1: Overview of Medical Information Sources.

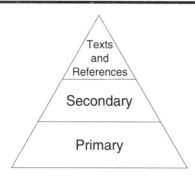

uate the medical information published in primary literature to facilitate access by students and practitioners. An efficient search method is to begin at the top of the pyramid with the compiled information and work down. This approach recognizes that textbooks and reference books, while providing excellent accumulated data, are not as current as more recently published reviews, editorials, and clinical trials.

Table 3–3 lists the most helpful references and is organized by the 9 major categories of drug information inquiries as listed on page 3–1. Reference entries under each category are listed in descending order from most likely to contain the information to least likely.

WHEN SHOULD I SEARCH THE PRIMARY LITERATURE?

>> If the questioner asks for primary literature references.

>> If the answer is not in text and references.

>> If the information found in text and references appears to be out of date.

HOW DO I USE SECONDARY SOURCES TO DO A LITERATURE SEARCH?

Secondary sources are all organized quite differently. Some secondary sources provide only the citation (defined as the journal article's author(s), title, journal title, year, volume, issue and page numbers), while others provide the citation along with an abstract. Frequency of publication (e.g., monthly, quarterly), format of publication (e.g., computer access, hard-bound book, section of a journal), and indexing format are additional differences in secondary sources.

Indexing large databases is difficult and large databases, such as Medlars (see Table 3–4), standardize medical terms or phrases to facilitate the process. If standardized terms are used, the secondary source publishes a list of synonyms in a *thesaurus* and the secondary source's *thesaurus* must be accessed in order to use the reference efficiently and accurately. Table 3–4 lists 7 commonly used secondary sources including their available format(s), how often they are updated, the type of information included, the type and number of journals indexed, and whether a published thesaurus is available. Computerized databases can often be searched by the standardized (thesaurus) term and by free text or *key words*. Key words are any words which appear in the citation or

TABLE 3–3: Drug Information Sources: Text and References Organized by Drug Information Categories

Category	Reference Choices[a]
Adverse Drug Reactions	AHFS DI/DrugDex/USP DI Martindale's: The Extra Pharmacopoeia Side Effects of Drugs Textbook of Adverse Drug Reactions Goodman and Gilman's: The Pharmacologic Basis of Therapeutics
Doses	Drug Facts and Comparisons AHFS DI/DrugDex/USP DI Physicians Desk Reference(s) Martindale's: The Extra Pharmacopoeia AMA Drug Evaluation
Pediatric	Pediatric Drug Handbook Harriet Lane Heandbook Current Pediatric Diagnosis and Treatment
Drug Administration	See **Doses** *If IV/IM* see Handbook of Injectable Drugs
Drug Identification Marketed	Drug Facts and Comparisons PharmIndex Identidex AHFS DI/DrugDex/USP DI Physicians Desk Reference(s) American Drug Index Handbook of Nonprescription Drugs American Druggist Blue Book Drug Topics Red Book
Investigational	PharmIndex Martindale's: The Extra Pharmacopoeia DrugDex USAN Unlisted Drugs Merck Index
Foreign	Martindale's: The Extra Pharmacopoeia Unlisted Drugs Index Nominum Diccionaria de Especialidades Farmaceuticas USAN
Drug Interactions Drug-drug	Drug Interactions & Updates Drug Interactions Facts Evaluation of Drug Interactions AHFS DI/DrugDex/USP DI
Side Effects of Drugs Drug-food	Drug Interactions & Updates USP DI Vol. II: Advice for the Patient

(Continued)

TABLE 3–3: Drug Information Sources: Text and References Organized by Drug Information Categories *(Continued)*

Category	Reference Choices[a]
Side Effects of Drugs *(Continued)*	
Drug-laboratory	Handbook of Clinical Drug Data Clinical Guide to Laboratory Tests Interpretation of Diagnostic Tests
Indications	Pharmacotherapy AMA Drug Evaluations AHSF DI/DrugDex/USP DI Applied Therapeutics: The Clinical Use of Drugs Current Medical Diagnosis and Treatment Current Pediatric Diagnosis and Treatment Manual of Medical Therapeutics Scientific American Harrison's: Principles of Internal Medicine
Infectious diseases	Mandell's: Principles and Practice of Infectious Disease Medical Letter Handbook of Antimicrobial Therapy Sanford's Guide to Antimicrobial Therapy
IV or IM Compatibilities	Handbook of Injectable Drugs King's Guide to Parenteral Admixtures Martindale's: The Extra Pharmacopoeia
Pharmacokinetics	Applied Pharmacokinetics: Priniciples of Therapeutic Drug Monitoring Basic Clinical Pharmacokinetics AHSF DI/DrugDex/USP DI Handbook of Clinical Drug Data Goodman and Gilman's: The Pharmacologic Basis of Therapeutics Martindale's: The Extra Pharmacopoeia
Teratogenicity	Physicians Desk Reference Drugs in Pregnancy and Lactation Catalog of Teratogenic Agents AHSF DI/DrugDex/USP DI

[a] Under each category, the references are listed roughly in the order they would most likely provide the

TABLE 4–4: Drug Information Sources: Secondary References

Secondary References	Format	Updates	Focus	Type of Journals Reviewed	Number of Journals Reviewed	Published Thesaurus
Clin-Alert. Scheible-Jacobs R ed. Medford, NJ: Clin-Alert, Inc.	Abstracting service as a newsletter edition	Semi-monthly	Adverse drug reactions	Medicine, pharmacy	600	No
Current Contents: Clinical Practice. Garfield E. Philadelphia, PA: Institute for Scientific Information Inc.	Table of contents indexed by author and key works in either a soft cover edition or on floppy disk	Weekly	Clinical practice	Medicine, pharmacy	850	No
Iowa Drug Information Service (IDIS). Seaba H, ed. Iowa City, IA: The University of Iowa.	Citation and whole article on microfiche; citation only on CD-ROM	Monthly	Clinical practice	Medicine, pharmacy	170	Yes
InPharma. Covich K ed. Langhorne, PA: Australian Drug Information Services.	Abstracting service as a newsletter edition or online searching	Weekly	Clinical practice	Medicine, pharmacy	1800	No
International Pharmaceutical Abstracts (IPA). Tousignaut D ed. Bethesda, MD: American Society of Hospital Pharmacists.	Abstracting service as a soft cover edition; CD-ROM and online searching available also	Monthly, quarterly	Pharmacy	Pharmacy practice	800	Yes

(Continued)

TABLE 4–4: Drug Information Sources: Secondary References *(Continued)*

Secondary References	Format	Updates	Focus	Type of Journals Reviewed	Number of Journals Reviewed	Published Thesaurus
Medlars **Index Medicus.** Lindberg DAB ed. Washington, DC: Superintendent of Documents, US Government Printing Office.	Citations as a soft cover edition	Monthly	Biomedical research, medicine, pharmacy, nursing	Research, clinical practice	2700	Yes
Compact Cambridge and other vendors.	Abstracting service on CD-ROM	Quarterly	As above	As above	3200	Yes
NLM, Grateful Med, Dialog, BRS and other vendors.	Abstracting service as online searching	Quarterly	As above	As above	3200	Yes
Reactions. Wright T ed. Langhorne, PA: Australian Drug Information Service.	Abstracting service as a newsletter edition	Weekly	Adverse drug reactions	Medicine, pharmacy	1800	No

abstract. A detailed explanation of how to use these sources is beyond the scope of this manual. Therefore, you are encouraged to find out which ones are available to you in the medical or pharmacy libraries and/or drug information center nearest you.

HOW DO I CONSTRUCT A SEARCH STRATEGY FOR A COMPUTERIZED LITERATURE SEARCH?

Each computerized secondary source, whether accessed from a personal computer connected to a CD-ROM reader or a modem access to a mainframe, utilizes different commands and nomenclature. Consult the specific source's user manual for detailed instructions. In general, the user types in a *search statement (SS)*. A simple search could be as follows:

> SS
>
> [1]mesalamine

The secondary source will respond with the number of citations (postings) containing the word/index term *mesalamine*.

> postings: 56

Search strategies can be combined to expand or limit the postings. Combinations are made by using the Boolean connecting words *"and," "or," "not."* The Boolean operator *"and"* limits posting retrievals (see Figure 3–2i). The Boolean operator *"or"* widens retrievals (see Figure 3–2ii). While the Boolean operator *"not"* limits retrieval, results can be unpredictable. For now, avoid the use of *"not"* (see Figure 3–2iii). Boolean operators can be combined in series. Figure 3–3i on page XX shows the theoretical retrieval if three statements are all combined with an *"and"*: A *"and"* B *"and"* C. Figure 3–3ii on page 3–13 shows the results when (A *"or"* B) *"and"* C are combined.

The following four steps are used to efficiently develop a search strategy:

1) Break the question into component parts or word sets labeling each set with the heading A, B, etc.

2) Write down all potential thesaurus and key word terms under each heading.

3) Combine each term listed together under a heading with the Boolean operator "or."

4) Combine each word set with the Boolean operator "and."

FIGURE 3–2: Overview of Medical Information Sources.

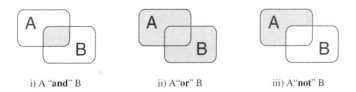

i) A "and" B   ii) A"or" B   iii) A"not" B

Example: Computerized Literature Search

Question: How effective is mesalamine (Rowasa) for the rectal treatment of ulcerative colitis?

Step One: Break the question into component parts or word sets, labeling each set A, B, etc.

How effective is mesalamine for the rectal treatment of ulcerative colitis?

   A. mesalamine
   B. rectal treatment
   C. ulcerative colitis

Note the concept of efficacy is not searchable.

Step Two: Write down all potential thesaurus and key word terms under each heading.

A	B	C
mesalamine[a]	ulcerative colitis[c]	rectal administration[d]
Rowasa	ulcerative	rect[e]
5-asa	colitis	enema
5-aminosalicyl[b]	ileitis	topical

a. If the word is a thesaurus term, it can be typed in without any special symbol. If used as a key word, some computerized databases require a special symbol (e.g., *) or a special word (e.g., all) to allow a word to be searched as a key word.

b. This is a truncation of 5-aminosalicylic acid and 5-aminosalicylate. Most computerized data-bases will allow truncation using a special symbol (e.g., an asterisk * or a colon :).

c. Check the database's thesaurus. The term may be colitis ulcerative.

d. Check the database's thesaurus. The term may be administration rectal.

e. This is a truncation (see note b). This truncation would also retrieve key words such as rectify, and rectangle, causing "false hits."

Step Three: Combine each term listed together under a heading with the Boolean operator "or."

SS

[1] mesalamine or Rowasa or 5-asa or 5-aminosalicyl:

[2] ulcerative colitis or ulcerative or colitis

[3] rect: or enema or topical or rectal administration

Step Four: Combine each word set with the Boolean operator "and."

[4] #1 and #2

[5] #3 and #4

FIGURE 3–3: Representation of Search.

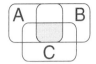

i) A "and" B "and" C

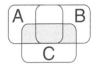

ii) A "or" B "and" C

Be patient. Rarely can a perfect search strategy be constructed the first time.

If too few citations were retrieved, you may need to think of additional terms or you may have typed "and" instead of "or" (a common mistake), or not many citations on the topic exist. To come up with more terms, type the command to review the thesaurus terms used by the indexer on the citations already retrieved. Perhaps they will provide a clue for other terms to use. Usually two word sets are sufficient for most questions although the example used three word sets. If you had actually used the example, more relevant postings would been found if SS #1 was combined with SS #3 and the disease state was not included.

Conversely, if too many citations were retrieved, limiting the search by requesting only English language and human studies may decrease the number of citations. Retrieval can also be limited, if relevant to your question, by requesting studies by age group, gender, reviews, comparative studies. If only two word sets were used, adding a third word set may limit the number of retrievals.

HOW DO I EVALUATE CLINICAL TRIALS?

Whole college courses are devoted to this topic and detailed review of drug literature evaluation is beyond this manual's objectives. A simplified approach follows.

In general, you, as the evaluator, are trying to determine if biases are apparent in how the study was written, designed, and completed. If biases are evident, the next step is to determine whether these biases are serious enough to invalidate the study's results.

Written Clinical Trials: Four Basic Sections

The four basic sections of a written clinical trial other than the abstract are: 1) introduction, 2) methodology, 3) results, and 4) discussion. Analyze each section or subsection to answer the evaluative questions.

Introduction.

>> Was a statement of the study's objective(s) clearly provided?

Methods.

>> Was the study design explained in sufficient detail to determine: how subjects were included or excluded; the number of subjects included; and the subject parameters that might influence the results?

>> Were the data collected retrospectively or prospectively?

>> Did the study use acceptable controls (i.e., placebo, standard drug, historical)?

>> Were subjects randomly assigned to treatment groups?

>> If the study involved a crossed-over treatment regimen, was the drug-free interval before cross-over of sufficient duration?

>> Did the design include blinding of subject or investigator (single blind); subject and investigator (double blind); the observer?

>> Were the test methods used to measure results subjective or objective, reliable, sensitive, and specific?

Results.

>> Were all pertinent results presented in sufficient detail for adequate analysis?

>> Were the tabular, graphic, and written presentations accurate, distorted, or misleading?

>> Was the statistical method used appropriate for the data collected?

>> Did a statistically significant difference support a clinically significant difference?

Discussion.

>> Were the authors' conclusions accurately based upon the results presented?

>> Were the authors' conclusions in keeping with the study's stated objectives?

HOW DO I COMPILE THE FACTS TO ANSWER THE QUESTION?

At this point, you have collected bits and pieces of information from text/references and the primary literature. The hardest part of providing drug information is summarizing and applying the information to a clinical situation. You must apply the knowledge from all your didactic courses to put the retrieved information in perspective with your clinical knowledge and to synthesize an answer.

To return to our previous example, the question was how effective is mesalamine for the rectal treatment of ulcerative colitis. We found that mesalamine is used for the treatment of mild to moderate distal ulcerative colitis from researching AHFS DI, DRUGDEX, USP DI, and Martindale's. A literature search found 13 relevant clinical trials. These clinical trials varied as to design, patient selection, doses used, and how efficacy was assessed. Now, the challenge is to summarize these results. In general, the following six steps will assist in sorting clinical trial information: *Step 1* list the specific disease state; *Step 2* list the extent of illness; *Step 3* list the study design; *Step 4* list the doses used; *Step 5* list the efficacy measurements; and *Step 6* list the results.

This method provides a framework for organizing and summarizing the clinical trial information to more easily see differences and similarities. The following is an example using this method.

1) Specific disease state: distal ulcerative colitis

2) Extent of illness: mild-to-moderate

3) Study design: single blind, double blind, crossover

4) Doses used: 1, 2, 3, or 4 gm rectally

5) Efficacy measurements: clinical symptoms, histology

6) Results: symptomatic improvement in 62% to 93%

HOW DO I FORMULATE AN ANSWER?

Answers to drug information questions must summarize the results of the literature search and be presented with a logical progression of facts to support the answer. Providing the questioner with an unorganized series of facts is unacceptable. For the busy clinician, start your summary with one phrase or sentence clearly stating your answer. Follow this with the supporting reasons for your answer. Formal or published answers to drug information questions usually start with in-depth background information followed by the summary of clinical data and end with the answer.

HOW CAN I BE SURE MY ANSWER IS CORRECT?

Prevent errors by carefully making notes from your information sources and rechecking numbers. If a concept or fact does not fit into what you have been taught, recheck the information with other references.

The best way to determine the accuracy of your answer is to recontact the questioner and find out if they used the information. If not, why not? If so, what happened? This feedback measures whether the provided information was relevant, timely, or useful.

Physical Examination

Michael Madalon
Randolph W. Hurley

This chapter provides an overview of adult physical examination (PE). It is not intended to teach the reader how to perform a physical examination, but rather it describes the key components of the diagnostic physical examination and relates the influence of drugs to this process.

4

The positive and negative findings noted during the physical examination of a patient are important. Likewise, the subjective and objective information gleaned from the physical examination and from the interview of a patient are crucial to the assessment of efficacy and toxicities associated with drug therapy. A basic understanding of human physiology and gross anatomy are required before the intricacies of a diagnostic examination can be truly appreciated and such reference texts should be accessible.

MEDICAL HISTORY

When a patient is admitted to the hospital or undergoes a detailed medical evaluation, the physician typically obtains a thorough medical history before physically examining the patient. The history describes the events in the life of the patient that are relevant to the patient's mental and physical health. The components of the medical history usually follow a standardized format as follows:

>> Identifying data (ID),

>> Chief complaint (CC),

>> History of present illness (HPI),

>> Past medical history (PMH),

>> Family and social history (FH/SH), and

>> Review of systems (ROS).

TECHNIQUES IN THE PHYSICAL EXAMINATION

Physical examination utilizes four main techniques: inspection, palpation, percussion, and auscultation. *Inspection* is visual observation of the patient with unaided eyes, although instruments are often used. *Palpation* is the use of touch to detect normal and abnormal physical findings. *Percussion* is the tapping of a body surface with a fingertip to produce sounds that help determine whether underlying structures are air-filled, fluid-filled, or solid. *Auscultation*, often with the aid of a stethoscope, is listening for normal and abnormal sounds.

SIGNS AND SYMPTOMS

When interpreting a history and physical examination, clinical signs and symptoms are often described. A *sign* refers to objective information gathered by the examiner during the PE (e.g., heart murmur, ankle edema, rales). A *symptom* refers to subjective information gathered from the patient while obtaining the history (e.g., nausea, pain). The patient's descriptions of symptoms are further scrutinized, clarified, and quantified by questioning the patient on the specific characteristics of symptoms as follows:

Characteristic	Question
Location	Where is it located in the body?
Chronology/Duration	When does it occur and for how long?
Quality/Intensity	How often does it occur and how intense is it? What does it feel like?
Aggravating/Alleviating factors	What makes it better or worse?
Related symptoms	What other symptoms are present?

ORGANIZATION OF THE PHYSICAL EXAMINATION

Recorded physical examinations are typically arranged in the following order:

>> General appearance

>> Vital signs

>> Skin and nails

>> Lymph nodes

>> HEENT (head, eyes, ears, nose, throat)

>> Neck

>> Back

>> Chest (general, lung, and breast exam)

>> Cardiovascular system (CV)

>> Gastrointestinal system (GI)

>> Genitourinary and rectal system (GU)

>> Peripheral vascular system (PVS)

>> Musculoskeletal system (MSK)

>> Neurological system (Neuro)

>> Mental status

General Appearance

This portion of the physical examination provides a brief description of the patient's overall appearance and may reflect the individual's general health, nutritional status, and level of distress. The patient's posture, facial expressions, hygiene, and mental status may be noted here as well. Typical observations might include:

>> This is a thin young female in NAD (No Apparent Distress).

>> This is a pale, tearful, male who is otherwise alert and oriented.

>> This is a WDWNWM (Well Developed, Well Nourished, White Male).

Vital Signs

Just as the name implies, a patient's vital signs are critical in assessing the clinical status of the patient and the acuity of a given problem. Vital signs include the temperature, pulse, blood pressure, and respirations. In addition, height and weight are typically recorded in this section.

Temperature (T). Body temperature is measured in the mouth, rectum, or axilla and identification of route is essential for interpretation of the result. Normal adult body temperatures are 35.8–37.3 °C (96.4–99.1 °F) when measured in the mouth; 35.3–36.8 °C (95.9–99.6 °F) when measured in axillae; and 36.3–37.8 °C (94.9–99.6 °F) when measured rectally. Temperatures greater than 37.8 °C (>100 °F) indicate fever.

Pulse (P). Physicians typically assess the rate, rhythm, and strength of the pulse. Normal heart rate (HR) is 60 to 100 beats per minute (BPM). Deviation from normals, particularly tachycardia (HR >100 BPM), is a sensitive indicator of disease. Bradycardia (HR <60 BPM) can be normal in a well-conditioned athlete or could be abnormal in a patient with hypothyroidism. A HR <60 BPM can also indicate increased vagal tone, cardiac conduction defects, or the effect of drugs with a negative chronotropic effect (e.g., beta blockers, digoxin). Tachycardia has a much broader differential diagnosis encompassing a myriad of conditions including pain, anxiety, volume depletion, and pulmonary embolism. Tachycardia can also be a side effect of drugs (e.g., sympathomimetic and anticholinergic medications).

Rhythm is difficult to accurately assess without the aid of electrocardiographic monitoring; however, the pulse's regularity or irregularity can be assessed. A pulse characterized as "irregularly-irregular" may indicate atrial fibrillation, whereas occasional "regularly irregular" beats may indicate premature atrial or ventricular contraction (PAC or PVC). An apical pulse is the preferred palpation approach for determination of a patient's heart rate because not all of the beats in atrial fibrillation may be conducted to the peripheral pulses.

Blood Pressure (BP) can vary according to age, race, and gender. It can even vary from minute to minute in any given patient. An appropriate cuff size and careful attention to proper technique for blood pressure measurement are critical to accurate assessment (e.g., a small cuff on a large patient's arm could overestimate the true blood pressure).

Adult blood pressure >140/90 mm Hg on more than one occasion, is considered abnormal. An increase in either the diastolic or systolic pressure has been correlated with cardiovascular morbidity and mortality. Orthostatic blood pressure and pulse are defined as the change in BP and pulse when the patient changes from a sitting to a standing position. A systolic BP drop of >10 mm Hg or a pulse rise of >10 to 20 BPM can reflect intravascular volume depletion, autonomic dysfunction, antihypertensive drug therapy, or a side effect of medications (e.g., anticholinergics and antidepressants).

Pulsus paradoxus originally described the decreased amplitude of the peripheral pulse with inspiration; however, it is now more accurately assessed with a blood pressure cuff and reflects the decrease in systolic BP with inspiration. A normal change is ≤10 mm Hg, but this value can be accentuated in pericardial tamponade, airways obstruction (such as asthma), or superior vena cava obstruction.

Respiratory Rate (RR). The rate and pattern of breathing are assessed and can reflect cardiopulmonary or neurological disease. A normal adult breathes at a rate of 12 to 18 respirations/min. Tachypnea (RR >20 respirations/min) can be caused by anxiety, pain, and a number of cardiac and pulmonary disease states. Bradypnea (RR <10 respirations/min) can be a sign of drug-induced respiratory depression such as that associated with opiates.

A number of normal and abnormal patterns of breathing have been described. Cheyne-Stokes breathing is a form of periodic breathing characterized by periods of apnea (absent respirations) alternating with a series of respiratory cycles in which the rate and amplitude increase to a maximum (i.e., hyperpnea or deep rapid breathing). Cheyne-Stokes breathing occurs in patients with brain damage (e.g., trauma or cerebral hemorrhage), CHF, and in normal persons at high altitude. Kussmaul's respirations are deep regular respirations that occur independent of the rate. Kussmaul breathing occurs in diabetic ketoacidosis and signals hyperventilatory respiratory compensations for the metabolic acidosis.

Height and Weight. Although not classical vital signs, height and weight are typically recorded in this section. Height and weight can be used together to calculate body surface area (BSA) and lean body weight (LBW). Day-to-day variation in body weight reflects changes in total body water (TBW) which is important in assessing the hydration and fluid status of the patient or for assessing response to diuretic therapy.

Skin, Hair, Nails

Skin. The integumentary system is perhaps one of the most assessable organ systems and skin rashes are a common form of adverse drug reactions. A notation of the skin examination in the medical record is typically brief, yet contains a number of descriptive terms and phrases. A more complete description would include details regarding color (e.g., brownness, cyanosis, yellowness or jaundice), vascularity (including "bruising" or purpura), edema, temperature, texture, mobility and turgor, and the presence of lesions.

Skin lesions are described in terms of primary and secondary lesions (see Figure 4–1). Primary lesions may arise from previously normal skin and can be divided into three categories:

1) Circumscribed, flat, nonpalpable changes in skin color (macules and patches);

2) Palpable solid elevations in the skin (nodules, plaques, papules, cysts, and wheals); and

3) Circumscribed superficial elevations of the skin formed by free fluid within the skin layers (vesicles, bulla, and pustules).

Secondary lesions result from changes in a primary lesion and include the development of erosions, ulcers, fissures, crusts, and scales.

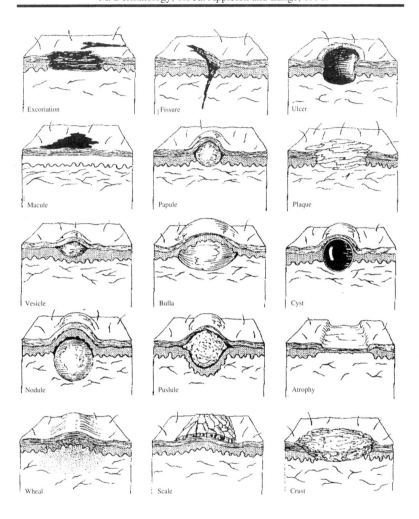

These descriptive terms can be combined in the record. For example, an erythematous maculopapular eruption (a common manifestation of drug-induced dermatologic
toxicity) could be described as circumscribed, flat, red, macules in combination with
palpable, solid, raised papules. See Table 4–1 and Figure 4–2 for more information
on descriptive dermatological terms and examples.

Drug-induced cutaneous eruptions occur in many different forms. These include
acneiform or pustular, eczematous, generalized erythroderma, exfoliation, fixed drug
eruptions, maculopapular, lupus-like, photosensitivity, and vesiculobullous lesions.
For a more complete list of drugs which cause eruptions, consult suggested references listed on page 4–21.

TABLE 4–1: Descriptive Dermatologic Terms and Examples

Lesion	Description	Example
Acneiform	Erythematous pustules	Acne
Annular	Ring shaped	Ringworm
Confluent	Lesions run together	Viral exanthems
Discoid	Disc shaped without central clearing	Lupus erythematosus
Eczematoid	An inflammation with a tendency to vesiculate and crust	Eczema
Erythroderma	Diffuse red color	Sunburn
Exfoliative	Sloughing of skin layers	Toxic epidermal necrolysis
Grouped	Clustered lesions	Vesicles of Herpes simplex
Iris	"Bulls eye" or target type lesions	Erythema multiform
Keratotic	Thickening	Psoriasis
Linear	In lines	Poison ivy
Papulosquamous	Raised papules or plaques with scaling	Psoriasis
Urticarial	Raised local edema of the skin (wheal)	Hives
Zosteriform	Linear arrangement along a dermatome	Herpes zoster

Hair is considered a skin appendage. It is described according to texture (e.g., dry and coarse as in hypothyroidism) and distribution (facial or upper body). Hirsutism (the growth of hair in women in a characteristically male pattern), can be due to androgen excess syndromes, corticosteroids and Cushing's syndrome, oral contraceptives, and androgenic medications. Hypertrichosis (increased hair growth, particularly on the face) is an adverse effect of medications such as minoxidil and cyclosporine.

Nails are also considered a skin appendage. A variety of nail changes have been described; perhaps the most important is clubbing (see Figure 4–3). Clubbing is the selective bullous enlargement of the distal segment of the digit due to an increase in soft tissue and is associated with flattening of the angle between the nail and nail base from 160° to 180°. Clubbing can be hereditary or idiopathic and is associated with a variety of conditions, including cyanotic heart disease and pulmonary disorders. Pitting and ridging of the nails is another common finding and is characteristic of psoriasis.

Lymph Nodes

Lymph nodes are not usually palpable, unless enlarged. (See Figure 4–4 for the location of lymph node groups.) Enlargement can be due to a variety of disorders including infections, neoplasia (lymphomas and metastatic malignancies), immunological

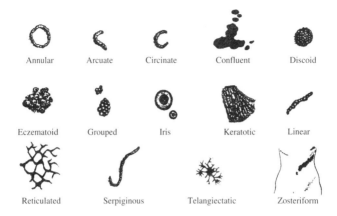

disorders (rheumatoid arthritis, systemic lupus erythematous), and other illnesses. Rarely, phenytoin produces a pseudolymphomatous enlargement of the lymph nodes.

Lymph nodes are described according to their size, location, firmness, mobility, and tenderness. Tender nodes suggest infection, whereas firm, nontender, immobile nodes suggest malignancy. Shotty nodes are small nodes that feel "like buckshot" underneath the skin and are not necessarily pathologic.

HEENT (Head, Eyes, Ears, Nose, Throat)

Head. When the head is described, its shape is noted using the terms normocephalic (occasionally abbreviated NC), hydrocephalic, or microcephalic. Evidence of trauma is discovered by inspection and palpation. Absence of trauma (atraumatic) is occasionally abbreviated AT.

Several disorders have characteristic facial features including the moon facies of Cushing's syndrome (or corticosteroid use), exophthalmos of Grave's disease, and the masked facies of scleroderma or parkinsonism. Several skin disorders and rashes

FIGURE 4–3: **Clubbing of the Finger.** Reprinted with permission.
Malasanos L et al. Health Assessment, The CV Mosby Co.

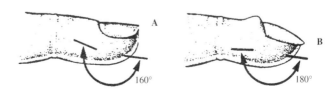

A. Normal angle of the nail.
B. Abnormal angle of the nail seen in late clubbing.

FIGURE 4–4: Location of Lymph Nodes in the Body.

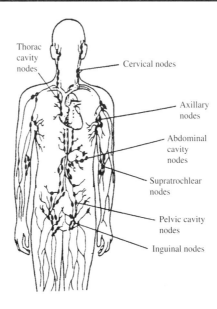

Thorac
cavity
nodes

Cervical nodes

Axillary
nodes

Abdominal
cavity
nodes

Supratrochlear
nodes

Pelvic cavity
nodes

Inguinal nodes

affect the face, including acne vulgaris, acne rosacea, the purplish heliotrope rash surrounding the eyelids in dermatomyositis, the butterfly-pattern malar rash over the cheeks in SLE, and the zosteriform rash of Herpes zoster.

Eyes. Routine bedside examination of the eyes includes observations of visual acuity (VA), visual fields (VF), the external eye, the extraocular muscles (EOM), pupillary responses, and a funduscopic examination. If an ophthalmologic problem is suspected, visual acuity is always checked first with a hand-held Snellen chart. Visual fields can only be grossly tested at the bedside. The conjunctiva of the external eye is examined for inflammation (conjunctival infection or conjunctivitis), mattering, and exudate. The presence of conjunctival pallor may indicate anemia. Abnormalities of the sclera include scleral icterus (a yellowish pigment overlying the sclera) that signifies jaundice in a patient with a bilirubin serum concentration >2 to 3 mg/dL. Arcus senilis (a white discoloration at the periphery of the cornea) is present to some degree in most people over 60 years of age. It was previously thought to be a marker of atherosclerosis, but arcus senilis now is considered to be a degenerative change and of little clinical significance.

The function of the extraocular muscles is described as intact (EOMI), if the patient can follow the examiner's finger through the normal directions of gaze. Thus, a muscle palsy or cranial nerve problem could be detected if the patient is unable to follow the examiner's finger when directed up-down or left-right. Strabismus is the lack of parallelism of the eyes' visual axes. Nystagmus is an abnormal rapid rhythmic spontaneous movement of the eyes (i.e., under conditions of fixation, the eyes drift slowly vertically or horizontally and is corrected by a quick movement to the original position). Nystagmus can indicate inner ear and brain disease and is also part of the triad of findings for Wernicke's encephalopathy. Nystagmus also can be a sign of drug toxicity [e.g., phenytoin, lithium, phencyclidine (PCP)].

In examining the pupillary response, the clinician tests the afferent function of the optic nerve along with the efferent pupillary response of the third cranial nerve. Normally, if a light is shone in one eye, both pupils will constrict (both a direct and consensual response). PERRLA (pupils equal, round, reactive to light and accommodation) is a typical mnemonic description in the medical record. A number of processes, both normal and abnormal, can produce anisocoria (a difference in the size of the pupils). Likewise, a number of drugs can classically affect pupillary size (e.g., barbiturates produce mydriasis or pupillary dilatation; opiates produce miosis or pinpoint pupils).

An ophthalmoscope is used in the funduscopic examination to view the optic fundus, retinal vessels, and optic disc. The retinal vessels are some of the few small sized vessels that can be readily seen in detail. Characteristic changes in the vessels are observed in a number of vascular diseases (See Chapter 6: Diagnostic Procedures, page 6–45.). Hypertension produces graded changes based on the severity and duration of the elevated blood pressure. Arteriovenous narrowing is one of the early changes in hypertension. Hemorrhages, exudates, and papilledema signify more extensive hypertensive retinopathy. Diabetic retinopathy is characterized by early microaneurysm and exudates that can progress to proliferation of blood vessels, retinal detachment, and vitreal hemorrhage.

Ophthalmologists utilize several additional instruments in the evaluation of eye complaints. These instruments include planometry to detect glaucoma; slit lamp examination which can identify a number of lesions including corneal opacities due to drug toxicity; and visual field testing which is important to monitor for hydroxychloroquine toxicity.

Ears. Bedside examination of the ear includes observation with the aid of an otoscope and gross tests of hearing with or without the aid of a tuning fork. Otitis externa (swimmer's ear) is typified by an inflamed external ear canal that is tender to the touch. Otitis media (middle ear infection) occurs behind the tympanic membrane (TM) and is common in children. The ear drum can be retracted if eustachian tube dysfunction is present. Bulging of the drum suggests fluid or pus in the middle ear. Pus in the ear canal might suggest tympanic membrane perforation, whereas blood could suggest basilar skull fracture in a patient with head trauma.

A conical shaped light reflex is observed on the normal TM due to the reflection of light from the otoscope. Distortion of the reflection's shape is also seen in otitis media. In addition, a device is available to insufflate air into the external ear canal through the otoscope. By insufflating air, the TM's ease of mobility can be assessed. Decreased mobility is seen in otitis media and eustachian tube dysfunction.

Nose. The nose is examined for deformities, swelling, septal defects, and discharge. Epistaxis, a nose bleed, may represent an adverse effect of anticoagulant therapy. Nasal polyps are associated with asthma in patients with aspirin hypersensitivity. Rhinitis medicamentosus, a side effect of prolonged nasal vasoconstrictor therapy, may manifest as mucosal swelling and edema.

Mouth and Oropharynx. Visual examination of the mouth and oropharynx can identify a number of diseases and adverse drug manifestations. Cyanosis of the lips might indicate hypoxemia. Gingival hyperplasia can be caused by phenytoin. Stomatitis (mouth sores) is a common complication of cytotoxic drugs or gold. Xerostomia (dry mouth) is observed as a lack of saliva and can be caused by a variety of connective tissue diseases (e.g., SLE, rheumatoid arthritis, Sjogren's syndrome) and medications (e.g., anticholinergics). Infectious disease manifestations include pharyngitis, erythema (with or without exudates), oral thrush/candidiasis (e.g., in immunocompromised patients or infants), and herpetic lesions. Aphthous stomatitis is a common nonspecific painful ulceration of the buccal mucosa. Hairy leukoplakia, a common manifestation of AIDS, appears as a white, raised lesion on the lateral margins of the tongue.

Neck

Structures examined in the neck include the trachea, carotid artery, jugular veins, and thyroid gland. The presence of masses or adenopathy is noted. A deviation of the trachea can occur to one side due to collapse or hyperexpansion of one lung (pneumothorax) or displacement by masses. Diffuse thyroid enlargement (goiter) and the presence of nodules is also noted. If appropriate, the neck's resistance to passive motion [e.g., in a patient with cervical arthritis (motion limited) or meningitis (neck stiffness detected)] is noted. Additional maneuvers that classically suggest meningeal irritation include Kernig's sign (resistance to extension of the knee after passive flexion at the hip), and Brudzinski's sign (flexion of the hips after passive flexion of the neck).

Jugular venous distention (JVD) reflects central venous pressure as shown in Figure 4–5; height of distention is measured in centimeters. JVD will be decreased in patients who are hypovolemic, and increased in conditions such as CHF, right-ventricular dysfunction, cardiac tamponade, and cor pulmonale. By applying pressure over the liver, the hepatojugular reflex (HJR) test (i.e., application of pressure over the liver and subsequent neck vein distention) assesses liver congestion and right ventricular function.

The carotid artery pulse is examined for duration and amplitude. A delayed upstroke is characteristic of aortic stenosis. A bounding pulse is characteristic of high-stroke volume states such as aortic regurgitation (waterhammer pulse). Auscultation of the carotid arteries can detect bruits (sounds or murmurs caused by blood flowing past an obstacle or an atherosclerotic narrowing).

FIGURE 4–5: Hepatojugular Reflex: Measuring the Jugular Venous Pressure. Reprinted with permission. Judge AC et al. Clinical Diagnosis, Little Brown and Co.

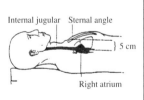
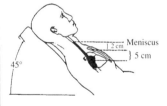

Jugular venous pressure cannot be measured (in supine patient)

Jugular venous pressure is 7 cm of water

Measuring the jugular venous pressure. The sternal angle (angle of Louis) is a bony ridge palpable between the manubrium and the body of the sternum at the level of the second intercostal space. It is always 5 cm vertically above the mid-right atrium. In any position, therefore, one may measure the distance from the sternal angle to the meniscus of the internal jugular vein and add 5 cm to obtain the jugular venous pressure.

Back

Examination of the back discloses any spinal deformities (e.g., scoliosis, kyphosis) or tenderness. Conditions of endogenous or exogenous corticosteroid excess can produce a "buffalo hump" over the upper back. Costovertebral angle (CVA) tenderness in the posterior flank is a classic sign of pyelonephritis.

Chest

General. Examination of the chest includes inspection, palpation, percussion, and auscultation. The chest is inspected for sternal deformities (e.g., pectus excavatum, pectus carinatum). (See Figure 4–6.) An increased anterio-posterior (AP) diameter (i.e., barrel chest) is seen in chronic obstructive airways disease (COAD). Vigorous use of the accessory muscles of respiration (sternocleidomastoid muscle, intercostal muscles) or retraction between the rib spaces on inspiration accompanies severe airways obstruction.

Palpation of the chest detects masses, tenderness, and fremitus. Fremitus is the normal vibration that can be felt on the thoracic wall during phonation. The patient is asked to repeat a word or phrase ("ninety-nine") while the chest wall is examined with the fingertips. Characteristic changes are noted with consolidation of the lung, pleural effusion, or bronchial obstruction.

FIGURE 4–6: Chest Wall Contours. Reprinted with permission. Judge AC et al. Clinical Diagnosis, Little Brown and Co.

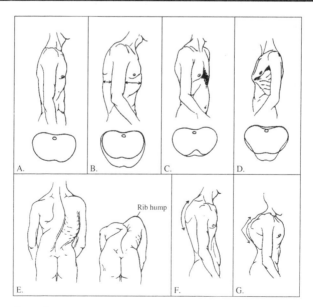

Chest wall contours. A. Normal. B. Barrel chest (emphysema). C. Pectus excavatum (funnel chest). D. Pectus carinatum (Pigeon breast). E. Scoliosis. F. Kyphosis. G. Gibbus (extreme kyphosis).

Percussion of the chest produces hyperresonant, high-pitched sounds over the air-filled lungs. Lower-pitched notes are heard over fluid or solid structures such as the heart or liver. High-pitched hyperresonant, tympanic sounds are observed in emphysema or pneumothorax. Dull, low pitched sounds are characteristic of pleural fluid or consolidation that might occur with congestive heart failure (CHF) and pneumonia.

A stethoscope is used to auscultate the anterior and posterior (AP) lung fields. Normal breath sounds are classified according to intensity, pitch, and duration of inspiration/expiration. Abnormal sounds include rales, rhonchi, wheezes, and rubs (see Figure 4–7). Rales are fine crackles emitted from the small airways and alveoli in conditions such as CHF, interstitial pulmonary disease, or pneumonia. Rhonchi are much more coarse and suggest secretions in the larger airways. Wheezes are caused by air movement through narrowed airways as in asthma or COAD. Rubs are "creaking" type noises often caused by inflamed pleura.

Voice sounds discerned with the aid of a stethoscope include bronchophony, whispered pectoriloquy, and egophony. Bronchophony is an increase in the clarity of spoken voice sounds. Whispered pectoriloquy is an increase in clarity of whispered voice sounds. Egophony is a nasal bleating sound detected when the spoken letter "E" sounds more like "A." These voice alterations can occur when a lung is consolidated by pneumonia or compressed by a pleural effusion.

Breasts. Since breast cancer occurs in one of nine women, breast examination is an important component of the physical examination. Inspection might disclose changes in skin texture or coloration or alterations in the contour of the breast. The nipple might become retracted or a discharge may be present. Palpation discloses the pres-

FIGURE 4–7: Schema of Breath Sounds. Reprinted with permission. Seidel HM et al. Mosby's Guide to Physical Examination, The CV Mosby Co.

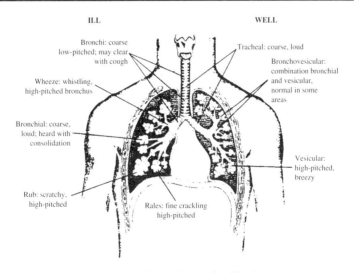

Schema of breath sounds in the well and ill patient.

ence of breast and axillary masses or tenderness. Galactorrhea, an abnormal milky discharge, can occur in either sex as a result of complex neurohumoral regulation. Dopaminergic antagonists, phenothiazines, and butyrophenones can also cause galactorrhea. Gynecomastia sometimes occurs in alcoholic men (due to testicular atrophy and hyperestrogenemia) and as a side effect of numerous medications (e.g., cimetidine, spironolactone, estrogens).

Cardiovascular (CV) System

Cardiac examination includes inspection, palpation, auscultation, and less commonly, percussion. For reference, the apex of the heart is the tip of the left ventricle; the base corresponds to the connections with the great vessels.

Inspection and palpation of the chest wall detects the point of maximal impulse (PMI) corresponding to systole at the apex of the heart. Typically the PMI lies in the fifth intercostal space medial to the midclavicular line (a line drawn down the body perpendicular to the middle of the clavicle). A diffuse or laterally displaced PMI is associated with left ventricular enlargement as in CHF. "Heaves," sustained precordial impulses noted by palpation, reflect ventricular hypertrophy. "Thrills" are palpable vibrations due to turbulent flow across an abnormal heart valve. A heart murmur with an associated thrill suggests more severe valve disease.

Auscultation with a stethoscope detects normal physiologic heart tones (S_1, S_2) and the presence of gallops (S_3, S_4), murmurs, or rubs. The rate and rhythm of the heart tones [regular rate and rhythm (RRR), normal sinus rhythm (NSR), or "irregularly irregular" in atrial fibrillation] are noted. Closure of the atrioventricular valves (tricuspid, mitral valves) produces the first heart sound, S_1. Closure of the aortic and pulmonic valves creates the second heart sound, S_2. The S_3, an abnormal diastolic filling sound created early in diastole after opening of the atrioventricular valves, is associated with CHF. S_4, an abnormal gallop occurring in diastole just before systole (presystolic), originates in the ventricle during the latter half of diastole when the atria contract to complete ventricular filling. It suggests poor compliance of the ventricular wall as in left ventricular hypertrophy from hypertension or aortic stenosis and can be a normal finding in otherwise healthy young adults. Murmurs are sounds made by turbulent blood flow, often across a structurally abnormal valve. Either narrowing (stenosis) or insufficiency (regurgitant flow back across a valve that should be closed) can occur. Murmurs are graded by severity from 1 to 6 (see Table 4–2).

Pericardial friction rubs are grating sounds caused by the rubbing together of inflamed pericardial surfaces. A relatively normal heart exam is often abbreviated S_1 S_2, no M/G/R (i.e., normal S_1 and S_2 and the absence of any murmurs, gallops, or rubs).

TABLE 4–2: Grading of Heart Murmurs

Grade	Description of Heart Murmur
I/VI	Heard only after special maneuvers
II/VI	Very faint, but can be observed
III/VI	Loud, without a thrill
IV/VI	Associated with a thrill; stethoscope must be on chest wall
VI/VI	Heard without a stethoscope; palpable thrill

Gastrointestinal (GI) System

Abdomen. The usual orderly sequence of inspection, palpation, percussion, and auscultation is altered when examining the abdomen and various organs (see Figure 4–8). Auscultation is performed after inspection so that the quality of the bowel sounds (BS) is not altered by palpating. The abdomen is inspected for contour (distended, scaphoid), skin rashes, abnormal venous pattern, and masses. Auscultation is performed to detect bruits and listen to bowel sounds. Mid-abdominal or flank bruits suggest atherosclerotic disease in the abdominal aorta or renal arteries, respectively. Bowel sounds are diminished in advanced stages of bowel obstruction, ileus due to a variety of reasons (e.g., postoperative, opioid drugs), or peritonitis. Hyperactive BS are noted in early stages of bowel obstruction and in diarrheal-type illnesses. High pitched "tinkles" and "rushes" suggest small bowel obstruction.

Percussion is performed to elicit tenderness and to detect organ size, masses, and abdominal distention. Gaseous abdominal distention produces a higher-pitched tympanic percussion note, while a fluid filled abdomen (e.g., in ascites) elicits a dull percussion note. Additionally, a fluid wave or succussion splash (i.e., a splashing sound) can be noted by tapping one side of the abdomen and palpating the transmitted vibration on the opposite abdominal wall. Percussion can detect fluid "dullness" that shifts when the patient is rolled from the supine position on to his side (e.g., "shifting dullness" of ascites). Liver and spleen enlargement can be detected by both percussion and palpation. Percussion also detects a distended bladder as in bladder outlet obstruction or neurogenic bladder dysfunction.

Palpation determines organ size, the presence of masses, and the degree of abdominal tenderness. The right upper quadrant is palpated for liver size, texture, and tenderness. Hepatomegaly is occasionally quantitated by the degree of distention (in centimeters) below the right costal margin (RCM). A normal sized liver generally does not distend more than 1 to 2 cm below the right costal margin. Percussion is an additional method used to measure the liver size with a span of 4 to 8 cm being normal. An enlarged liver can be associated with hepatitis, right-sided heart failure, infil-

FIGURE 4–8: Superficial Topography of the Abdomen: A Four-Quadrant System. Reprinted with permission. Judge AC et al. Clinical Diagnosis, Little Brown and Co.

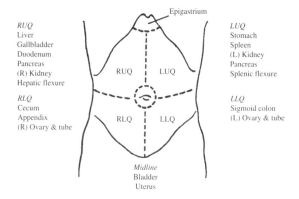

RUQ
Liver
Gallbladder
Duodenum
Pancreas
(R) Kidney
Hepatic flexure

RLQ
Cecum
Appendix
(R) Ovary & tube

LUQ
Stomach
Spleen
(L) Kidney
Pancreas
Splenic flexure

LLQ
Sigmoid colon
(L) Ovary & tube

Epigastrium

Midline
Bladder
Uterus

trating diseases, and cancer. The liver is enlarged early in cirrhosis but shrinks and is smaller at later stages when the fibrosis occurs. Normally, the spleen is not palpable, unless it is enlarged. Splenomegaly can be due to portal hypertension, leukemias and lymphomas, hemolytic anemia, and infections. The kidneys are also difficult to palpate unless they are enlarged (e.g., polycystic kidney disease). An enlarged pulsating mass suggests an aortic aneurysm. The gallbladder is not palpable unless enlarged. A tender gallbladder suggests cholecystitis, while a nontender gallbladder suggests bile duct obstruction from cancer. Abdominal tenderness in specific locations suggests involvement of the various organs as outlined in Figure 4–8. Rebound tenderness and guarding (involuntary spasm of the abdominal wall muscles) are considered "peritoneal signs" that indicate peritoneal inflammation due to conditions such as appendicitis, diverticulitis, pancreatitis, or cholecystitis.

Murphy's sign and McBurney's point are two eponyms pertinent to the abdominal exam that may occur in the medical record. Murphy's sign is positive in cholecystitis: during right upper quadrant (RUQ) palpation, as the patient inspires, the inflamed gallbladder descends due to the downward motion of the diaphragm and thus comes in contact with the examiner's fingers. The patient experiences pain and abruptly halts inspiration. Rebound tenderness over McBurney's point (a point on the abdominal wall lying between the umbilicus and the anterior superior iliac spine) suggests acute appendicitis.

Genitourinary (GU) System and Rectal Examination

Male. The male GU exam is performed with the patient in the upright position. The penis is examined for skin lesions (e.g., syphilitic ulcers, chancroid, herpetic lesions, condyloma) and urethral discharge (suggesting a sexually transmitted disease). Phimosis is the inability to retract the foreskin. The inguinal area is examined for skin rashes (e.g., tinea cruris, candida). Hernias present as inguinal or scrotal masses. An incarcerated hernia cannot be "reduced" by pushing the contents back through the defect in the abdominal wall musculature. Other scrotal masses include varicoceles (dilated scrotal veins) and hydroceles (fluid collections that are translucent on transillumination with a bright light). Testicular size and masses are noted. Testicular self-examination is important for early diagnosis of cancer in men. Testicular atrophy can accompany alcoholism. Testicular tenderness is noted in testicular torsion (an acute genitourinary emergency) or orchitis. Epididymal tenderness is present in epididymitis.

Female. The female pelvic exam is typically performed in the "dorsal lithotomy" (supine with legs in stirrups) position on a specialized examination table. The exam consists of an examination of the external genitalia, a speculum exam, and a bimanual examination of the pelvic organs. The speculum exam allows direct visualization of the vagina and cervix. Appropriate specimens are obtained to evaluate vaginitis or sexually transmitted diseases; the Papanicolaou (Pap) smear is taken to detect cervical cancer. The bimanual exam is so-named because both hands are used to examine the pelvic organs (one internally and the other externally, on the abdominal wall). The cervix is examined for cervical motion tenderness (CMT), suggesting pelvic inflammatory disease. The uterus and ovaries (adnexa) are examined for size, tenderness, and the presence of masses.

Rectal Exam. The rectal exam includes an examination of the prostate gland in men to screen for malignancy or enlargement. The prostate is examined for nodules (suggesting cancer) and tenderness (suggesting prostatitis). Rectal masses can be palpated and the stool can be tested for occult blood (as a screen for malignancy or occult GI bleeding). Hemorrhoids, both internal and external, are also noted. Altered anal sphincter tone is a clue to neurologic dysfunction.

Peripheral Vascular System (PVS)

The peripheral arterial pulses are evaluated to determine occlusion and flow. Typically, a description of the carotid pulse and presence of bruits is found in the neck or cardiovascular section. Similarly, description of the abdominal aorta (if palpable) and abdominal bruits is noted in the abdomen section. Several different grading systems are used to characterize the other peripheral pulses. One such system describes a gradation of pulse intensity from 0 to 4+, with 0 being the absence of a pulse, 3+ being normal, and 4+ denoting a bounding pulse. Diminished pulses (0 to 1+) might indicate atherosclerotic occlusion. (See Table 4–3 for an example.)

Extremities

If not specifically recorded in other sections, examination of the extremities might include notation of skin, nail, hair, and joint abnormalities. The presence of venous disease including varicosities, venous insufficiency, and evidence of thrombophlebitis is noted. Calf swelling and tenderness may indicate a deep venous thrombosis (DVT). Homans' sign (calf pain produced on passive dorsiflexion of the foot) is a relatively insensitive indicator of DVT.

"Dependent edema" can occur in the pretibial area in an ambulatory patient. In a bedridden patient, the sacral area is the most dependent portion of the body and thus early edema might initially manifest in this location. Edema may be pitting or nonpitting. Pitting refers to a noticeable, transient indentation in the tissue subsequent to firm pressure with the fingertips over a bony surface and reflects displacement of the excess interstitial fluid. Pitting is arbitrarily graded depending on severity from trace to 4+. Obviously, diuretics can speed the resolution of edema, while corticosteroids or nonsteroidal anti-inflammatory medications can hasten the development of edema.

Musculoskeletal System (MSK)

The musculoskeletal system comprises the supporting structures of the body such as bones, joints, tendons, ligaments, and musculature. Joints are examined for the presence of deformities, swelling, effusions, warmth, redness, and tenderness. Two common types of arthritis, osteoarthritis (OA) and rheumatoid arthritis (RA), have differing patterns of joint involvement. Osteoarthritis often affects the large weight-bearing

TABLE 4–3: Sample Recording System for Peripheral Pulses

Pulse	R	L
Carotid	2/4	2/4
Brachial	2+	2+
Radial	3+	3+
Femoral	3+	3+
Popliteal	2+	2+
Dorsalis pedis (DP)	1+	0
Post tibial (PT)	1+	1+

joints: the knees, hips, and spine with bony proliferation causing swelling with nodules. In the hands, osteoarthritis affects the proximal and distal interphalangeal (PIP and DIP) joints and is known as Bouchard's and Heberden's nodes, respectively. Although RA can also affect weight-bearing joints, it classically causes symmetrical small joint arthritis, particularly of the hands, wrists, elbows, and feet. In contrast to OA, rheumatoid arthritis affects the metacarpophalangeal joints (MCP) and PIP joints of the hands and spares the DIP joints. A joint's range of motion can become limited by a number of diseases that affect the joint.

The musculature or motor system is examined for bulk, strength, tone, tenderness, and the presence of abnormal spontaneous movements (e.g., fasciculations). Examination of the motor system is part of the neurologic exam and is discussed in that section.

Neurological System

Examination of the nervous system includes evaluation of the mental status, cranial nerves, motor and sensory function, coordination, deep tendon reflexes (DTRs), and gait. The medical record contains various levels of detail regarding the neurological examination depending on the clinical situation.

Mental Status. A patient's mental status examination consists of a variety of at least twenty psychic characteristics. The mnemonic "como estas" (Spanish for "how are you") summarizes these characteristics (see Table 4–4). See the appendix on page 4–22 of this chapter for an example of a mental status examination.

TABLE 4–4: Psychic Characteristics

Cognitive functions (i.e., calculation, concentration, insight, and judgment)

Overview (i.e., appearance, attitude, level of consciousness, and movements)

Memory (i.e., recent and remote)

Orientation (i.e., to person, place, and time)

Emotion (i.e., affect and mood)

Speech (i.e., fluency, form, and comprehension)

Thought (i.e., process, content, and perceptual disturbances)

Attention (i.e., abstract thinking, recall, and intelligence)

Something else that the practitioner has forgotten that might be important for the patient

Cranial Nerves. The function of the 12 cranial nerves (CN I to XII) is described in Table 4–5. A common mnemonic utilizes the first character in each of the following words in the sentence "On Old Olympus' Towering Tops, A Finn And German Viewed Some Hops" to identify the 12 cranial nerves.

TABLE 4–5: Cranial Nerves and Their Functions

Cranial Nerves	Function
Olfactory (I)	*Sensory:* smell reception and interpretation
Optic (II)	*Sensory:* visual acuity and visual fields
Oculomotor (III)	*Motor:* raise eyelids, most extraocular movements, changes of lens shape and pupillary constriction
Trochlear (IV)	*Motor:* inward and downward eye movement
Trigeminal (V)	*Motor:* chewing, mastication, jaw opening and clenching *Sensory:* sensation to facial skin, ear, tongue, nasal and mouth mucosa, cornea, iris, lacrimal glands, conjunctiva, eyelids, forehead, and nose
Abducens (VI)	*Motor:* lateral eye movement
Facial (VII)	*Motor:* movement of facial expression muscles except jaw, close eyes, labial speech sounds (M, b, W and rounded vowels) *Sensory:* taste, anterior two thirds of tongue, sensation to pharynx *Parasympathetic:* secretion of tears and saliva
Acoustic (VIII)	*Sensory:* hearing and balance or equilibrium
Glossopharyngeal (IX)	*Motor:* voluntary muscles for phonation or swallowing *Sensory:* sensation of nasopharynx, gag reflex, taste posterior one third of tongue *Parasympathetic:* secretion of salivary glands, carotid reflex
Vagus (X)	*Motor:* voluntary muscles of phonation (guttural speech sounds) and swallowing *Sensory:* sensation behind ear and part of external ear canal *Parasympathetic:* secretion of digestive enzymes, peristalsis, carotid reflex, involuntary action of heart, lungs, and digestive tract
Spinal accessory (XI)	*Motor:* turn head, shrug shoulders, some actions for phonation and swallowing
Hypoglossal (XII)	*Motor:* tongue movement for speech sound articulation (l, t, n) and swallowing

Motor Exam. The motor exam includes evaluation of bulk, strength, tone, tenderness, and the presence of abnormal movements. Both primary muscle diseases and diseases of nerves innervating muscles can cause weakness and atrophy.

Muscle strength is graded on a scale of 0 (no movement) to 5 (normal strength). (See Table 4–6.)

Muscle tone can be decreased (flaccid) or increased (spasticity). The phenothiazines and butyrophenones can cause dystonias which are characterized by sustained increased muscle tone and contraction, particularly in the head and neck. The extrapyramidal tract is a system consisting of the basal ganglia and nigrostriatal pathways in the brain. It is involved with initiation of movements, and diseases of these areas cause movement disorders such as Parkinson's disease and Huntington's chorea. The phenothiazines and butyrophenones can have extrapyramidal side effects including dystonias, tremors, and cogwheel rigidity (passive range of motion of an affected muscle group elicits a sensation as if one was pulling on a ratchet or cogwheel).

A number of abnormal movements can be seen in muscles. Fasciculations are miniscule uncoordinated contractions of muscle fibers often due to denervation of the muscle. Tremors are more obvious and a number of drugs can cause tremors (e.g., antipsychotics, lithium, cyclosporine).

Sensory. Conventionally, the primary sensations include pain, touch, vibration, joint position sense (JPS), and thermal sensation. Pain sensation is conveyed by small unmyelinated fibers and is tested with a pinprick (PP). Light touch (LT) is mediated by a combination of small and larger nerve fibers; this is tested with a wisp of cotton. Vibration and JPS (also called proprioception) are mediated by large myelinated fibers. Vibration sensation is tested with a tuning fork. Peripheral neuropathies often begin distally affecting the longest nerve fibers first. This gives rise to the term "stocking and glove" distribution to denote abnormalities in the hands and feet. As peripheral nerves convey information back to the spinal cord (and ultimately the brain), the nerve fibers segregate and the dorsal roots and enter the dorsal horn of the spinal cord. This allows for a topographically coherent pattern of information entering the spinal cord: each dorsal root receives information from a particular topographical region of the body called a dermatome. In evaluating a sensory abnormality, the clinician tests whether a deficit fits a dermatomal distribution, indicating dorsal root involvement (see Figure 4–9) or the distribution of a collection of spinal segments constituting a peripheral nerve (peripheral neuropathy).

TABLE 4–6: Muscle Strength Grading

Grade	Muscle Strength
0	No muscle contraction
1	Flicker or trace of contraction
2	Movement possible, but not against gravity
3	Moves against gravity, but not against resistance
4	Can move against resistance
5	Normal strength

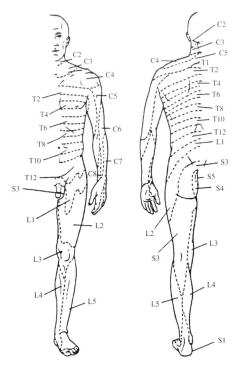

Sensory Dermatones

Coordination and Vestibulocerebellar Testing. Coordination of movement is a complex process involving both sensory afferent information regarding proprioception and muscle efferent stimuli. Muscle efferent stimuli causes contraction in certain muscle groups and inhibits muscle contraction in the opposing muscle groups. The Romberg test (testing balance with the patient standing, feet together, eyes closed) evaluates proprioception and cerebellar function. Ataxia (the inability to coordinate voluntary muscle movements) can be tested by asking the patient to alternately point from his nose to the clinician's finger [finger-to-nose test (FTN)]. Coordination in the lower extremities is evaluated with the heel-to-shin (HTS) test. The ability to perform rapid alternating movements (RAM) can also be impaired.

Deep Tendon Reflexes (DTRs). Evaluation of DTRs examines the spinal reflex arc. When an already partially stretched tendon is tapped briskly with a reflex hammer, stretch receptors in the tendon send an impulse to the spinal cord that elicits a contraction of the corresponding muscle. The spinal reflex arc is modified by control from the brain via descending corticospinal tracts. Typically, this often has an inhibitory influence. With damage to those higher centers, as in stroke or descending nerve tracts (i.e, the upper motor neurons), the spinal reflex arc is uninhibited and the DTRs are hyperactive. With damage to the peripheral nerve or particular dorsal roots

FIGURE 4–10: Example of Deep Tendon Reflex (DTR) Recording.

Grading Scale. 0 = No Response; + = Diminished; ++ = Normal;
+++ = Hyperactive; ++++ = Hyperactive, often with clonus.

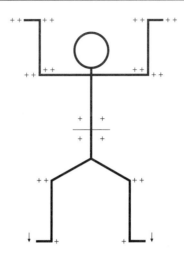

(i.e., low motor neurons) the reflex arc is interrupted and the DTRs are diminished. Reflexes are graded on a scale from 0 to 4. A stick figure typically appears in the chart to designate the elicited reflexes (see Figure 4–10).

The plantar reflexes refer to the reflex motion of the great toe after a noxious stimuli is applied to the bottom of the foot. An upgoing toe, Babinski's Sign, is suggestive of an uppermotor neuron lesion (but can be normal in infants). A downgoing toe is normal.

SUGGESTED REFERENCES

1. Malasanos L et al. Health Assessment. 4th Edition. St Louis: The C.V. Mosby Co, 1989.

2. Swartz MH. Textbook of Physical Diagnosis. Philadelphia: W.B. Saunders Co, 1989.

3. Judge RD et al. Clinical Diagnosis: A Physiologic Approach. 5th Edition. Boston: Little, Brown and Co, 1988.

4. Bowers AC, Thompson JM. Clinical Manual of Health Assessment. St. Louis: The CV Mosby Co, 1988.

5. Seidel HM et al. Mosby's Guide to Physical Examination. St. Louis: The CV Mosby Co, 1987.

6. Bates B. A Guide to Physical Examination and History Taking. 5th Edition. Philadelphia: J B Lippincott Co, 1990.

7. Sapira JD. The Art and Science of Bedside Diagnosis. Baltimore: Urban and Schwarzenber, 1989.

8. Orkin M. Dermatology. 1st Edition. Norwalk: Appleton and Lange, 1990.

APPENDIX 4–1: Mini-Mental Status Exam

Maximum Score	Patient Score	Assessment	Questions
		Orientation	
5	_____	What is the (year)? (season)? (date)? (day)? (month)?	Ask for the date. Then ask specifically for parts omitted (e.g., "Can you also tell me what season it is?"). One point for each correct answer.
5	_____	Where are we: (state)? (country)? (town)? (hospital)? (floor)?	Ask in turn "Can you tell me the name of this hospital?" One point for each correct answer.
		Registration	
3	_____	Name 3 objects (1 second to say each). Then ask the patient to name all 3 after you have said them.	Ask the patient if you may test his memory. Then say the names of 3 unrelated objects, clearly and slowly, about one second for each.
#/Trials	_____	Give 1 point for each correct answer. Then repeat them until he learns all 3. Count trials and record.	After you have said 3, ask him to repeat them. This first repetition determines his score (0 to 3) but keep saying them until he can repeat all 3, up to 6 trials. **Note:** If he does not eventually learn all 3, recall cannot be meaningfully tested.
		Attention and Calculation	
5	_____	Serial 7's. (1 point for each correct.) Stop after 5 answers.	Ask the patient to begin with 100 and count backwards by 7. Stop after 5 subtractions (93, 86, 79, 72, 65). Score the total number of correct answers.

Maximum Score	Patient Score	Assessment	Questions
		***Attention and Calculation*(Continued)**	
5	_____	Alternatively spell "world" backwards.	If the patient cannot or will not perform this task, ask him to spell the word "world" backwards. The score is the number of letters in correct order, e.g. dlrow = 5, dlorw = 3.
		Recall	
3	_____	Ask the patient if he can recall the 3 words you previously asked him to remember. Score 0 to 3.	Ask for the 3 objects repeated above. Give 1 point for each correct.
		Language	
2	_____	Name a pencil and a watch (2 points)	*Naming:* Show the patient a wrist watch and ask him what it is. Repeat for pencil. Score 0 to 2.
1	_____	Repeat the following: "No ifs, ands, or buts." (1 point)	*Repetition:* Ask the patient to repeat the sentence after you. Allow only one trial. Score 0 or 1.
3	_____	Following a 3-stage command: "Take a paper in your right hand, fold it in half, and put it on the floor"(3 points)	*3-State Command:* Give the patient a piece of plain blank paper and repeat the command. Score 1 point for each part correctly executed.
1	_____	Read and obey the following: Close your eyes. (1 point)	*Reading:* On a blank piece of paper print the sentence "close your eyes" in letters large enough for the patient to see clearly. As him to read it and do what it says. Score 1 point only if he actually closes his eyes.
			Continued

Maximum Score	Patient Score	Assessment	Questions
		Language	
1	_____	Write a sentence (1 point)	*Writing:* Give the patient a blank piece of paper and ask him to write a sentence for you. Do not dictate a sentence, it is to be written spontaneously. It must contain a subject and verb and be sensible. Correct grammar and punctuation are not necessary.
1	_____	Copy a design (1 point)	*Copying:* On a clean piece of paper, draw intersecting pentagons, each side about 1 inch, and ask him to copy it exactly as it is. All 10 angles must be present and 2 must intersect to score 1 point. Tremor and rotation are ignored.
TOTAL SCORE:	_____	**A score of 27 to 30 is generally considered acceptable.** *ASSESS level of consciousness along a the following continuum: Alert, Drowsy, Stupor, Coma. Estimate the patient's level of sensorium, from alert to coma.*	

Clinical Laboratory Tests

Richard C. Christopherson
Karen E. Vick Smith

INTERPRETATION OF CLINICAL LABORATORY TESTS

A clinical laboratory test can provide a useful diagnostic clue, assist with a therapeutic assessment, or have programmatic implications. This chapter contains many of the most commonly encountered laboratory tests used in clinical medicine. Each section contains a specific format aimed at quickly providing the user with: 1) normal values and the SI (Systeme international) units; 2) a description of the specific test; and 3) the clinical implications of abnormal findings.

If specific tests are not described or a more detailed review of clinical laboratory tests is required, see the most recent edition of F.K. *Widmann's Clinical Interpretation of Laboratory Tests* published by F.A. Davis Company (Philadelphia) or John B. Henry's *Clinical Diagnosis and Management by Laboratory Methods* published by W.B. Saunders (Philadelphia). Before using this chapter, it is important to review several general principles regarding the use of laboratory tests. A brief review of these principles follows.

Normal Values

In determining normal values, a variety of factors and the interrelationship of these factors must be considered. Normal values will vary depending on a patient's age, gender, weight, and height. Changes from normal will also occur when certain medications are being used that may either falsely elevate or lower the results of a specific test. Other factors that affect normal values include: the timing of the sample; relationship to a meal; the method of analysis; and the disease state itself. Similarly, abnormal values are not always significant and occasionally normal values can be viewed as abnormal in some diseases. Therefore, it is always important to refer to published normals or reference standards used by the clinical laboratory performing the test and any documentation concerning interferences with the particular assay being performed.

Laboratory Error

Laboratory error is generally an uncommon occurrence. When it does occur, the consequences can have serious implications for patient care. As a practitioner you should suspect laboratory error when 1) a particularly low or high value occurs or 2) when you receive an unexpected value based upon the patient's clinical status. Examples of potential causes of laboratory errors include:

>> A spoiled specimen (e.g., contaminated, wrong container, exposed to improper temperature or light conditions).

>> Specimen taken at the wrong time.

>> Incomplete specimen.

>> Faulty reagents.

>> Technical error.

>> Medication (e.g., due to interference with the assay) that can falsely lower or elevate the result.

>> Diet (e.g., elevated blood sugar that was obtained soon after eating).

>> Specimen from wrong patient.

>> Diagnostic or therapeutic procedures [e.g., digital stimulation of the prostate or a prostate biopsy may increase the prostate specific antigen (PSA)].

Sensitivity/Specificity

The accuracy and reliability of laboratory tests are based upon the sensitivity and specificity of each test. The *sensitivity* of a particular test is the likelihood of a *positive* test result in a person with a disease (a true-positive rate). *Specificity* refers to the likelihood of a *negative* test result in a person without a disease (a true-negative rate). Therefore, the clinical implications of these two factors are that test performance can change as the test is more widely utilized. Further, the selection bias of individuals may affect the measurement of a test's sensitivity and specificity. For example, selecting all healthy volunteers may over-estimate the specificity of a test, while selecting individuals with extensive disease may overestimate the sensitivity of the method. In any case, it is important to remember the following points when evaluating laboratory values:

>> Test values represent probability values (probability that a disease or abnormality is in fact present).

>> Many laboratory values are expressed as continuous variables and provide only an indication that normality or an abnormality is present.

Common Laboratory Orders

Laboratory tests are frequently ordered in groups or as panels of tests to simplify the task. The cost of these panels is often less expensive than the cost of each test ordered individually. The following are descriptions of some of the more commonly used laboratory test panels and associated abbreviations.

>> **Chemistry Survey (Chem Survey).** Glucose, blood urea nitrogen (BUN), creatinine (Scr), calcium (Ca^{++}), phosphate (PO_4^-), uric acid, magnesium (Mg^{++}), cholesterol, and total serum protein (TSP).

>> **SMA-6**. Sodium (Na^+), potassium (K^+), chloride (Cl^-), carbon dioxide (CO_2), BUN, and glucose.

>> **SMA-12.** SMA-6 plus albumin (Alb), TSP, bilirubin (T. Bil), alkaline phosphatase (Alk Phos), calcium (Ca^{++}), and Scr.

>> **Electrolytes (Lytes).** Na^+, K^+, Cl^-, and CO_2.

>> **Complete Blood Count (CBC) with Differential (diff).** White blood cell count (WBC) and differential (segmented neutrophils, bands, eosinophils, basophils, lymphocytes, atypical lymphocytes, and monocytes).

>> **Arterial Blood Gases (ABGs).** pH, pCO_2, pO_2, and base excess and bicarbonate (HCO_3).

>> **Hematology Panel (Heme panel).** WBC, red blood cells (RBCs), hemoglobin (Hgb), hematocrit (Hct), RBC indices, and red cell distribution width (RDW).

>> **Enzymes.** Alanine aminotransferase (ALT), aspartate aminotransferase (AST), amylase, lipase, gamma glutamyltransferase (GGT), lactic acid dehydrogenase (LD), and creatine kinase (CK).

>> **Isoenzymes.** CK (MM, MB, BB bands) and LD (LD_1, LD_2).

>> **Urine Electrolytes.** Na^+ and K^+.

In addition to these abbreviations, test results are frequently recorded in a patient's chart using a variety of formats. It is usually easy to identify particular laboratory tests just by knowing the normal values. A commonly used format is described below.

$$\text{General Format} \quad \frac{Na}{K} \left| \frac{Cl}{CO_2} \right. \underset{\diagdown BUN}{\overset{\diagup Cr}{\longleftarrow Glu}}$$

Chapter RoadMap

Continued

Continued

LABORATORY TESTS

ROUTINE HEMATOLOGY

Hematocrit (Hct)

Normal Values	Male: 40%–50%	SI units = 0.4–0.5
	Female: 35%–45%	SI units = 0.35–0.45

Description
The hematocrit (or packed cell volume) describes the space occupied by packed red blood cells (RBCs). It is expressed as a percentage of red cells in volume of whole blood and represents a calculated value.

Clinical Implications

- **Decreased Values** are seen in anemia (various causes), hemolytic reactions, leukemia, cirrhosis, massive blood loss, and hyperthyroidism.

- **Increased Values** are seen in erythrocytosis, dehydration, COAD, polycythemia, and shock.

- The Hct lacks clinical validity immediately after moderate blood loss or transfusion. It can appear normal after acute hemorrhage.

- The Hct usually parallels the RBC count when erythrocytes are of a normal size (i.e., as the number increases, so does the Hct) unless the anemia is macrocytic or microcytic.

- If the patient has iron-deficiency anemia with small RBCs, the Hct decreases because microcytic cells pack into a smaller volume. However, the RBC count may appear normal.

- The hematocrit is approximately three times the hemoglobin (Hgb) value.

- One unit of blood will increase the Hct by 2%–4%.

Hemoglobin (Hgb)

Normal Values	Male: 13–18 gm/dL	SI units = 8.1–11.2 mmol/L
	Female: 12–16 gm/dL	SI units = 7.4–9.9 mmol/L

Description
Hemoglobin is the compound that serves as the transportation vehicle of oxygen (O_2) and carbon dioxide (CO_2). It consists of globin (a single protein-tetramer composed of two alpha and two beta units) and heme (which contains iron atoms and porphyrin, a red pigment). The iron pigment of hemoglobin combines with oxygen. When hemoglobin carries oxygen, blood is scarlet (arterial) and when it loses oxygen, the blood becomes dark red (venous). One gram of hemoglobin carries 1.34 mL of oxygen. This oxygen carrying capacity correlates with the amount of Hgb present, not the number of RBCs.

Hemoglobin (Hgb) *(Continued)*

Description (Continued)   A decrease in the normal Hgb protein types A_1, A_2, F (fetal), and S is associated with sickle cell anemia. Hgb also serves as a buffer by shifting chloride in and out of RBCs according to the level of O_2 in plasma (for each chloride entering the RBC, one anion of HCO_3 is released).

The definition of anemia based upon a specific hemoglobin value varies because of varying body adaptations (e.g., to high altitudes, pulmonary disease, exercise); however, a hemoglobin value of 12 gm/dL generally suggests an anemic condition. The total amount of circulating hemoglobin is more important than the number of erythrocytes in determining anemia.

Clinical Implications
- The Hgb concentration is decreased in anemia (especially iron-deficiency anemia), hyperthyroidism, cirrhosis, hemorrhage, hemolytic reactions, increased fluid intake, and pregnancy.

- The Hgb concentration is increased in hemoconcentration (polycythemia, burns), COAD, CHF, and in people who live at high altitudes.

- Hgb concentration fluctuates in patients with hemorrhages and burns because of fluid replacement and blood transfusions.

- The Hgb concentration can be used to assess the severity of anemia, response of anemia to treatment, or progression of disease(s) associated with anemia.

Red Blood Cell (RBC or Erythrocyte) Count

Normal Values   *Male:* 4.4–5.6 10^6 SI units = 4.4–5.6 x10^{12}
            cells/mm^3 cells/L
        Female: 3.8–5.0 10^6 SI units = 3.5–5.0 x10^{12}
            cells/mm^3 cells/L

Description   The main function of the RBC is to carry oxygen from the lungs to body tissue and to transfer CO_2 from tissues to the lungs by hemoglobin. RBCs are shaped like biconcave disks which increase the surface area so more oxygen can combine with Hgb. Biconcavity also allows the cell to change its shape to more easily pass through small capillaries. Erythrocyte production is stimulated by the hormone erythropoietin in response to decreased oxygen.

With a life span of 120 days, the erythrocyte is the major cell released into circulation. If the demand for erythrocytes is high, immature cells will be released

Red Blood Cell (RBC or Erythrocyte) Count *(Continued)*

Description (Continued) into the circulation. At the end of their life span, older erythrocytes are removed from circulation by phagocytes in the spleen, liver, and bone marrow (reticuloendothelial system or RES).

Erythropoiesis. In bone marrow, the erythrocyte develops in the following sequence: 1) hemocytoblast (precursor of all blood cells); 2) prorubricyte (synthesis of Hgb); 3) rubricyte (nucleus shrinks, Hgb synthesis increases); 4) metarubricyte (nucleus disintegrates, Hgb synthesis increases); 5) reticulocyte (nucleus absorbed); and 6) erythrocyte (mature red cell without nucleus/reticulum).

Clinical Implications
- Generally the Hgb or Hct values are used for monitoring the associated quantitative changes of the RBCs.

- The RBC count is decreased in anemias and systemic lupus erythematosus (SLE).

- RBCs are increased in polycythemia vera, secondary polycythemia (hormone secreting tumors), diarrhea/dehydration, vigorous exercise, burns, and high altitudes.

Red Cell Indices

Mean Corpuscular Volume (MCV)

Calculation

$$MCH = \frac{(Hgb)\,(10)}{(RBC)\,(10^{-6})}$$

Normal Values 82–98 μ^3/cell SI = 82–98 fl

Description
- The MCV is an index for classifying anemia based upon counting erythrocytes. It expresses the volume (or size) of a single red cell as being normocytic (normal size), microcytic (small size <75 μ^3/cell), or macrocytic (large size >105 μ^3/cell).

Clinical Implications
- **Decreased Values** are seen in iron-deficiency anemia, pernicious anemia, and thalassemia. These anemias are, therefore, "microcytic anemias."

- **Increased Values** are seen in liver disease, alcoholism, antimetabolite therapy, folate/B_{12} deficiency, and valproate therapy; and these anemias are "macrocytic anemias."

- In sickle cell anemia, the MCV is of questionable value since the Hct is unreliable due to the abnormal erythrocyte shape.

Red Cell Indices *(Continued)*

Clinical Implications
(Continued)

- MCV is a calculated value; therefore, it is possible to have a wide variation in macrocytes/microcytes and still have a normal MCV.

- MCV is almost universally increased secondary to Zidovudine (AZT) treatment and often can be used as an indirect measure of compliance.

Mean Corpuscular Hemoglobin (MCH)

Calculation

$$MCH = \frac{(Hgb)\,(10)}{(RBC)\,(10^{-6})}$$

Normal Values

28–34 pg/cell   SI = 28–34 pg/cell

Description

The MCH index is a calculated value that indicates the average weight of Hgb in the RBC, and hence the amount of color (i.e., normochromic, hypochromic, hyperchromic) in the RBC. It is useful in the diagnosis of anemia.

Clinical Implications

- An increase in MCH indicates macrocytic anemia.

- A decrease in MCH indicates microcytic anemia.

Mean Corpuscular Hemoglobin Concentration (MCHC)

Calculation

$$MCHC = \frac{(Hgb)\,(100)}{(Hct)}$$

Normal Values

32–36 gm/dL   SI = 320–360 gm/L

Description

The MCHC index measures the average concentration of Hgb in the RBC. For a given MCHC, the smaller the cell, the higher the concentration. This index relies on the Hgb and Hct for calculation of MCHC and is a better index of red cell hemoglobin because cell size affects MCHC in contrast to the MCH.

Clinical Implications

- MCHC is decreased in iron deficiency, microcytic anemia, pyridoxine-responsive anemia, thalassemia, and hypochromic anemia.

- MCHC is increased in spherocytosis, *not* pernicious anemia.

Reticulocytes

Normal Values

0.5%–2.0% red cells   SI = 0.005–0.02 red cells

Description

Reticulocytes are young, non-nucleated cells of the erythrocyte series formed in the bone marrow. An increase in the reticulocyte count indicates that RBC production is accelerated; a decrease in the number indicates that bone marrow red cell production is reduced.

Reticulocytes *(Continued)*

Clinical Implications

- The reticulocyte count differentiates anemias due to bone marrow failure from those due to hemorrhage or hemolysis (red cell destruction) because hemorrhage or hemolysis should stimulate reticulocytosis in patients with competent bone marrow function.

- The reticulocyte count should be increased in hemolytic anemias, sickle cell disease, and metastic carcinoma.

- If the reticulocyte count is not increased when the patient is anemic, it implies that the bone marrow is not producing enough erythrocytes (e.g., iron-deficiency anemia, aplastic anemia, untreated pernicious anemia, chronic infection, radiation therapy).

- Following treatment of anemias, an increase in "retics" reflects the effectiveness of treatment. After adequate doses of iron in iron-deficient anemia, the reticulocyte count increases by about 20%; it increases proportionally when pernicious anemia is treated by transfusion. A maximum increase may be expected to occur in 7 to 14 days after appropriate treatment (i.e., iron supplement).

White Blood Cell, Leukocyte (WBC)

Normal Values

3200–10,000/mm^3 SI = 3.2–10.0 x10^9 L

Description

The main functions of the WBC are to fight infection, defend the body by phagocytosis of foreign organisms, and produce or transport/distribute antibodies. There are two major types of white blood cells:

1) Granulocytes: neutrophils, eosinophils, and basophils

2) Agranulocytes: lymphocytes and monocytes.

Leukocytes are formed in the bone marrow (myelogenous), stored in lymphatic tissue (spleen, thymus, tonsils), and transported via blood to organs or tissues. The average life span of a leukocyte is 13 to 20 days. Vitamins, folic acid, and amino acids are needed for leukocyte formation. The endocrine system regulates the production, storage, and release of leukocytes.

Granulocyte development begins with myeloblasts (immature cells in the bone marrow) that mature progressively to become promyelocytes, myelocytes (found in the bone marrow), metamyelocytes, bands (neutrophils in early stages of maturity), and ulti-

White Blood Cell, Leukocyte (WBC) *(Continued)*

Description (Continued)

mately, polymorphonuclear segmented neutrophils (also called "polys" or "segs"). Lymphocyte development begins with lymphoblasts (immature) that mature to prolymphoblasts and finally to lymphocytes (mature cell). Monocyte development begins with monoblasts (immature) that mature to become promonocytes and then to monocytes (mature cell).

Clinical Implications

- **Leukocytosis.** 20,000 (slight); 30,000 (moderate); 50,000 (high).

    ° Usually due to an increase of only one cell type (neutrophilia).

    ° Absence of anemia helps to distinguish infection from leukemia.

    ° Hemorrhage, trauma, drugs (e.g., mercury, epinephrine, corticosteroids), necrosis, toxins (eclampsia), and leukemia are other causes.

    ° Food, exercise, emotion, menstruation, stress, seizures, and cold baths can also increase the WBC count.

- **Leukopenia** is a decrease to <4000. Causes of leukopenia include:

    ° Viral infections, hypersplenism, leukemia.

    ° Drugs (antimetabolites, antibiotics, anticonvulsants, chemotherapy).

    ° Pernicious/aplastic anemia.

    ° Multiple myeloma.

- **Staining Procedures**

    ° Neutral reaction for neutrophils.

    ° Acid stain for eosinophils.

    ° Basic stain for basophils.

- The concentration of leukocytes follows an hourly rhythm with low levels in early morning and peak levels in the late afternoon.

- **Age.** The normal concentration of leukocytes in newborns and infants is 10,000 to 20,000 and decreases until age 21.

WBC Differential (Diff)

Normal Values

See Table 5–1.

WBC Differential (Diff) *(Continued)*

Description
- Neutrophils combat bacterial infection and inflammatory disorders.
- Eosinophils combat allergic disorders and parasitic infections.
- Basophils combat blood dyscrasias and myeloproliferative disease.
- Lymphocytes combat viral infections and bacterial infections.
- Monocytes combat severe infections.

Neutrophils (PMNs, Polys, Segs)

Normal Values
Segs: 36%–73%   SI = 0.36 – 0.73
Bands: 0%–12%   SI = 0.00 – 0.12

Description
The neutrophil is the most abundant leukocyte. Neutrophils primarily defend against microbial invasion by phagocytosis. These cells also play a major role in the tissue damage associated with noninfectious diseases such as rheumatoid arthritis, asthma, and inflammatory bowel disease.

Clinical Implications
- **Neutrophilia.** An increased percentage of circulating neutrophils. Causes include bacterial or parasitic infections, metabolic disturbances, hemorrhage, or myeloproliferative disorders.

- **Neutropenia.** A decreased percentage of circulating neutrophils. Causes include decreased neutrophil production, increased cell disappearance, viral infection, blood diseases, hormonal disorders, toxic agents, and a massive infection.

- **"Shift to Left"** or an increase in bands (immature cells) occurs when immature neutrophils are released into the circulation. This left shift can be caused by infection, chemotherapeutic agents, a cell production disorder (leukemia), or hemorrhage.

TABLE 5–1: Normal Values: WBC Differential

	Segs	Bands	EOS	Basos	Lymph	Alymph	Mono
Percentage (%)	36–73	0–12	0–6	0–2	15–45	0–10	0–11
Absolute count[a]	1260–7300	0–1440	0–500	0–150	800–4000	0	100–800

[a] Absolute neutrophil count (ANC) calculation = WBC x % (Segs + Bands).

Clinical Implications
(Continued)

- **"Shift to Right"** or an increase in "segs" (mature cells) occurs in liver disease, megaloblastic anemia due to B_{12} or folic acid deficiency, hemolysis, tissue breakdown, surgery, or certain drugs (e.g., corticosteroids).

- Typically, an increase in the percentage of neutrophils parallels the severity of an infection.

- If the neutrophil count is increased to a notably greater extent than the total WBC count, it often indicates the presence of a severe infection.

- The degree of neutrophilia is proportionate to the amount of tissue involved in inflammation. Neutrophils will leave the blood to migrate to areas of inflammation, however, marrow storage release usually overcompensates, resulting in neutrophilia.

- In cases of tissue necrosis or destruction (e.g., crush injuries, burns, MI, surgeries), neutrophilia may occur via a neutrophilic promoting substance and other poorly understood mechanisms.

Eosinophils (EOS)

Normal Values

0%–6%

Description

Eosinophils are capable of phagocytosis. They are active in later stages of inflammation where they ingest antigen-antibody complexes. These cells are also active in allergic reactions and parasitic infections where an increase serves as a useful diagnostic or monitoring tool.

Clinical Implications

- Eosinophilia represents an increase in the number of eosinophils of more than 6% or an absolute count of more than 500. Causes include the body's response to *n*eoplasm, *A*ddison's disease, *a*llergic reactions, *c*ollagen vascular disease, or *p*arasitic infections. The mnemonic NAACP is helpful to remember these causes.

- Eosinopenia is a decrease in the numbers of circulating eosinophils. Eosinopenia can be encountered when glucocorticosteroids are produced in response to bodily stress (e.g., infectious mononucleosis, Cushing's disease).

- Eosinophils disappear early in pyogenic infections.

- The eosinophil count is lowest in the morning and increases from noon to midnight.

- Eosinophilia can be masked by steroid use and can be substantially increased by L-tryptophan (i.e., eosinophilic-myalgia syndrome).

Basophils

Normal Values 0%–2%

Description The function of basophils is not clearly understood. Basophils are phagocytic cells that contain heparin, histamine, and serotonin. A high basophil count is often noted when the serum concentration of histamine is high. Tissue basophils are also called mast cells.

Clinical Implications
- **Basophilia** (increased basophils) is associated most commonly with granulocytic and basophilic leukemia, myeloid metaplasia, and allergic reactions.

- **Basopenia** (decreased basophils) is associated with acute infection, stress reactions, and following prolonged steroid therapy.

Monocytes (Monomorphonuclear Monocytes)

Normal Values 0%–11%

Description Monocytes are the largest cells in the blood and serve as the body's second line of defense. The histiocyte, a fixed tissue macrophage, is capable of phagocytosis and performs scavenger functions. Monocytes also produce interferon.

Clinical Implications
- **Monocytosis** is associated with certain viral, bacterial, and parasitic infections and collagen, vascular, and hematological disorders.

- **Monocytopenia** or a decreased number of monocytes is not usually identified with a disease, but secondary to stress, glucocorticoids, or myelotoxic or immunosuppressive drugs.

Lymphocytes (Monomorphonuclear Lymphocytes)

Normal Values 15%–45%

Description Lymphocytes are the second most common white cell. They are small, motile cells that migrate to the inflammatory site during the early and late stages of inflammation. These cells are the source of serum immunoglobulins and are important in the body's cellular immune response. The majority of lymphocytes are located in the spleen, lymphatic tissue, and lymph nodes. Only about 5% of total lymphocytes are present in the circulation.

Clinical Implications
- **Lymphocytosis** is associated with viral diseases (e.g., mumps, mononucleosis, upper respiratory infections), bacterial diseases, and hormonal disorders.

- **Lymphopenia** is associated with Hodgkin's disease, SLE, burns, and trauma.

- **Virocytes** (stress lymphocytes, Downy type cells, atypical lymphocytes) are atypical cells that can also appear in viral, fungoid, and paratoxoid infections; after transfusions; and as a response to stress.

Clinical Implications
(Continued)
- Transformed lymphocytes are used as a measure of histocompatibility.

- Absolute lymphocyte counts <1000 reflect anergy.

Platelets (PLT)

Normal Values   170–380 10^3/mm^3 SI = 170–380 10^9/L

Description   Platelets (thrombocytes), the smallest of the formed elements in the blood, are necessary for blood clotting. Platelets are activated after contact with non-endothelial surfaces and subsequently adhere to subendothelial components (e.g., collagen). During the adhesion/aggregation phase, the coagulation mechanism is activated and thrombin is formed. Platelets then become interdispersed with RBCs and WBCs to form a clot. Formation of platelets occurs primarily in the bone marrow. The life span of a platelet is approximately 7.5 days. Two-thirds of all platelets are circulating in the blood, while one-third are located in the spleen.

Clinical Implications
- **Increased platelets** (thrombocythemia/ thrombocytosis) are associated with cancer, polycythemia vera, splenectomy, trauma, cirrhosis, myelogenous/granulocytic leukemia, stress, and active rheumatoid arthritis.

- **Decreased platelets** (thrombocytopenia) are associated with idiopathic thrombocytopenic purpura (ITP); pernicious, aplastic, and hemolytic anemia; allergic reactions; and bone marrow lesions.

- Many drugs (e.g., amrinone, antineoplastic agents, heparin, penicillins, gold salts, penicillamine) can cause thrombocytopenia.

- Decreases below 20,000 may be associated with spontaneous bleeding, prolonged bleeding time, petechiae, or ecchymosis.

- The precise number of platelets necessary for hemostasis is not firmly established. Patients with platelet deficits require observation for signs/ symptoms of GI bleeding, petechiae, hematuria, and episodes of spontaneous bleeding.

- Valproic acid decreases platelet count that is dose dependent. It also decreases platelet adhesiveness resulting in an increased bleeding time with a normal PT and aPTT.

- Aspirin and NSAIDs primarily affect platelet function rather than the actual platelet count.

ELECTROLYTES AND CHEMISTRY SURVEY

Sodium (Na+)

Normal Values 135–144 mEq/L   SI = 135–144 mmol/L

Description Sodium is the most abundant cation in extracellular fluid. It maintains osmotic pressure and acid-base balance, and aids in the sequence of transmission of nerve impulses. Sodium serum concentrations are regulated by the kidneys, the central nervous system (CNS), and the endocrine system. (See Chapter 8: Fluid and Electrolyte Therapy for a more detailed discussion of daily requirements.)

Clinical Implications
- **Hyponatremia** generally reflects excess body water rather than low total body sodium. Predisposing factors include burns, diarrhea/vomiting, and excessive use of fluids that do not contain electrolytes, Addison's disease, nephritis, and diabetic acidosis.

- SIADH (syndrome of inappropriate antidiuretic hormone) leads to increased body water and hyponatremia. It may be caused by certain tumors and some drugs (e.g., thiazide diuretics, chlorpropamide, carbamazepine, clofibrate, cyclophosphamide) and may be associated with some pulmonary disorders (e.g., tuberculosis, pneumonias). Patients with SIADH usually have a high urine sodium concentration and the urine osmolality is inappropriately high compared to serum osmolality.

- Cystic fibrosis patients may become hyponatremic due to increased loss of sodium in sweat.

- Clinical signs of acute saline depletion include nausea, fatigue, cramps, psychosis, seizures, and coma (Table 5–2).

- **Hypernatremia.** Predisposing factors include dehydration, aldosteronism, diabetes insipidus, and the use of osmotic diuretics. Generally, hypernatremia is an uncommon manifestation since thirst is the primary defense mechanism used to prevent hypertonicity. Therefore, hypernatremia primarily occurs in patients who are unable to ingest adequate fluids (e.g., comatose patients, infants).

- **IV Therapy Considerations.** A patient receiving >400 mg/day of sodium (e.g., 3 L/day of normal saline containing 155 mEq/L of sodium) usually will have difficulty with fluid balance and should be checked for signs of edema or elevated blood pressure. Healthy subjects can accommodate large increases in sodium intake as long as thirst mechanisms and renal function are intact.

Sodium (Na⁺) *(Continued)*

Clinical Implications (Continued)

- Numerous drugs affect sodium concentrations directly (sodium content) or indirectly by affecting urinary excretion of sodium.

- Total body water deficit = 1 liter for each 3 mmol of Na⁺ > normal.

Potassium (K⁺)

Normal Values

0–17 yr: 3.6 – 5.2 mEq/L	SI = 3.6 – 5.2 mmol/L
≥18 yr: 3.6 – 4.8 mEq/L	SI = 3.6 – 4.8 mmol/L

Description

Potassium is the principle intracellular fluid cation which (with bicarbonate) serves as the primary buffer within the cell. Approximately 80% to 90% of potassium is excreted in the urine by the kidneys. The mineralocorticoid activity of adrenocorticosteroids also regulates potassium concentration within the body. Only about 10% of the total body concentration of potassium is extracellular and about 50 mmol are in extracellular fluid. Therefore, the serum concentration of potassium is a poor measure of total body potassium. Nevertheless, the serum potassium concentration correlates well with its physiological effects on nerve conduction, muscle function, acid/base balance, and heart muscle contraction.

Clinical Implications

- **Hyperkalemia.** Predisposing factors are reduced excretion of potassium as seen with some types of renal failure, cell damage (e.g., burns, surgery), acidosis, Addison's disease, uncontrolled diabetes, and RBC transfusions.

TABLE 5–2: Clinical Signs of Water Depletion

Magnitude of Deficit (Adults)	Clinical Features
≤1.5 L	Thirst
1.5–4.0 L	Marked thirst Dry mouth Urine specific gravity increased Hematocrit, skin turgor, and blood pressure normal
≥4.0 L	Intolerable thirst Marked hypernatremia Oliguria Body weight decreased Slightly increased hematocrit Apathy, stupor If not corrected: hyperosmolar coma, death

Potassium (K+) *(Continued)*

Clinical Implications
(Continued)

• **Hypokalemia.** A serum potassium concentration of less than 3.5 mmol/L is usually defined as hypokalemia. As with many laboratory tests a falling trend (e.g., 0.1–0.2 mmol/L/day) is more worrisome than just one low laboratory result. Predisposing factors include vomiting/diarrhea, severe burns, primary aldosteronism, renal tubular acidosis, diuretics, steroids, cisplatin, ticarcillin, chronic stress, liver disease with ascites, and amphotericin therapy.

• Potassium values do not vary with circulatory volume. Potassium is an intracellular ion and its serum concentration should not be affected by circulatory volume.

• The chloride salt of potassium (KCl) is preferred for the treatment of hypokalemia. The optimal replacement dose of KCl depends upon the degree of hypokalemia and whether ECG changes are present. Adults usually ingest 60 to 120 mmol/day of potassium and hospitalized patients not receiving food by mouth often receive 10 to 30 mEq K+/L of IV fluids. (See Chapter 8: Fluid and Electrolyte Therapy for more detailed potassium administration guidelines.)

• Hypokalemia enhances the effects of digitalis preparations and may result in digitalis toxicity.

• As a very rough guideline, potassium blood levels rise about 0.6 mmol/L for every 0.1 decrease in blood pH from normal (pH 7.4).

• Specific ECG changes are associated with changes in serum potassium levels.

• Hypokalemia may be difficult to correct with KCl supplementation if the patient is also hypomagnesemic.

• Neuromuscular function is affected in both hyper- and hypokalemia.

• Glucose tolerance testing or large ingestions of glucose can decrease potassium blood levels by shifting potassium intracellularly.

• If the WBC is greater than 50,000/mm^3, the laboratory report of the serum potassium concentration can be spuriously decreased due to an intracellular shift of potassium into the leukocytes if the serum sample remains in the laboratory test tube for a long period of time.

Potassium (K+) *(Continued)*

Clinical Implications
(Continued)

- Calculation of total body potassium deficit is not well defined. Each 1 mmol/L decrement in the serum potassium represents a 100–200 mmol/L potassium deficit. When the serum level falls below 3 mmol/L, each 1 mmol/L decrement represents an additional 200–400 mmol deficit in total body stores.

- Protein synthesis is decreased with a potassium deficiency.

Chloride (Cl⁻)

Normal Values

97–106 mEq/L SI = 97–106 mmol/L

Description

The chloride anion resides predominantly in the extracellular space. It participates in the maintenance of acid/base and water balance through its influence on osmotic pressure. Although an alteration in the serum concentration of chloride is seldom a clinical problem, the chloride concentration is monitored because it is helpful in the diagnosis of acid/base disorders.

Clinical Implications

- **Decreased serum chloride concentrations** can be caused by vomiting, gastric suctioning, aggressive diuresis, burns, heat exhaustion, diabetic acidosis, and acute infection. A decreased chloride concentration is frequently associated with a metabolic alkalosis.

- **Increased serum chloride concentrations** can result from dehydration, hyperventilation, metabolic acidosis, and kidney disorders.

- Chloride values are useful in assessment of acid-base disturbances accompanying renal dysfunction. The plasma concentration of chloride, however, can be maintained near normal even in the presence of renal failure.

- Serum concentrations of sodium, bicarbonate, and chloride can be used to calculate the anion gap (AG) as follows:

$$AG = (Na^+) - [HCO_3^- + Cl^-]$$

An anion gap of greater than 12 indicates the presence of unmeasured anions such as methanol, urea, ketones, lactate, and ethylene glycol. See Chapter 8: Fluid and Electrolyte Therapy for a more detailed discussion.

Carbon Dioxide (CO₂) Content

Normal Values

22–32 mEq/L SI = 22–32 mmol/L

Carbon Dioxide (CO_2) Content *(Continued)*

Description	In normal plasma, 95% of total CO_2 is present as bicarbonate (HCO_3) ions and the other 5% as dissolved CO_2 gas and carbonic acid (H_2CO_3).
	There is often confusion by use of the term CO_2. The plasma CO_2 content is mainly bicarbonate, a base that is in solution and regulated by the kidneys. Dissolved CO_2 gas is mainly acid and is regulated by the lungs. Therefore, laboratory values of plasma CO_2 reflect bicarbonate concentrations.
Clinical Implications	• **Elevated CO_2** has been associated with severe vomiting, emphysema, and aldosteronism.
	• **Decreased CO_2** has been associated with acute renal failure, diabetic acidosis, and hyperventilation.
	• Increased or decreased levels can be caused by nitrofurantoin or salicylates.

Glucose [Fasting Blood Sugar, (FBS)]

Normal Values	70–100 mg/dL (≥7 yr)	SI = 3.89–5.55 mmol/L
	60–100 mg/dL (12 months–6 yr)	SI = 3.33–5.55 mmol/L
Description	Glucose is formed from the digestion of carbohydrates and by conversion of glycogen in the liver. Testing of the blood for glucose is primarily a screening procedure that indicates inability of the islet cells of the pancreas to produce insulin; inability of intestines to absorb glucose; inability of cells to utilize glucose efficiently; or the inability of the liver to accumulate and breakdown glycogen.	
Clinical Implications	• Elevated blood sugar (hyperglycemia) or glucose intolerance (fasting values >120 mg/dL) can accompany Cushing's disease, acute distress, pheochromocytoma, chronic liver disease, potassium deficiency, chronic illness, and bacterial sepsis.	
	• Lowered blood sugar concentration (hypoglycemia) can result from insulin overdose or Addison's disease.	
	• Many drugs such as glucocorticosteroids and anesthetic agents can increase the blood sugar concentration in excess of 200 mg/dL.	
	• When the serum glucose concentration is repeatedly >140 mg/dL, diabetes mellitus must be considered.	
	• Correlating the serum concentrations with the presence of urine glucose is useful for determining a patient's renal glucose threshold.	

Blood Urea Nitrogen (BUN)

Normal Values   7–20 mg/dL (≥6 yr)   SI = 2.5–7.4 mmol/L
                    5–18 mg/dL (1–5 yr)   SI = 1.8–6.4 mmol/L

Description   Urea is a non-protein nitrogenous end-product of protein catabolism. It is formed in the liver, carried by the blood to the kidneys, and excreted in urine. The BUN, therefore, provides an index of glomerular filtration. The BUN concentration can be affected by tissue necrosis, protein catabolism, and the state of hydration. It is not as sensitive an indicator of renal function as creatinine or creatinine clearance.

Clinical Implications
- **Increased BUN** is most commonly caused by inadequate excretion secondary to kidney disease/urinary obstruction. Decreased renal function caused by shock, dehydration, infection, or diabetes mellitus, can increase the BUN. Major gastrointestinal bleeding, with subsequent catabolism of blood to nitrogen or an increased protein intake also could increase the BUN.

- **Decreased BUN.** The BUN is decreased with end stage liver failure because the liver is unable to convert ammonia to urea. It is decreased by overhydration because of a dilutional effect, and by impaired absorption disorders because of an inability to absorb nitrogen subsequent to the digestion of protein.

- The elderly may have an increased BUN because of renal impairment.

- Nephrotoxic drugs (e.g., tetracycline, gentamicin) can increase the BUN.

- **BUN/Cr Ratio.** A ratio of >20 indicates pre-renal azotemia, while a ratio <20 is associated with intrinsic renal disease and azotemia.

Creatinine

Normal Values   1 yr: 0–0.6 mg/dL   SI = 0–53 µmol/L

                    2–3 yr: 0–0.7 mg/dL   SI = 0–62 µmol/L

                    4–7 yr: 0–0.8 mg/dL   SI = 0–72 µmol/L

                    8–10 yr: 0–0.9 mg/dL   SI = 0–81 µmol/L

                    11–12 yr: 0–1 mg/dL   SI = 0–88 µmol/L

                    13–17 yr: 0.6–1.2 mg/dL   SI = 53–106 µmol/L

                    ≥18 yr: 0.6–1.3 mg/dL   SI = 53–115 µmol/L

Description   Creatinine is a breakdown by-product of muscle creatine and phosphocreatine and is excreted renally. Creatinine production is constant as long as muscle mass remains constant. A reduction in kidney function reduces excretion of creatinine.

Creatinine *(Continued)*

Clinical Implications

- The serum creatinine concentration is increased with impaired renal function, regardless of whether the renal dynfunction is caused by nephritis, urinary tract obstruction, muscle disease, or severe dehydration.

- The serum creatinine concentration can be decreased as the result of muscular dystrophy, atrophy (e.g., spinal cord injury), malnutrition, or decreased muscle mass of aging.

- Drugs such as ascorbic acid, cimetidine (Tagamet), levodopa (Larodopa), and methyldopa (Aldomet) can interfere with the laboratory test measurement of creatinine independent of their effects on renal function.

- Creatinine values may be normal despite impaired renal function in elderly and malnourished patients due to decreased muscle mass.

- Creatinine has a serum half-life of about one day. Therefore, significant improvement in renal function requires several days before a new steady state level of creatinine is truly reflective of renal function.

- A serum creatinine of 2 and 3 mg/dL indicates a very general sense that renal function is about 50% and 30% of normal, respectively.

- Creatinine of 10 mg/dL = essentially no renal function and the patient will require dialysis.

- Creatinine serum concentrations also are dependent upon the patient's weight, age, and muscle mass.

Calcium (Ca^{++})

Normal Values

8.8–10.4 mg/dL SI = 2.2–2.6 mmol/L

Description

The calcium cation is involved in muscle contraction, cardiac function, transmission of nerve impulses, and blood clotting. Approximately 98% to 99% of the body's calcium is stored in the skeleton and teeth. Of the calcium in the blood, 50% is ionized and the remainder is protein bound. Only ionized calcium can be utilized in functional processes. A decrease in the serum albumin concentration of 1 gm/dL will decrease the total calcium serum concentration by about 0.8 mEq/dL (see Chapter 11: Common Pharmaceutical Calculations).

Clinical Implications

- **Hypercalcemia** is most commonly the result of hyperparathyroidism or neoplasms. Other causes include parathyroid adenoma or hyperplasia (associated with hypophosphatemia), Hodgkin's disease, multiple myeloma, leukemia, Addison's disease, Paget's disease, respiratory acidosis, bone metastasis, immobilization, and therapy with thiazide diuretics.

Calcium (Ca⁺⁺) *(Continued)*

Clinical Implications
(Continued)

- **Hypocalcemia** can result from hyperphosphatemia, alkalosis, osteomalacia, hypermagnesemia, inadequate calcium replacement, laxative use, and furosemide and calcitonin administration. Pseudohypocalcemia is sometimes encountered when the serum albumin concentration is low because of the association of calcium with albumin as described above.

- The following factors influence calcium levels:

  ○ Parathyroid hormone acts on bone to release calcium into the blood, increases intestinal calcium absorption, and enhances renal calcium reabsorption.

  ○ Vitamin D stimulates intestinal calcium absorption.

  ○ Estrogens increase calcium deposits in bone.

  ○ Androgens, glucocorticoids, and excessive thyroid hormone can lead to hypocalcemia and bone decalcification.

  ○ When requesting ionized calcium levels, blood pH should be measured concurrently.

Phosphorus, Inorganic (PO₄)

Normal Values			
Male: 0–5 yr:	4–7 mg/dL	SI = 1.29–2.25 mmol/L
	6–13 yr:	4–5.6 mg/dL	SI = 1.29–1.80 mmol/L
	14–16 yr:	3.4–5.5 mg/dL	SI = 1.09–1.78 mmol/L
	17–19 yr:	3–5 mg/dL	SI = 0.97–1.61 mmol/L
	≥20 yr:	2.6–4.6 mg/dL	SI = 0.89–1.48 mmol/L
Female: 0–5 yr:	4–7 mg/dL	SI = 1.29–2.25 mmol/L
	6–10 yr:	4.2–5.8 mg/dL	SI = 1.35–1.87 mmol/L
	11–13 yr:	3.6–5.6 mg/dL	SI = 1.16–1.8 mmol/L
	14–16 yr:	3.2–5.6 mg/dL	SI = 1.03–1.8 mmol/L
	≥17 yr:	2.6–4.6 mg/dL	SI = 0.84–1.48 mmol/L

Phosphorus, Inorganic (PO₄) *(Continued)*

Description	Phosphate, an anion, is required for generation of bony tissue, metabolism of glucose and lipids, maintaining acid/base balance, and storage and transfer of energy within the body. Approximately 85% of the body's total phosphorus is combined with calcium. When evaluating phosphate levels, the serum calcium values must also be checked.
Clinical Implications	• **Hyperphosphatemia** is associated with kidney dysfunction, uremia, excessive phosphate intake, hypoparathyroidism, hypocalcemia, excessive Vitamin D intake, bone tumors, respiratory acidosis, lactic acidosis, and diphosphonate therapy.
	• **Hypophosphatemia** can be associated with hyperparathyroidism, rickets, diabetic coma, hyperinsulinism, continuous IV glucose administration in a non-diabetic, antacids, diuretic phase of severe burns, and respiratory alkalosis.

Uric Acid

Normal Values	Male ≥15 yr: 3.6–8.5 mg/dL	SI = 214–506 µmol/L
	Female ≥18 yr: 2.3–6.6 mg/dL	SI = 137–393 µmol/L

Description	Uric acid is formed from the breakdown of nucleic acids. Serum concentration of urate increases when there is excessive production/destruction of cells (e.g., psoriasis, leukemia) or an inability to excrete urate renally.
Clinical Implications	• Hyperuricemia is associated with leukemia, lymphomas, shock, chemotherapy, metabolic acidosis, and significant renal dysfunction because of either increased production or decreased excretion.
	• Values below normal are not significant.
	• Drugs that increase urate blood levels include thiazides, salicylates (<2 gm/day), ethambutol, niacin, and cyclosporine.
	• Drugs that decrease blood levels include allopurinol (Zyloprim), probenecid (Benemid), sulfinpyrazone (Anturane), and salicylates (>3 gm/day).

Magnesium (Mg⁺⁺)

Normal Values	1.7–2.3 mg/dL SI = 0.85–1.15 mmol/L
Description	Magnesium is required for the utilization of adenosine triphosphate (ATP) as an energy source. It also has a role in carbohydrate metabolism, protein syn-

Magnesium (Mg⁺⁺) *(Continued)*

Description (Continued)   thesis, nucleic acid synthesis, and muscle contraction. Magnesium deficiency in a normal diet is rare; however, high phosphate diets suppress magnesium absorption. Magnesium also regulates neuromuscular irritability, the clotting mechanism, and calcium absorption.

Clinical Implications

- **Hypermagnesemia** is associated with renal dysfunction, diabetic acidosis, large doses of magnesium antacids in the presence of renal insufficiency, hypothyroidism, and dehydration.

- **Hypomagnesemia** can be associated with diarrhea, hemodialysis, malabsorption syndromes, drugs (e.g., thiazides, amphotericin B, cisplatin), lactation, acute pancreatitis, and chronic alcoholism.

- Magnesium deficiency may cause apparently unexplained hypocalcemia and hypokalemia resulting in severe neuromuscular irritability.

- Increased magnesium can act as a sedative and can depress cardiac and neuromuscular activity.

- To prevent arrhythmias, magnesium sulfate IV should not exceed 2 gm/hr.

- Hypomagnesium may cause ventricular arrhythmias.

Cholesterol

Normal Values   *Desirable:* 0–199 mg/dL   SI = 0–5.17 mmol/L
Borderline: 200–239 mg/dL   SI = 5.2–6.21 mmol/L
High Risk: ≥240 mg/dL   SI = ≥6.22 mmol/L

Description   Cholesterol exists in muscle, RBCs, and cell membranes. It is used by the body to form steroid hormones, bile acids, and cell membranes. Elevated cholesterol concentrations are associated with atherosclerosis and an increased risk of coronary artery disease.

Clinical Implications

- **Increased levels** of >200 mg/dL are considered to be high and require a triglyceride evaluation. Associated conditions include cardiovascular disease, atherosclerosis, Type II familial hypercholesterolemia, and obstructive jaundice.

- **Decreased levels** are associated with malabsorption, liver disease, sepsis, and pernicious anemia.

- A patient must fast for 12 hours before blood is obtained to measure the serum concentration of cholesterol, and should maintain a "normal" diet for 7 days prior. Alcohol should not be consumed 24 hours before testing and all lipid-lowering drugs should be withheld.

Total Serum Protein (TSP)

Normal Values	0–2 yr: 4.5–7.5 gm/dL SI = 45–75 gm/L
	≥3 yr: 6.3–8.0 gm/dL SI = 63–80 gm/L
Description	The three major protein categories are: 1) tissue or organ proteins; 2) plasma proteins and; 3) hemoglobin. The plasma proteins (albumin and globulins) reflect nutritional status and also serve as buffers in the maintenance of acid-base balance.
Clinical Implications	• **Hyperproteinemia** may be due to hemoconcentration secondary to dehydration. In this case, both albumin and globulin increase. If TSP increases but the albumin serum concentration is unchanged, the albumin/globulin (A/G) ratio falls. Collagen diseases, SLE, acute liver disease, and multiple myeloma are associated with hyperproteinemia.
	• **Hypoproteinemia** (decreased total protein) is usually associated with a low albumin and a small change in globulin *yielding* a low A/G ratio. It is normally associated with increased loss of albumin in the urine, decreased formation in the liver, insufficient protein intake, or severe burns.

Arterial Blood Gases (ABG)

Description	Arterial blood gas concentrations are analyzed to evaluate the exchange of oxygen and carbon dioxide to assess acid-base status. Arterial blood can be obtained by either an arterial puncture or from an indwelling arterial line to assess pH, pCO_2, pO_2, and SaO_2.

Common indications for the use of arterial gases include:

- **Gas Exchange Abnormalities**
  - ° acute and chronic pulmonary disease
  - ° acute respiratory failure
  - ° cardiac disease
  - ° rest and exercise pulmonary testing
  - ° monitoring O_2 therapy
  - ° sleep disorder studies

- **Acid-Base Disturbances**
  - ° metabolic acidosis
  - ° metabolic alkalosis

Oxygen Saturation (SaO_2)

Normal Values 95%–99% oxygen (O_2)

Description The oxygen saturation (SaO_2) describes the amount of oxygen carried by hemoglobin expressed as a total percentage of the total capacity of oxygen to combine with hemoglobin.

Clinical Implications
- SaO_2 is used with pO_2 to evaluate the extent of oxygenation of hemoglobin and the adequacy of tissue oxygenation.
- The partial pressure of O_2 dissolved in plasma determines the amount of oxygen bound to hemoglobin. The large pool of oxygen carrying hemoglobin allows blood to transport 65 times the amount of oxygen dissolved in the plasma. This relationship is determined by pH, temperature, the concentration of 2,3 DPG (diphosphoglycerate), and the molecular species of hemoglobin.

Partial Pressure of Oxygen (PaO_2)

Normal Values 75–100 mm Hg SI = 10–13.3 kPa
(room air, age dependent)

Description PaO_2 is a measure of the partial pressure exerted by the amount of O_2 dissolved in the plasma. It provides an estimate of the lung's ability to oxygenate blood.

Clinical Implications
- **Decreased PaO_2 values** are associated with chronic obstructive airways disease (COAD), restrictive airway disease, anemia, hypoventilation due to physical or neuromuscular impairment, and compromised cardiac function. PaO_2 values <40 mm Hg are a major concern.
- **Increased values** are associated with increased O_2 delivery by artificial means (e.g., nasal prongs, mechanical ventilation), hyperventilation by the patient, and polycythemia (increase in red blood cell mass and oxygen carrying capacity).

Partial Pressure of Carbon Dioxide ($PaCO_2$)

Normal Values 35–45 mm Hg SI = 4.7–6.0 kPa

Description $PaCO_2$ reflects the pressure exerted by the CO_2 dissolved in the plasma. It can be used to evaluate the effectiveness of alveolar ventilation and to determine the acid-base status of the blood.

Clinical Implications
- **Decreased $PaCO_2$** is usually associated with hypoxia, anxiety/nervousness, and pulmonary embolism. Values <20 mm Hg are a major concern.
- **Increased $PaCO_2$** is usually associated with obstructive lung disease or reduced function of the respiratory center. $PaCO_2$ values >60 mm Hg are a major concern.

Clinical Implications ***(Continued)***	• In general, a rise in $PaCO_2$ is associated with hypoventilation while a decrease reflects hyperventilation.
	• Typically, for each mEq decrease in HCO_3, the $PaCO_2$ will decrease by 1.3 mm Hg.

pH

Normal Values	7.35–7.45 *Panic Values:* < 7.25 or >7.55
Description	The serum pH reflects the chemical balance of acids and bases within the body. Hydrogen ion sources within the body include volatile acids and fixed acids (i.e., lactic acid, ketoacids).
Clinical Implications	• pH is generally decreased in acidemia (due to increased formation of acids).
	• pH is generally increased in alkalemia (due to acid loss).
	• When evaluating a pH value, pCO_2 and HCO_3 should also be obtained to estimate the respiratory or metabolic component contributing to the patient's acid-base status.

Anion Gap (AG)

Normal Values	13–17 mEq/L
Description	The anion gap is used clinically in the diagnosis of metabolic acidosis. Calculations using available electrolyte information assist in quantification of unmeasured cations and anions. The unmeasured cations include Ca^{++} and Mg^{++}; unmeasured anions include protein, phosphate, sulfate, and organic acids.

The anion gap can be calculated using two different approaches:

$$Na^+ - (Cl^- + HCO_3^-) \quad or \quad Na + K - (Cl + HCO_3) = AG$$

See Chapter 11: Pharmaceutical Calculations and Chapter 8: Fluid and Electrolytes Therapy for further discussion.

Clinical Implications	• A high anion gap (with a high pH) may indicate extracellular volume contraction or administration of penicillins in large doses.
	• A high anion gap (with a low pH) is demonstrated with "MULEPAK" (**M**ethanol ingestion, **U**remia, **L**actic acidosis, **E**thylene glycol ingestions, **P**araldehyde ingestion, **A**spirin intoxication, and **K**etoacidosis).

Anion Gap (AG) *(Continued)*

Clinical Implications
(Continued)

- A low anion gap has been associated with hypoalbuminemia, dilution, hypernatremia, marked hypercalcemia, or lithium toxicity.

- A normal anion gap can occur with metabolic acidosis as the result of diarrhea, renal tubular acidosis, or hypercalcemia.

Bicarbonate Buffer System

Normal Values

21–28 mEq/L

Description

The bicarbonate buffer system consists of carbonic acid (H_2CO_3) and bicarbonate (HCO_3). Quantitatively it is the major buffer system in the extracellular body fluid. It reflects the following relationship:

$$\text{Total } CO_2 \text{ content} = \text{carbonic acid} + \text{bicarbonate}$$

Clinical Implications

- **Increased bicarbonate** may indicate respiratory acidosis due to decreased ventilation.

- **Decreased bicarbonate** may indicate respiratory alkalosis due to increased alveolar ventilation and removal of CO_2 and water *or* metabolic acidosis due to accumulation of body acids or a loss of bicarbonate from the extracellular fluid.

URINALYSIS (UA)

Normal Values

See Table 5–3.

Description

The UA provides valuable information in the evaluation of patients with renal disease.

Clinical Implications

- **Specific Gravity.** A specific gravity >1.025 in the morning indicates good concentrating ability; 1.010–1.012 indicates the urine is isotonic with plasma (285–295 mOsm). Glucosuria, iodinated contrast media, and massive proteinuria (>2 gm/24 hr) also can increase the specific gravity of urine.

- **Appearance**
  - *Red-Brown color* indicates urine contains hemoglobin, myoglobin, bile pigments, blood, or dyes.
  - *Yellow-Red color* indicates the presence of vegetables, phenazopyridine, or phenophthalein cathartics.
  - *Blue-Green color* indicates the patient consumed beets.
  - *Dark or Black color* indicates the presence of porphyrins.

URINALYSIS (UA) *(Continued)*

Clinical Implications
(Continued)

- **Appearance***(Continued)*

  ° *Turbid urine* is secondary to presence of urates/phosphates or WBCs.

  ° *Foamy urine* contains protein or bile acids.

- **Alkaline pH.** Urea splitting organisms such as Proteus, Klebsiella, or *E. coli* or renal tubular acidosis caused by amphotericin therapy can alkalinize urine.

- **Protein.** A trace amount can be noted when a patient stands for prolonged periods of time. To quantitate the urinary protein a 24 hr urine is collected.

- **Proteinuria** (with dipstick method) may be false-positive in patients with alkaline urine. The urinary protein may be: a) normal, indicating increased glomerular permeability or a renal tubular disorder or b) abnormal because of multiple myeloma and Bence-Jones proteins.

- **Glucose.** The correlation of urine glucose with serum glucose can be helpful in monitoring and adjusting antidiabetic medications.

- **Ketones.** Starvation, poorly controlled diabetes mellitus, and alcoholism can result in the appearance of ketones in the urine.

- **Sediment.** No particular type of urine cast is pathognomonic for a specific renal disorder; however, the presence of red cell casts and white cell casts is ominous.

TABLE 5–3: Normal Values: Urinalysis

Parameter	Normal Value
Specific gravity	1.001–1.035
Appearance	Straw-colored, yellow
pH	4.5–8.5
Protein	0–trace (Tr); <50 mg/dL or (<0.5 gm/L)
Glucose	Negative
Ketones	Negative
Blood	Negative
Sediment analysis	Cell count for RBC, WBC (see Table 5–4)
Gram's stain	Negative

LABORATORY TESTS BY ORGAN SYSTEM

CARDIAC DIAGNOSTIC TESTS
Cardiac Isoenzymes
Creatine Kinase (CK)

Normal Values	*Male:* <200 U/L	SI = <3.33 µkat/L
	Female: <150 U/L	SI = <2.50 µkat/L
	CK isoenzymes MM 97%–100%	
	MB 0%–3%	
	BB 0%	

Description Creatine kinase (formerly known as creatine phosphokinase) is an enzyme found in high concentrations in heart and skeletal muscle. It is used as a specific test for the diagnosis of a myocardial infarction (MI) and as a reliable measure of skeletal muscle diseases (e.g., muscular dystrophy, polymyositis).

TABLE 5–4: Cell Types in the Urine Sediment

Cell Type	Normal	Clinical Considerations
RBC	0–3/hpf[a]	*Cystitis* is the most frequent cause of hematuria, although slight hematuria often occurs secondary to exertion, trauma, or febrile illness
		Yeast cells may be confused with RBCs. To distinguish between the two, acetic acid administration will result in a lysis of the RBC, but not yeast cells
Epithelial	0–2/hpf	*Epithelial cells* increase with tubular damage or heavy proteinuria
Bacteria		Presence of bacteria on Gram's stain of unspun specimen correlates well with culture growth of ≥10⁵ organisms (i.e., indicates presence of urinary tract infection). A culture and sensitivity (C&S) is useful to confirm the presence of bacteria
WBC	0–5/hpf	*Polymorphonuclear leukocytes* are the most common form of WBCs observed. If seen, and two routine cultures are negative, the culture should be tested for tubercle bacilli
Casts	0–occasional per low power field	Red cell casts usually signify active glomerular disease. Fatty and waxy casts may be seen with inflammatory or degenerative renal disease. Leukocyte casts are usually associated with pyelonephritis. Hyaline or granular casts may be more commonly seen and are less significant

[a] hpf = High Powered Field.

Description ***(Continued)***	CK can be divided into three isoenzymes: MM or CK_3, BB or CK_1, and MB or CK_2. Skeletal muscle contains primarily MM; cardiac muscle primarily MM and MB; and brain tissue primarily BB. Normal CK is virtually 100% MM.
Clinical Implications	• Myocardial Infarction (MI). The CK begins to rise 4 to 6 hours after myocardial injury, reaches a peak serum concentration within 30 hours, and returns to normal 2 to 3 days after infarction. If there is a negative CK-MB within 48 hours of onset of pain, the patient probably has not had an MI.
	• Other diseases that can cause increased CK levels include cerebrovascular disease, muscular dystrophy, polymyositis, dermatomyositis, delirium tremens (DTs), chronic alcoholism, subarachnoid hemorrhage, and CNS trauma.
	• Elevated MM enzymes occur in muscle trauma, IM injections, shock, MI, and following surgery.
	• Elevation of the MM level is an indication of skeletal muscle injury; elevation of MB provides a more definitive indication of myocardial injury.
	• Elevated MB enzymes occur in MI, myocardial ischemia, and muscular dystrophy.
	• Elevated BB enzymes occur in biliary atresia, brain trauma, and certain other brain injuries or tumors.

Lipoprotein Panel

Includes cholesterol, low density lipoprotein (LDL) cholesterol, triglycerides, and high density lipoprotein (HDL) cholesterol.

Cholesterol
See page 5–26.

Low Density Lipoproteins (LDL)

Normal Values	*Desirable:* <130 mg/dL	SI = <3.36 mmol/L
Adult	*Borderline:* 130–159 mg/dL	SI = 3.36–4.11 mmol/L
	High Risk: ≥160 mg/dL	SI = >4.13 mmol/L
Description	LDL are beta cholesterol esters.	
Clinical Implications	• **High LDL values** are associated with coronary vascular disease or familial hyperlipidemia. Levels may also be elevated in samples taken from non-fasting subjects. Levels may also be elevated in types IIa and IIb hyperliproteinemia, diabetes mel-	

Clinical Implications
(Continued)

litus, hypothyroidism, obstructive jaundice, nephrotic syndrome, familial and idiopathic hyperlipidemia, and with the use of estrogens or estrogen-containing oral contraceptives.

• **Decreased LDL levels** may occur in patients with hypoproteinemia or abetalipoproteinemia.

High Density Lipoproteins (HDL)

Normal Values

Adult: 30–70 mg/dL SI = 0.78–1.81 mmol/L

Description

HDL are the products of liver and intestinal synthesis and triglyceride catabolism.

Clinical Implications

• There is an inverse relationship between HDL-cholesterol levels and the incidence of coronary artery disease.

• **Increased HDL** can occur in chronic alcoholism, primary biliary cirrhosis, and subsequent to exposure to industrial toxins or polychlorinated hydrocarbons. Patients taking clofibrate, estrogens, nicotinic acid, oral contraceptives, and phenytoin may have increased HDL levels.

• **Decreased HDL** can occur in patients with cystic fibrosis, severe hepatic cirrhosis, diabetes mellitus, Hodgkin's disease, nephrotic syndrome, malaria, and some acute infections. Patients receiving probucol, hydrochlorothiazide, progestins, and prolonged parenteral nutrition may have decreased HDL levels.

Triglycerides

Normal Values

Male: 40–160 mg/dL   SI = 0.45–1.80 mmol/L

Desirable Adult

Female: 35–135 mg/dL   SI = 0.4–1.53 mmol/dL

Description

Triglycerides are found in plasma lipids as chylomicrons and very low density lipoproteins (VLDL).

Clinical Implications

• Triglycerides are increased in patients with alcoholic cirrhosis, alcoholism, anorexia nervosa, biliary cirrhosis, biliary obstruction, cerebral thrombosis, chronic renal failure, diabetes mellitus, Down's syndrome, hypertension, idiopathic hypercalcemia, hyperlipoproteinemia (types I, IIb, III, IV and V), glycogen storage diseases (types I, III, and VI), gout, ischemic heart disease, hypothyroidism, pregnancy, acute intermittent porphyria, respiratory distress syndrome, thalassemia major, viral hepatitis, and Werner's syndrome.

*Triglycerides (**Continued**)*

Clinical Implications
(Continued)

- Cholestyramine, corticosteroids, estrogens, ethanol, high carbohydrate diets, intravenous miconazole, oral contraceptives, and spironolactone can increase triglycerides.

- Decreased triglycerides may be seen with chronic obstructive lung disease, hyperparathyroidism, hyperthyroidism, hypolipoproteinemia, intestinal lymphangiectasia, severe parenchymal liver disease, malabsorption, and malnutrition.

- Ascorbic acid, asparaginase, clofibrate, and heparin can decrease triglyceride serum concentrations.

RENAL DIAGNOSTIC TESTS
Creatinine, Urine (Cl_{Cr})

Normal Values

Male: 1–2 gm/24 hr

Adult

Female: 0.8–1.8 gm/24 hr

Description

Creatinine is formed as a result of dehydration of muscle creatine and functions solely as a waste product of creatine. Since creatinine is freely filtered by renal glomeruli and is not appreciably tubularly reabsorbed under normal conditions, serum creatinine and creatinine clearance provide a reflection of glomerular filtration.

Clinical Implications

- Creatinine production decreases with advanced age as muscle mass diminishes.

- An accurate 24 hr-urine collection is desirable. The concentration of urine creatinine in conjunction with urine volume and duration of collection (minutes) provide a good estimate of true renal function. (See Chapter 11: Common Pharmaceutical Calculations.)

Na^+/K^+ Ratio, Urine

Normal Values

0.9–3.88

Description

The Na^+/K^+ ratio in urine is useful in evaluating kidney function, fluid and electrolyte balance, acid/base balance, and extent of aldosterone effects on electrolyte composition of the urine.

Clinical Implications

- Diurnal variation occurs.

- Timed collection is required for an accurate measurement. A single collection may be used to assess responses to spironolactone therapy. The urine Na^+/K^+ ratio >1 with effective spironolactone therapy.

Urine Sodium (Na⁺)

Normal Values   27–287 mEq/L/24 hr SI = 27–287 mmol/24 hr

Description   The urine sodium concentration is useful in assessing fluid balance, aldosterone effects, and renal concentrating ability. The wide range of normal values reflects dietary variations.

Clinical Implications
- In cases of hyponatremia, urine sodium of <10 mmol/L may indicate dehydration, congestive heart failure, liver disease, or nephrotic syndrome.
- Urine sodium >4 mmol/L may indicate diuretic use, Addison's Disease, or SIADH.
- Urine sodium >40 mmol/L and oliguria may suggest renal tubular necrosis.
- Wide range for normal values reflect diet, posture, stress, and endocrine effects.

Urine Chloride (Cl⁻)

Normal Values   110–250 mEq/L/24 hr SI = 110–250 mmol/24 hr

Description   Used in workup of acid-base status to determine whether metabolic alkalosis is chloride-responsive. Normal values are diet- and perspiration-dependent.

Clinical Implications   The chloride value only has meaning if Na^+, K^+ intake and output are also known. It can serve as a guide in monitoring individuals on salt restricted diets.

Urine Potassium (K⁺)

Normal Values   26–123 mEq/L/24 hr SI = 26–123 mmol/24 hr

Description   Concentration is diet-dependent. It is used in workup of aldosteronism, renal tubular acidosis, and alkalosis.

Clinical Implications
- Renal losses in a hypertensive patient not on diuretics suggest possible aldosteronism, adrenal carcinoma, or renal tubular acidosis.
- Elevated levels of urinary potassium are seen in patients with chronic renal failure, diabetes mellitus, renal tubular acidosis, dehydration, primary aldosteronism, and Cushing's disease.
- Decreased levels of urinary potassium are seen in acute renal failure, excessive ingestion (or production) of mineralocorticoids, and in malabsorption/diarrhea syndromes.
- Urine pH is decreased in patients who have decreased potassium levels (hydrogen secreted in exchange for sodium) because less potassium is available for exchange.

Creatinine Clearance, Calculated (Cl$_{Cr}$)

Normal Values	See Table 5–5.
Description	Creatinine clearance measures the rate at which creatinine is cleared from the body by the kidney, essentially a measure of the glomerular filtration rate (GFR).
Clinical Implications	• The measured creatinine clearance can provide a more accurate assessment. (See Chapter 11: Common Pharmaceutical Calculations.) Also see Urine Creatinine on page 5–35.
	• Note lower creatinine clearances in children (presumably resulting from less muscle mass).

GASTROINTESTINAL/HEPATIC DIAGNOSTIC TESTS

Amylase, Serum

Normal Values	20–100 U/L SI = 0.33–1.66 μkat/L
Description	Amylase is an enzyme that converts starch to sugar. It is produced in the salivary glands, pancreas, liver, and fallopian tubes. If there is an inflammation of the pancreas or salivary glands, more of the enzyme enters the blood.
Clinical Implications	• **Increased levels** are associated with acute pancreatitis; acute exacerbation of chronic pancreatitis; carcinoma of the lung, esophagus, or ovaries; partial gastrectomy; obstruction of pancreatic duct; perforated peptic ulcer; mumps; obstruction or inflammation of salivary duct or gland; acute cholecystitis; cerebral trauma; burns; traumatic shock; diabetic ketoacidosis; dissected aortic aneurysm; and morphine administration.
	• **Decreased levels** are associated with acute pancreatitis subsidence, hepatitis, cirrhosis of liver, or toxemia of pregnancy.

TABLE–5-5: Calculated Creatinine Clearance[a]

Age	Male (mL/min)	Female (mL/min)
0–6 months	40–60	40–60
7–12 months	50–75	50–75
13 months–4 yr	60–100	60–100
5–8 yr	65–110	65–110
9–12 yr	70–120	70–120
≥13 yr	80–130	75–120

[a] Degree of Impairment: Severe = <10 mL/min; Moderate = 10–30 mL/min; Mild = 30–70 mL/min.

Lipase

Normal Values	4–20 U/dL SI = 0.67–4.00 µkat/L (Kinetic method) (values may vary with methodology)
Description	Lipase converts fatty acid to glycerol. The major source of lipase is the pancreas; therefore lipase appears in the bloodstream following damage to the pancreas.
Clinical Implications	• Increased levels are associated with pancreatitis, obstruction of the pancreatic duct, pancreatic carcinoma, acute cholecystitis, cirrhosis, severe renal disease, morphine administration, and inflammatory bowel disease.
	• When secretions from the pancreas are blocked, serum lipase rises. Elevation may not occur until 24 to 36 hours after onset of illness.
	• Lipase may be high when amylase levels are normal.
	• Lipase persists longer in the serum than amylase in patients with pancreatitis.

Alanine Aminotransferase (ALT)

[Formerly Serum Glutamic Pyruvic Transaminase (SGPT)]

Normal Values	0–35 U/L SI = 0–0.58 µkat/L
Description	High concentrations of the ALT enzyme are present in the liver. It is also found in heart, muscle, and kidney. ALT is relatively more abundant in hepatic versus cardiac tissue and is more liver specific than AST. ALT is utilized in the diagnosis of liver disease and to monitor the course of treatment for hepatitis, postnecrotic cirrhosis, and hepatotoxic effects of drugs.
Clinical Implications	• Increased levels are found in hepatocellular disease, active cirrhosis, obstructive jaundice/biliary obstruction, and hepatitis.
	• Many drugs can increase levels.
	• A twofold increase is significant.

Alkaline Phosphatase (Alk Phos)

Normal Values	See Table 5–6.
Description	This enzyme originates mainly in the bone, liver, and placenta. High concentrations can be found in the biliary canaliculi with some located in the kidney and intestines. The release of this enzyme, as an index of bone disease, is related to bone cell production and

Alkaline Phosphatase (Alk Phos) *(Continued)*

Description *(Continued)*	deposition of calcium in the bone. In liver disease, the alkaline phosphatase blood level rises when its excretion is impaired as a result of biliary tract obstruction. Fractionation by heat can differentiate the origin of alkaline phosphatase (i.e., liver or bone). The terms "liver lives" (heat stable) and "bone burns" (heat labile) are useful to help remember common reporting terms.
Clinical Implications	• **Elevated levels** are associated with obstructive jaundice, liver lesions, hepatocellular cirrhosis, Paget's disease, metastatic bone disease, osteomalacia, hyperparathyroidism, total parenteral nutrition, and hyperphosphatemia. • **Reduced levels** are associated with hypophosphatemia, malnutrition, and hypothyroidism. • After intravenous administration of albumin, there is often a moderate increase of alkaline phosphatase that can last for several days. • Note the higher normal values during ages of rapid bone growth listed in Table 5–6 .

TABLE 5–6: Normal Values: Alkaline Phosphatase

	Age (yr)	U/L
Male	0–9	75–375
	10	150–350
	11–13	150–450
	14	150–400
	15–16	50–300
	17	50–225
	18	50–175
	≥19	35–130
Female	0–10	75–375
	11	150–425
	12	150–375
	13	50–325
	14	50–250
	15	50–175
	16–17	50–150
	≥18	35–130

Ammonia (NH₃)

Normal Values	12–55 µmol/L SI = 15–55 µmol/L
Description	Ammonia is formed by bacterial metabolism of proteins in the intestine. Normally ammonia is removed from the blood by the liver and converted to urea. Urea is then excreted by the kidney. Generally, ammonia levels vary with protein intake. Exercise can increase ammonia levels.
Clinical Implications	• Increased levels are associated with liver disease, pericarditis, severe heart failure, acute bronchitis, pulmonary emphysema, urinary tract obstruction, hepatic coma, azotemia, and Reye's syndrome.
	• Measurements of blood ammonia levels are used to evaluate metabolism as well as the progress of severe liver disease and response to treatment.
	• In Reye's syndrome, elevated ammonia levels and encephalopathy may occur.

Aspartate Aminotransferase (AST)
[Formerly Serum Glutamic Oxaloacetic Transaminase (SGOT)]

Normal Values	*Male:* 0–50 U/L	SI = 0–0.83 µkat/L
	Female: 0–40 U/L	SI = 0–0.67 µkat/L
Description	AST, an enzyme of high metabolic activity, is found in heart, liver, skeletal muscle, kidney, brain, spleen, pancreas, and lung. Any disease that causes change in these highly metabolic tissues, or any injury or death of these cells, will release the enzyme into the circulation.	
Clinical Implications	• **Increased levels** occur in MI, liver disease, acute pancreatitis, trauma, acute hemolytic anemia, acute renal disease, severe burns, and with the use of various drugs.	
	• **Decreased levels** occur in the acidotic patient with diabetes mellitus.	
	• Normal serum concentrations (0–80 U/L) can be slightly higher in infants 1 to 60 days of age.	

Bilirubin (Bili, T. Bili)

Normal Values	*Total:* ≤1.4 mg/dL	SI = <24 µmol/L
	Direct: ≤0.40 mg/dL	SI = <7 µmol/L
Description	Bilirubin is a breakdown of hemoglobin and a by-product of hemolysis. It is primarily removed by the liver and excreted into the bile with a small amount found in the serum. A rise in the bilirubin occurs if there is excessive RBC destruction or if the liver is unable to secrete the amount produced.	

Bilirubin (Bili, T. Bili) *(Continued)*

Description
(Continued)

There are two forms of bilirubin: 1) indirect or un-conjugated (which is protein bound) and 2) direct or conjugated that circulates freely in the serum. An increase in conjugated bilirubin is more frequently associated with increased destruction of RBCs, while an increase in unconjugated bilirubin is more likely in dysfunction or blockage of the liver.

Bilirubin is important in evaluating liver function, hemolytic anemias, and hyperbilirubinemia (in newborns).

Clinical Implications

- Bilirubin elevations accompanied by jaundice may be due to hepatocellular injury, disease of parenchymal cells, bile duct obstruction, or red cell hemolysis.

- Elevations of unconjugated bilirubin levels occur in hemolytic anemia, trauma with evidence of a large hematoma, and pulmonary infarcts.

- Elevations of conjugated bilirubin levels occur in pancreatic cancer and cholelithiasis.

- Both levels increase in hepatic metastasis, hepatitis, cirrhosis, and cholestasis secondary to drugs.

- Hemolyzed blood falsely elevates bilirubin.

Gamma Glutamyl Transferase (GGT)

Normal Values

0–1 months: 0–200 U/L	SI = 0–3.33 μkat/L
1–2 months: 0–120 U/L	SI = 0–2.00 μkat/L
2–3 months: 0–100 U/L	SI = 0–1.67 μkat/L
4–17 months: 0–50 U/L	SI = 0–0.83 μkat/L
18 months–15 yr: 0–30 U/L	SI = 0–0.50 μkat/L
≥16 yr male: 0–65 U/L	SI = 0–1.08 μkat/L
≥16 yr female: 0–40 U/L	SI = 0–0.67 μkat/L

Description

GGT is present mainly in the liver, kidney, prostate, and spleen. The liver is considered the source of normal serum activity despite the fact the kidney has the highest level of the enzyme. The enzyme is believed to function in the transport of amino acids and peptides. Men have higher levels due to the concentrations found in the prostate.

Monitoring GGT values may be of benefit to detect acute or chronic alcohol drinkers, obstructive jaundice, cholangitis, and cholecystitis.

Gamma Glutamyl Transferase (GGT) *(Continued)*

Clinical Implications   Increased GGT levels are associated with cholecystitis, cholelithiasis, cirrhosis, biliary obstruction, barbiturate use, hepatotoxic drugs (especially those which induce the cytochrome P450 system). GGT is very sensitive, but not *specific*. Elevations of just GGT (not AST, ALT) do not necessarily indicate liver damage.

Hemoccult (Guaiac or Benzidine Method)

Normal Values   Negative

Description   Commonly used to measure the presence of blood in stools, nasogastric output, and other bodily secretions.

Clinical Implications
- Presence of blood in stools requires further investigation.
- **False positives** are observed with large doses of iron, iodides, phenazopyridine, or red meat within 3 days of test.
- **False negatives** are observed with high doses of ascorbic acid.

Lactate Dehydrogenase (LD) [Formerly LDH]

Normal Values   42 days–11 months: 200–470 U/L   SI = 3.33–7.83 µkat/L

1–3 yr: 225–350 U/L   SI = 3.75–5.83 µkat/L

4–6 yr: 200–325 U/L   SI = 3.33–5.42 µkat/L

7–9 yr: 200–300 U/L   SI = 3.33–5.00 µkat/L

10–13 yr: 150–275 U/L   SI = 2.50–4.58 µkat/L

14–16 yr: 50–250 U/L   SI = 2.50–4.17 µkat/L

≥17 yr: 90–200 U/L   SI = 1.50–3.33 µkat/L

Description   An intracellular enzyme, LD is widely distributed in the tissues, particularly in the liver, kidney, heart, lungs, and skeletal muscle. This glycolytic enzyme catalyzes the interconversion of lactate and pyruvate. LD levels are nonspecific, but aid in confirmation of myocardial or pulmonary infarction in combination with other findings. The LD may also be helpful in diagnosing muscular dystrophy and pernicious anemia. More specifics can be determined if LD is broken down into isoenzymes. Therefore, specific isoenzymes can be requested [i.e., LD1:LD2 for myocardial infarction (MI)].

Lactate Dehydrogenase (LD) [Formerly LDH] *(Continued)*

Clinical Implications

- In an acute MI, the LD increases and the LD1:LD2 ratio usually "flips" to >1. Levels increase within 12 to 24 hours of infarction and peak usually 3 to 4 days after an MI.

- With a pulmonary infarction, the LD is usually increased within 24 hours after onset of pain.

- **Elevated levels** are associated with acute MI, acute leukemia, skeletal muscle necrosis, pulmonary infarct, skin disorders, shock, megaloblastic anemia, and lymphomas. Various drugs and disease states also increase levels.

- **Decreased levels** reflect a good response to cancer therapy.

ENDOCRINE DIAGNOSTIC TESTS
Thyroid: Thyroid Function Tests

T_4-RIA (Thyroxine Determination by Radioimmunoassay)

Normal Values	1–3 days: 8.2–19.9 µg/dL SI = 106.0–258.7 mmol/L
	4–7 days: 6–15.9 µg/dL SI = 78–206.7 mmol/L
	1–52 wk: 6.1–14.9 µg/dL SI = 79.3–193.7 mmol/L
	1–2 yr: 6.8–13.5 µg/dL SI = 88.4–175.5 mmol/L
	3–10 yr: 5.5–12.8 µg/dL SI = 71.5–166.4 mmol/L
	>10 yr: 5–11 µg/dL SI = 65–143 mmol/L

Description

The T_4 RIA test measures the level of total circulating thyroid using a radioimmunoassay procedure in the laboratory. It will provide an accurate result even if a contrast organic iodine has been used in a recent x-ray.

Clinical Implications

- **Increased values** are associated with hyperthyroidism, acute thyroiditis, pregnancy, early hepatitis, idiopathic TBG (thyroid-binding globulin) elevation, and the use of estrogens.

- **Decreased values** are associated with hypothyroidism, chronic thyroiditis, nephrosis, and idiopathic TBG decrease. Values will be decreased with use of anabolic steroids, salicylates, phenytoin, or propranolol.

- Administration of traces of radioactive iodine within 48 hours before testing will interfere with the results.

T_4 (Thyroxine Total)

Normal Values   5–12.5 µg/dL SI = 65–160 nmol/L

Description   Approximately 95% is bound to thyroxin-binding globulin (TBG) as well as prealbumin and albumin. About 5% of circulating T_4 is in the free or unbound form. The measurement of T_4 is a good index of thy-

T_4 (Thyroxine Total) **(Continued)**

Description (Continued)

roid function when the TBG is normal. Therefore, this test is commonly performed to rule out hyperthyroidism and hypothyroidism. Finally, the T_4 test also can be used as a guide in establishing and following maintenance doses of thyroid in the treatment of hypothyroidism.

Clinical Implications

• Values can be increased in hyperthyroidism, acute thyroiditis, subacute thyroiditis, hepatitis, the first trimester of pregnancy, and with the use of estrogens.

• Values can be decreased in creatinism, myxedema, hypothyroidism, thyroiditis, subacute thyroiditis, Simmond's disease, nephrosis, cirrhosis, hypoproteinemia, and malnutrition.

• Values are usually normal in T_3 toxicosis.

T_3 (Triiodothyronine)

Normal Values

1–3 days: 89–405 ng/dL	SI = 1.4–6.2 nmol/L
4–7 days: 91–300 ng/dL	SI = 1.4–4.6 nmol/L
1–4 wk: 88–275 ng/dL	SI = 1.4–4.2 nmol/L
1–12 months: 85–250 ng/dL	SI = 1.3–3.9 nmol/L
1–10 yr: 80–250 ng/dL	SI = 1.2–3.9 nmol/L
>10 yr: 80–160 ng/dL	SI = 1.2–2.5 nmol/L

Description

T_3 is more metabolically active than T_4, but has a shorter half-life. In the serum, there exists less T_3 than T_4 which is bound less firmly to thyroid-binding globulin. T_3 testing is of little value in diagnosing hypothyroidism. The T_3 test is a diagnostic test for hyperthyroidism and T_3 thyrotoxicosis (i.e., elevated T_3 levels will be seen with normal T_4 levels in T_3 thyrotoxicosis).

Clinical Implications

• **Increased values** are associated with hyperthyroidism, T_3 thyrotoxicosis, daily dosage of ≥ 25 μg (liothyronine), acute thyroiditis, idiopathic TBG elevation, daily dosage of 300 μg of levothyroxine (T_4), pregnancy, estrogen use, and oral contraceptives.

• **Decreased values** are associated with hypothyroidism (however some clinically hypothyroid patients will have normal levels), starvation, idiopathic TBG, acute illness, anabolic steroids, androgens, large doses of salicylates, and phenytoin.

T_3UR (Triiodothyronine Uptake Ratio)

Normal Values

T_3U = 24%–35%   SI = 0.25–0.35

T_3UR = 0.8–1.3 ratio between patient specimen and the standard control

T₃UR (Triiodothyronine Uptake Ratio) *(Continued)*

Description   The measurement of T_3UR is an indirect measurement of unsaturated thyroxin-binding globulin (TBG) in the blood. Low T_3UR levels are indicative of situations that result in elevated levels of TBG.

Clinical Implications
- **Increased levels** are associated with hyperthyroidism, nephrosis, severe liver disease, metastatic malignancy, pulmonary insufficiency, thyroxine and desiccated thyroid therapy, heparin, androgens, anabolic steroids, phenytoin, and large doses of salicylates.

- **Decreased levels** are associated with hypothyroidism, pregnancy, hyperestrogenic status, and T_3 treatment for hypothyroidism.

Thyroid Stimulating Hormone (TSH)

Normal Values   Adult: 2–11 μU/mL   SI = 2–11 mU/L

Description   The TSH is included in workup of a low T_4 (RIA) result. It can differentiate primary hypothyroidism from a euthyroid state and primary hypothyroidism from pituitary/hypothalamic hypothyroidism.

Clinical Implications
- TSH is increased in primary hypothyroidism.

- If clinical evidence for hypothyroidism is present and the TSH is not elevated, the implication of possible hypopituitarism exists.

Adrenal Gland

Plasma Cortisol

Normal Values   *Morning:* 6–24 μg/dL   SI = 165–662 nmol/L
Evening: 3–12 μg/dL   SI = 83–331 nmol/L

Description   Cortisol affects the metabolism of proteins, carbohydrates, and lipids and inhibits the effect of insulin. It stimulates gluconeogenesis by the liver and decreases the rate of glucose use by the cells.

In the healthy person (that awakens in the morning and sleeps at night), the secretion rate of cortisol is higher in the early morning (6 to 8 a.m.) and lower in the evening (4 to 6 p.m.).

Clinical Implications
- **Extreme increases** in the morning and no variation later in the day suggest carcinoma.

- **Decreased levels** are expected in liver disease, Addison's disease, anterior pituitary hyposecretion, and hypothyroidism.

- **Increased levels** are found in hyperthyroidism, stress (circadian variation less apparent in this setting), obesity, Cushing's syndrome, pregnancy, and the use of spironolactone and/or oral contraceptives.

Cosyntropin Test

> **Normal Cortisol Values**   *Rise:* >8 µg/dL   SI = >220 nmol/L
>   *Peak:* >20 µg/d   SI = >551 nmol/L

> **Description**   A test to detect adrenal insufficiency. Cosyntropin is a synthetic subunit of adrenocorticotropic hormone (ACTH) that exhibits the full corticosteroid stimulation effect of ACTH in normal persons. For a more detailed discussion of the diagnostic procedure and clinical implications, see Chapter 6: Diagnostic Procedures.

Dexamethasone Suppression Test (DST)

> **Normal Values**   Suppression of plasma cortisol to <5 µg/dL (SI = <138 nmol/L) in any sample after the first baseline or <0.5 µg/dL of baseline.

> **Description**   The DST identifies depressed persons who are likely to respond to antidepressants or electroconvulsive therapy (ECT). For a more detailed discussion of the procedure and clinical implications, see Chapter 6: Diagnostic Procedures.

Hemoglobin A_1C (HgbA$_1$C)

> **Normal Values**   4%–8% of total hemoglobin SI = 0.04–0.08 fraction of total Hgb

> **Description**   Glycosylated hemoglobin measures the blood glucose bound to hemoglobin. The more glucose the RBC is exposed to, the higher the percentage of glycosylated hemoglobin.
>
> Hemoglobin A_1 undergoes glycosylation by a slow non-enzymatic process within the RBC; has a life span of 120 days; and is dependent upon available glucose. The measure of hemoglobin A_1C reflects the average blood sugar level 2 to 3 months before the test and allows for assessment of blood glucose control during that time. An elevated hemoglobin A_1C indicates that glucose was not under good control over the 2 to 3 months before the time the level was obtained.

> **Clinical Implications**
> - A diabetic patient who has only recently come under good control may still have a high HbgA$_1$C.
> - Values vary with laboratory; therefore, assessments should be based on a single laboratory consistently performing the test.

HEMATOLOGIC DIAGNOSTIC TESTS
Anemias

Iron (Fe)

> **Normal Values**

Newborn: 100–250 µg/dL	SI = 18–45 µmol/L
Infant: 40–100 µg/dL	SI = 17–18 µmol/L
Child: 50–120 µg/dL	SI = 9–22 µmol/L
Adult male: 50–160 µg/dL	SI = 9–29 µmol/L
Adult female: 40–150 µg/dL	SI = 7–27 µmol/L

Description   Serum iron measures the amount of iron bound to transferrin.

Clinical Implications
- Serum iron is increased in pernicious anemia, aplastic anemia, hemolytic anemia, thalassemia, acute hepatitis, acute porphyria, hemochromatosis, pyridoxine deficiency, excessive iron therapy, repeated transfusions, and nephritis.

- Serum iron is decreased in iron-deficiency anemia, remission of pernicious anemia, cancer, nephrosis, kwashiorkor, some systemic infections, idiopathic pulmonary hemosiderosis, hypothyroidism, paroxysmal nocturnal hemoglobinuria, pregnancy, and rheumatoid arthritis.

- Treatment with ACTH may decrease serum iron.

- Treatment with dextran, chloramphenicol, and oral contraceptives may increase serum iron.

- Iron is a frequent cause of accidental poisonings, especially in children. Toxicity is associated with levels above 500 µg/dL within 6 hours of ingestion.

- Iron levels in many patients with iron-deficiency anemia may remain in the low normal range (false negatives). Diurnal and day-to-day variations of as much as 30% may occur, therefore the serum iron value alone is not useful. Better diagnostic information is obtained when serum iron is evaluated along with total iron binding capacity (TIBC).

Ferritin

Normal Values

Newborn: 25–200 ng/mL	SI = 25–200 µg/L
1 month: 200–600 ng/mL	SI = 200–600 µg/L
2–5 months: 50–200 ng/mL	SI = 50–200 µg/L
6 months–15 yr: 7–140 ng/mL	SI = 7–140 µg/L
Adult male: 15–200 ng/mL	SI = 15–200 µg/L
Adult female: 12–150 ng/mL	SI = 12–150 µg/L

Description   Ferritin is a measure of the body's iron stores and reflects storage of iron in the reticuloendothelial system.

Clinical Implications
- **Increased levels** are seen in hemochromatosis, hemosiderosis, liver diseases, malignancies, hyperthyroidism, non-iron-deficiency anemias, and chronic inflammation.

- **Decreased levels** are found in iron-deficiency anemia.

- Levels return to normal within a few days of the start of iron therapy unless the patient is noncompliant or continuing to lose iron.

Transferrin

Normal Values   200–400 mg/dL SI = 2–4 gm/L

Description   Transferrin is a serum protein (beta-globulin) which is synthesized in the liver and reticuloendothelial system. It functions to bind and transport ferric iron between tissues (primarily liver) and bone marrow where the iron is incorporated into the red blood cells' hemoglobin.

Clinical Implications
- Transferrin is increased in iron-deficiency anemia, estrogen therapy, pregnancy, and hypoxia.

- Transferrin is decreased in nephrotic syndrome, chronic renal failure, gastrointestinal losses, severe burns, chronic infections, malignancies, malnutrition, genetic deficiency (a transferrinemia), kwashiorkor, severe liver diseases, certain inflammatory conditions, and iron overdose.

- Transferrin is usually about 30% saturated with iron. The remaining 70% which is unsaturated reflects the body's total iron-binding capacity (TIBC).

- Transferrin is one of several proteins which may reflect nutritional status. Mild to moderate malnutrition is associated with levels from 100 to 200 mg/dL. With severe malnutrition transferrin levels may be ≤100 mg/dL.

Total Iron Binding Capacity (TIBC)

Normal Values   *Infant:* 100–400 μg/dL   SI = 17.9–71.6 μmol/L

                          Children and Adults: 250–400 μg/dL   SI = 44.8–71.6 μmol/L

Description   TIBC is an indirect measure of serum transferrin. It is determined by adding an excess of iron to plasma to saturate all transferrin with iron. By removing excess iron, the serum iron concentration is determined.

Clinical Implications
- TIBC is increased in iron-deficiency anemia, acute and chronic blood loss, acute liver damage, third trimester of pregnancy, and with estrogen use.

- TIBC is decreased in hemochromatosis, anemias (of chronic diseases and infections), nephrosis, thalassemia, other non-iron-deficiency anemias, and in therapy with chloramphenicol, corticotropin, and corticosteroids.

- TIBC is less sensitive to changes in iron stores than serum ferritin.

Glucose-6-Phosphate Dehydrogenase (G6PD) in Erythrocytes

Normal Values   8.6–18.6 U/gm Hgb SI = 8.6–18.6 U/gm Hgb

Description   G6PD in red blood cells functions to maintain re-duced glutathione in the hexose monophosphate shunt which prevents oxidation of hemoglobin to methemoglobin. Reduced levels of G6PD may cause hemolytic anemia.

Clinical Implications
- G6PD is decreased in about 13% of American black males, American black females (3% with about 20% carriers), and about 50% of Sardinians, Greeks, and Kurdish Jews. Decreased enzyme lev-els are also seen in Chinese.

- Increased G6PD may be seen in pernicious and other megaloblastic anemias, thrombocytopenia purpura, chronic blood loss, hyperthyroidism, and within seven days of a myocardial infarction.

- **Class I deficiency** is the most severe and presents as chronic hemolysis in the absence of oxidative stress.

- **Class II deficiency** has levels of G6PD <10% of normal; however, it is associated with severe episodic hemolysis rather than chronic hemolysis.

- **Class III deficiency** is associated with occasional hemolytic episodes with identifiable precipitating factors.

- **Class IV** is normal.

- Precipitating factors include 4- and 8-aminoquino-line antimalarials, para-amino salicylates, methyl-ene blue, aspirin, quinine, quinidine, large doses of ascorbic acid, nitrofurantoin, some sulfonamides and sulfones, fava beans, infections, and diabetic ketoacidosis.

- The degree of hemolysis is dependent upon the ex-tent of deficiency and the dose of the precipitating agent. Hemolysis generally occurs by the third day of drug exposure.

Coagulation Tests

Activated Partial Thromboplastin Time (aPTT) and Prothrombin Time (PT)

Normal Values   *aPTT:* 20–30 sec

  PT: 11–13 sec

Description   The aPTT is used to detect deficiencies of the com-ponents of the intrinsic thromboplastin system. It is used for monitoring heparin therapy.

Description
(Continued)

The PT is used to directly measure a defect in Stage II of the clotting mechanism and ability of prothrombin, fibrinogen, Factor V, Factor VII, and Factor X. It is used for monitoring warfarin therapy.

Clinical Implications

- **aPTT.** Prolonged in coagulation defects of Stage I von Willebrand's disease, hemophilia, liver disease, or disseminated intravascular coagulopathy (DIC).

- **PT.** Prolonged in prothrombin deficiency, vitamin K^+ deficiency, hemorrhagic disease of the newborn, liver disease, or salicylate intoxication.

- **aPTT** can also be used to determine the presence of circulating anticoagulants (antibodies induced in hemophiliacs by plasma transfusions).

- Heparin is used for the treatment of deep vein thrombosis (DVT) as a primary agent because it works rapidly and prevents fibrin clot formation, inhibits thrombosis formation, and may inhibit extension of existing thrombi.

- Warfarin may prolong the aPTT because of its effects on Factors II, IX, and X. However, this is usually not clinically significant and it is not used to monitor warfarin's efficacy.

- Warfarin acts in the liver to delay coagulation by interfering with the action of Vitamin K^+ dependent Factors (II, VII, IX, X). It is usual to perform a PT test each day when adjusting anticoagulant doses. Warfarin requires 16 to 48 hours to cause the desired change in the PT; although large warfarin doses can have a major impact on PT within hours because of its suppression of Factor VII. Effects on Factors IX, X, and II take 16 to 48 hours and more closely correlate with thrombus formation. For warfarin therapy the goal is usually to adjust the PT to 1.2 to 1.5 times the patient's control value.

- If the PT is >40 sec, it is necessary to evaluate for bleeding including lung auscultation, neurologic exam, and occult blood in urine.

- Green leafy vegetables contain Vitamin K^+ and can antagonize the effect of warfarin.

- Variations exist in reporting methods; check with your lab.

Fibrin Degradation Products (Fibrin Split Products, FDP, FSP)

Normal Values

Serum: <8 µg/mL (1:10 dilution)	SI = <8 mg/L
Urine: <0.25 µg/mL	SI = <0.25 mg/L

Fibrin Degradation Products (Fibrin Split Products, FDP, FSP) **(Continued)**

Description

Formed by the fibrinolytic action of plasmin on the abnormal fibrin deposition in the vasculature.

Clinical Implications

- Serum levels are elevated in 1) venous thrombosis and pulmonary embolus which indicate the clot has begun to dissolve; 2) disseminated intravascular coagulation (DIC); and 3) some snake bites.

- Elevated urine levels suggest renal disease or rejection crisis following renal transplant.

- False elevations are caused by exercise, stress, and traumatic venipuncture.

- Most interferences are caused by streptokinase, urokinase, or elevated rheumatoid factor.

- FDP is one of the most sensitive and specific tests for DIC.

- In DIC, FDPs usually begin to fall within one day. If levels are very high, it may take a week or longer to return to normal.

Thrombin Time (TT)

Normal Values

±3–5 seconds of control value (usual control range is 17.5–23.5 sec). 15–22 seconds (with the reptilase method).

Description

TT tests the fibrinogen to fibrin conversion, a late phase of coagulation. TT is affected by the concentration of fibrinogen and plasmin, and the presence of fibrin degradation products (FDP) and antithrombotic agents.

Clinical Implications

- **TT is elevated** in disseminated intravascular coagulation (DIC) in approximately 60% of cases. It is a less sensitive and specific test for DIC than other tests. TT is also elevated in deficiencies of fibrinogen and in the presence of inhibitors of thrombin or fibrinogen. Unfortunately, it will not differentiate DIC from primary fibrinolysis. It is also elevated with heparin (most methods), urokinase, streptokinase, and asparaginase therapy.

- **TT is not elevated** in the presence of heparin when assayed by the reptilase method. Furthermore, it is not elevated with warfarin, aspirin, dipyridamole, or sulfinpyrazone.

Factor V

Normal Values

50%–100% of control

Description

Factor V is one of the cofactors in the transformation of prothrombin to thrombin.

Factor V **(Continued)**

Clinical Implications
- Defects in Factor V result in increased PT and PTT values, but not bleeding time.

- Factor V is usually decreased in DIC, along with Factors VIII and XIII, but is not usually used for primary diagnosis of DIC due to time and technical difficulties.

- Circulating anticoagulants interfering with Factor V are associated with SLE and streptokinase or uro-kinase administration.

Factor VIII

Normal Values

60%–135% of normal or 60–135

Minimal Hemostatic Level: 15%–20% of normal or 15–20 AU

Minimal Level for Major Surgery: 25% of normal or 25 AU

Description

Factor VIII is one of the cofactors in the activation of Factor X by the intrinsic pathway. Hemophilia A (classic hemophilia) is the hereditary deficiency of Factor VIII. The gene for Factor VIII is located on the X-chromosome. Factor VIII has a serum half-life of 8 to 12 hours.

Clinical Implications
- Factor VIII levels may be decreased in DIC, along with Factors V and XIII. The consumption of these factors is due to the abnormal clot formation in the microvasculature. Factor VIII assays are not usually used for the primary diagnosis of DIC.

- Defects in factor VIII activity will result in increased PTT and coagulation time, but a normal PT and bleeding time.

- Circulating anticoagulants interfering with the Factor VIII activity are associated with the following conditions: systemic lupus erythematosus (SLE), rheumatoid arthritis, drug reaction, postpartum period, advanced age, and following replacement therapy for hereditary deficiency.

- Interferences occur with IV epinephrine, oral contraceptives, asparaginase, dextrothyroxine, vigorous exercise, and during the last trimester of pregnancy.

Antithrombin III (ATIII)

Normal Values

Reference ranges differ for the many methods available. Check with your lab.

Description

ATIII is a naturally occurring thrombin-inhibitor, which also inactivates the activated forms of factors XII, XI, IX, X, and probably VII.

Clinical Implications
- Heparin's anticoagulant activity results from accelerating the inhibitory activity of ATIII. A decrease in ATIII may predispose patients to thrombus formation as well as the failure of heparin anticoagulation.

- **Increased ATIII** may be seen in acute hepatitis, vitamin K^+ deficiency, following renal transplant, inflammation, and during menstruation.

- **Decreased ATIII** may be seen in DIC, congenital deficiency, following liver transplant and partial hepatectomy, cirrhosis, chronic liver failure and other liver diseases, nephrotic syndrome, carcinoma, during the last trimester of pregnancy and the early postpartum period, and mid-period of the menstrual cycle.

- Test interferences include anabolic steroids, warfarin, heparin, asparaginase, estrogens, and oral contraceptives.

- ATIII is 30% lower in serum than in plasma.

- The ATIII level does not influence routine coagulation tests.

IMMUNOLOGIC/RHEUMATOLOGIC DIAGNOSTIC TESTS
Acquired Immunodeficiency (AIDS) Antibody Tests

Description
This series of tests is commonly conducted in a patient possibly infected with the AIDS virus, Human Immunodeficiency Virus (HIV). Most patients with AIDS are anergic with: moderate anemia (Hgb of 7 to 12 gm/dL); moderate thrombocytopenia; moderate leukopenia (1,000 to 3,000/mm^3); and lymphocytes <1200/mm^3.

ELISA (Enzyme-Linked Immunosorbent Assay)

Description
An assay that is used to detect the presence of antibody to the HIV virus.

Clinical Implications
- A confirmed positive antibody test means that the patient is infected or potentially infectious and has a high probability of developing symptomatic illness within 7 years of infection.

- This test may result in false-positive and false-negative test results for HIV.

- The current sensitivity of a licensed ELISA test is 99% or greater. When used in conjunction with an appropriate confirmatory test (i.e., Western Blot), false results are potentially eliminated.

Western Blot

Description

A radioimmunoprecipitation assay is often used as a confirmatory assay to follow up on the results of an ELISA test.

Clinical Implications

In general, the results are similar to those of the ELISA test. Due to the expense associated with this test as compared to the ELISA, it is not used as the initial screening test for HIV but as a confirmatory test for a positive ELISA test.

Lymphocytes

Normal Values

Lymphocytes: $1.2–3.3 \times 10^3/\text{mm}^3$

T4 or CD_4: (helper/inducer lymphocytes) $(400–1185/\text{mm}^3)$

T8 or CD_8: (suppressor) $(180–865/\text{mm}^3)$

Description

Lymphocytes constitute the second most common white cell in circulating blood, though circulating lymphocytes represent <5% of the total lymphocyte pool. There are two major lymphocytes: 1) T-lymphocytes (thymic dependent), cell-mediated immune response and 2) B-lymphocytes (bone marrow derived), humoral antibody response.

Clinical Implications

- As the T_4 lymphocytes decrease, the patient has a greater chance of developing an opportunistic infection. Patients with HIV infections show increased T_8 and decreased T_4 levels. The T_4/T_8 ratio is less than 1.2 and often close to zero.

- It appears if the T_4 lymphocytes count is ≥ 400 cells/mm^3 (or $\geq 20\%$), an HIV positive person is less likely to develop AIDS. Whereas a T_4 <200 cells/mm^3 (or <10% total lymphocytes) may mean the person is at risk for developing an opportunistic infection such as *Pneumocystis carinii* (PCP) or *Mycobacterium avium-intracellular* (MAI).

- Prospective studies of HIV-infected patients have indicated that T_4 lymphocyte counts and T_4/T_8 ratio decline as a function of time.

Erythrocyte Sedimentation Rate (ESR, Sed Rate)

Normal Values

See Table 5–7.

Description

A nonspecific test that may be useful for monitoring infections and inflammatory diseases.

Clinical Implications

- **Increased ESR** is seen in conditions that have increased plasma fibrinogen, globulin or cholesterol, infections (e.g., tuberculosis), inflammatory diseases (e.g., rheumatoid arthritis), and tissue destruction (e.g., acute MI, neoplasms).

TABLE 5–7: Normal Values: Erythrocyte Sedimentation Rate (ESR)

Westergren Method

Child	0–10 mm/hr
Male (<50 yr)	0–15 mm/hr
Female(<50 yr)	0–20 mm/hr
Male(>50 yr)	0–20 mm/hr
Female (>50 yr)	0–30 mm/hr

Wintrobe Method

Male	0–15 mm/hr
Female	0–25 mm/hr

Erythrocyte Sedimentation Rate (ESR, Sed Rate) (Continued)

Clinical Implications (Continued)

- **Decreased ESR** may be seen in polycythemia vera, sickle cell anemia, hereditary spherocytosis, DIC, cachexia, hepatic necrosis, and excessive anticoagulation.

- ESR is useful for following certain diseases (e.g., myocardial infarction, rheumatic fever, rheumatoid arthritis, tuberculosis).

- The Westergren method is more accurate and preferred, but it is more time consuming to perform.

Beta$_2$-Microglobulin (B$_2$M)

Normal Values

Serum: 18–39 yr: 1.1–2 mg/   SI = 93.2–169.5 nmol/L

40–59 yr: 1.2–2.6 mg/L SI = 101.7–220.4 nmol/L

60–79 yr: 1–3 mg/L   SI = 84.8–254.3 nmol/L

Urine: <120 μg/24 hr   SI = <101.7 nmol/day

Description

B$_2$M is a cell membrane associated 100 amino acid protein that is increased during inflammatory reactions and in active chronic lymphocytic leukemia. This protein is readily filtered by the glomerular basement membrane and almost completely reabsorbed by the proximal renal tubular. Serum B$_2$M values depend upon glomerular filtration rate (GFR), whereas urinary B$_2$M values vary with the functional activity of proximal renal tubular cells. Therefore, in glomerular disease, B$_2$M is increased in the serum and decreased in the urine. In tubular dysfunction, the opposite is true. It is useful for evaluating kidney allograft rejection in transplant patients and will often change in advance of serum creatinine values.

Beta$_2$-Microglobulin (B$_2$M) **(Continued)**

Clinical Implications
- Serum B$_2$M monitoring may allow diagnosis of kidney rejection before changes in serum creatinine are seen, allowing for faster treatment.

- During the treatment of acute rejection, serum B$_2$M often drops faster than serum creatinine and may allow reducing corticosteroid doses faster than if creatinine values were used as the only index of rejection.

- Serum B$_2$M values may increase in HIV positive patients. This may be a sign of disease progression.

Alpha-Fetoprotein (AFP, α_1 Fetoglobulin)

Normal Values
Adult: <8.5 ng/mL   SI < 8.5 µg/L

Fetal: peak at 200–400 mg/dL or 2–4 gm/L in first trimester, is normally absent the first weeks after birth

Description
A protein synthesized in the liver (with a t $^1/2$ of 3.5 days) that is primarily used as a tumor marker. Some fetal AFP enters the maternal circulation.

Clinical Implications
- **AFP is mildly elevated or normal** in alcoholic liver disease, cirrhosis, viral and chronic active hepatitis, ataxia-telangiectasia, tyrosinemia, and inflammatory bowel diseases.

- **AFP is normal** in seminoma of testes, choriocarcinoma, adenocarcinoma and dermoid cyst of the ovary.

- **AFP is elevated** in:

  ° Hepatoma (50% to 100% of cases) levels may reach >1000–3000 ng/mL.

  ° Hepatic metastases from carcinoma of stomach, pancreas, colon, or lung (usually <1000 ng/mL).

  ° Embryonal carcinoma (27% to 90% of cases) or malignant teratoma (60% to 90% of cases) of ovary and testes.

  ° Neonatal hepatitis.

  ° Pregnancy (in serum and amniotic fluid) in cases of multiple pregnancy, intrauterine death, many congenital malformaties, and spontaneous abortion.

- Failure of markers to decrease after surgery suggests metastatic disease and the need for chemotherapy.

- AFP should decrease with intensive chemotherapy, although remains elevated. The rise of previously declined marker levels suggests recurrent tumor.

- AFP is recommended for any pregnant woman on valproic acid (in addition to amniocentesis).

MICROBIOLOGIC DIAGNOSTIC TESTS
Minimum Bactericidal Concentration (MBC) and Minimum Inhibitory Concentration (MIC)

Description

Varying concentrations of an antimicrobial are prepared in liquid growth medium or on solid medium. A standard number of organisms are added to each test tube or agar plate and incubated. After the appropriate incubation period, the test tubes or agar plates are examined for growth. The tube or plate that contains the lowest concentration of antibiotic that prevents visible growth is considered the MIC. The tubes that demonstrate no growth are then placed onto an antibiotic free agar and incubated for 24 hours. The MBC is the lowest concentration of drug that results in a 99.9% reduction in the initial bacterial count.

The MIC is a quantitative measure of a particular drug's activity against identified bacteria. This allows the comparison of antibiotics in order to choose the antibiotic with the lowest MICs for likely eradication of an infection by use of usual doses of an antimicrobial agent. The MBC can determine if the antibiotic will kill the organism (i.e., bactericidal).

Clinical Implications

- Although useful in selecting the antimicrobial agent, MICs are not reliable predictors of success or failure of drug therapy.

- Susceptible organisms are those with the lowest MICs that will be effectively treated by the antimicrobial.

- Moderately susceptible organisms are those less likely to be effectively treated and should therefore be treated with maximum doses of the antimicrobial.

- Resistant organisms are those with high MICs to the tested antimicrobial suggesting probable failure of treatment.

Gram's Stain

See Chapter 6: Diagnostic Procedures.

Schlicter's Test [Serum Bactericidal Titer (SBT)]

Desired Value

Bactericidal activity at >1:8 dilution

Description

This test is used to determine the maximum dilution of the serum or body fluid which is bactericidal for the patient's infecting organism. Other terms include cidal titer ratio and serum cidal test. It is frequently used in evaluating endocarditis and osteomyelitis therapy .

Schlicter's Test [Serum Bactericidal Titer (SBT)] *(Continued)*

Clinical Implications

- When a Schlicter's test is requested, information on current antibiotics (including date/time of last dose, route of administration, patient's clinical diagnosis, and the specimen collected) is necessary. A serum inhibitory titer might suggest an adequate therapeutic level, but yields no clue about the potential drug toxicity. The results will reflect combined in *vitro* effect of all antimicrobial agents present in a patient's serum or body fluid.

- Paired pre- (15 minutes before dose) and postdose (30 to 45 minutes after dose) specimens are preferred.

Hepatitis Panel

Normal Values

Negative.

Description

There are at least four different types of viral hepatitis. These forms are clinically similar but differ with respect to immunology, epidemiology, prognosis, and prophylaxis. The specific types of viral hepatitis are: 1) Hepatitis A: infectious hepatitis; 2) Hepatitis B: serum or transfusion hepatitis; 3) Hepatitis D: always associated with Hepatitis B; and 4) Hepatitis C (formerly nonA/nonB): viral hepatitis caused by Hepatitis C.

Patients at risk for hepatitis infection include: renal dialysis patients, hematology/oncology patients, hemophiliacs, IV drug abusers, and homosexuals.

Serological Markers

- Hepatitis A

  ○ The HAV-Ab/IgM is detected 4 to 6 weeks after the infection. It indicates acute stage Hepatitis A. It becomes negative 4 months after exposure.

  ○ The HAV-Ab/IgG is detected 8 to 12 weeks after infection. The presence indicates previous exposure/immunity to Hepatitis A.

- Hepatitis B

  ○ HBs-Ag Hepatitis B surface antigen occurs 4 to 12 weeks after infection. A positive result indicates acute stage Hepatitis B (acute and chronic infection).

  ○ HBe-Ag is present 4 to 12 weeks after infection. The presence indicates acute active stage (highly infectious); while the presence of the "e" antigen beyond 10 weeks is indicative of progression to a chronic carrier state.

Hepatitis Panel *(Continued)*

Serological Markers
(Continued)

- HBc-AB Hepatitis B core antibody occurs 6 to 14 weeks after infection. Its presence indicates past infection: it is a lifelong marker.

- HBe-AB antibody is present 8 to 16 weeks after infection. Its presence indicates resolution of acute infection.

- HBs-Ab Antibody. A positive result occurs 2 to 10 months after infection. It indicates previous exposure/ immunity to Hepatitis B, but not necessarily to other types. It is also an indicator of clinical recovery.

Infectious Mononucleosis (IM) Monospot

Normal Values   Negative.

Description   The IM monospot is a serologic test used for the diagnosis of infectious mononucleosis.

Clinical Implications

- A negative test indicates the absence of significant infectious mononucleosis specific heterophile antibodies. False negatives occur ≤2% of the time.

- A positive test correlates with a heterophile titer of ≥1:28. False positives occur 3% to 6% of the time and may be associated with hepatitis A or B, leukemia, lymphoma, or pancreatic carcinoma.

- Acute and convalescent (2 to 3 weeks after onset) titers should be obtained. A fourfold increase in titers from acute to convalescent titers is considered diagnostic.

- The highest incidence of infectious mononucleosis occurs in whites aged 15 to 24. Clinical infectious mononucleosis is associated with exposure to Epstein Barr Virus (EBV) in the teenage years. The incidence in whites is 30 times higher than in blacks, presumably because many blacks are exposed to EBV in early childhood.

Venereal Disease Research Laboratory (VDRL)

Normal Values   Negative.

Description   VDRL is a slide flocculation test used in the diagnosis and staging of syphilis.

Clinical Implications

- The test does not become positive until 4 to 6 weeks after infection (1 to 3 weeks after the development of chancres). Positive tests should be confirmed with fluorescent treponemal antibody absorbed (FTA-ABS) testing.

Venereal Disease Research Laboratory (VDRL) *(Continued)*

Clinical Implications
(Continued)

- False positives may occur in pregnancy, drug addiction, infectious mononucleosis, leprosy, malaria, and collagen diseases such as rheumatoid arthritis and systemic lupus erythematosus.

- Up to 25% of patients may be nonreactive in early primary, late latent, and late syphilis. It is negative in more than 25% of patients with syphilitic aortitis.

- Titers may be helpful in following disease. A decrease in titer may indicate response to treatment.

- Titers fall over 6 to 12 months with treatment of primary syphilis. Titers fall over 12 to 18 months with treatment of secondary syphilis. Some may remain positive for several years. Late latent or tertiary syphilis have titers which may gradually decrease only over years. Increased titers indicate relapse or reinfection.

- Titers >1:16 are high and usually indicate active disease. Titers ≤1:8 are usually false positives or occasionally, active disease.

- See Table 5–8.

- Some with primary or secondary syphilis may actually have high titers but undiluted serum is nonreactive. Diluted serum will be positive in these patients.

- Serial, quantitative VDRLs are helpful in the diagnosis and assessment of response of congenital syphilis.

- CSF samples tested for VDRL are used to determine the presence of neurosyphilis. These should always be quantified. Reactive or weakly reactive VDRLs almost always indicate active infection.

TABLE 5–8: Normal Values: Venereal Disease Research Lab

	% of Serum with + VDRL	Titers
Primary syphilis	76	<1:32
Secondary syphilis	100	>1:32
Early latent	95	Variable
Late latent	72	Variable
Late	70	Variable

NUTRITIONAL DIAGNOSTIC TESTS

Albumin

Normal Values`   *0–1 yr:* 3–5 gm/dL   SI = 30–50 gm/L
                     ≥1 yr: 3.5–5 gm/dL   SI = 35–50 gm/L

Description   Albumin is formed in the liver and helps maintain normal water distribution (colloidal osmotic pressure). It aids in the transport of blood constituents (e.g., ions, bilirubin, hormones, enzymes, and drugs).

Clinical Implications
- **Increased albumin levels** are generally not observed.

- **Decreased albumin levels** are associated with inadequate iron intake, severe liver disease, malabsorption, severe burns, excessive intravenous administration of glucose, valproic acid therapy, nephrotic syndrome, diabetes, and SLE.

- Albumin + Immunoglobins = Total Serum Protein (TSP)

- Decreased serum albumin may result in an increase in free drug (and increased effect) for those agents which are highly protein bound (i.e., phenytoin, aspirin, valproate).

Zinc, Serum

Normal Values   70–150 µg/dL SI = 10.7–22.9 µmol/L

Description   Approximately 80% of the total zinc in whole blood is in the erythrocytes. Zinc is a cofactor of many enzymes (e.g., alkaline phosphatase, lactic dehydrogenase).

Clinical Implications
- Decreased levels of zinc usually occur because of abnormal losses such as in Crohn's disease, pregnancy, fistulas, and malabsorption. Primary losses are in pancreatic and intestinal secretions. Decreased levels may be seen in alcoholics, fasting obese patients, renal disease, diabetics, liver disease, porphyria, proteinuria, trauma, sickle cell disease, infection, hypoalbuminemia, stress, prolonged parenteral nutrition, and corticosteroid treatment.

- Increased levels of zinc are rare but may be seen with tissue injury, hemolysis, and contaminated collection tubes.

- Signs of deficiency include dermatitis, hair loss, diarrhea, depression, and hypogeusia.

- Serum concentrations undergo circadian variations with peaks at about 9 a.m. and again at about 6 p.m.

- Serum concentrations of zinc may be 16% higher than plasma because of platelet destruction during clotting.

BODY FLUID ANALYSIS
Cerebrospinal Fluid (CSF) Examination

Normal Values	*Glucose:* 40–80 mg/dL SI = 2.22–4.44 mmol/L
	Appearance: clear, colorless, no clot
	Opening pressure: 70–180 mm water
	Protein:
	Ventricular: 5–15 mg/dL SI = 0.05–0.15 gm/L
	Cisternal: 10–25 mg/dL SI = 0.1–0.25 gm/L
	Lumbar: 15–45 mg/dL SI = 0.15–0.45 gm/L
	WBC: 0–10 mm^3

Description

Collection of CSF may be obtained via lumbar, cisternal, or ventricular puncture. The gross appearance as well as laboratory analysis of the fluid is important for differential diagnosis.

Clinical Implications

- The appearance may be purulent, opalescent, or turbid in cases of meningitis. Bloody CSF may be seen in cases of subarachnoid hemorrhage, traumatic tap, head trauma, and subdural hematoma.

- Opening pressure may be increased in cases of meningitis, encephalitis, brain tumor, head trauma, subarachnoid hemorrhage, and uremia.

- Protein may be increased in meningitis, encephalitis, tumor (brain and spinal cord), or a traumatic tap.

- Fasting glucose is usually normal in CSF. It may be increased in diabetic coma and sometimes in uremia.

- WBC may be increased in meningitis, encephalitis, and tumor (brain and spinal cord). WBC will be the same as that in the blood of patients with bloody CSF taps.

Glucose (in CSF)

Normal Values

40–80 mg/dL SI = 2.22–4.44 mmol/L

Description

The measurement of CSF glucose is helpful in determining impaired transport of glucose from plasma to CSF and increased use by CNS, leukocytes and microorganisms. CSF glucose varies with blood glucose levels and is usually 40% to 80% of blood glucose value.

Clinical Implications

- **Decreased glucose levels** are associated with infection, tuberculosis, and the spread of lymphomas or leukemias into the meninges. All types of organisms consume glucose and decreased glucose reflects bacterial activity.

- **Increased glucose levels** associated with diabetes.

- Glucose levels are usually in the normal range with aseptic meningitis.

REFERENCES

For a more detailed discussion on laboratory tests, see the following references.

1. Condon RE. Manual of Surgical Therapeutics, 7th ed. Boston: Little Brown & Co.; 1988.

2. Fischback F. A Manual of Laboratory Diagnostic Tests, 4th ed. Philadelphia: J.B. Lippincott Co.; 1992.

3. Henry JB. Clinical Diagnosis and Management by Laboratory Methods, 18th ed. Philadelphia: W.B. Saunders Co.; 1991.

4. Macklis RM. Manual of Introductory Clinical Medicine, 2nd ed. Boston: Little Brown & Co.; 1988.

5. Sacher RH, McPherson RA. Widmann's Clinical Interpretation of Laboratory Tests, 10th ed. Philadelphia: F.A. Davis Co.; 1991.

6. Scully RE et al. Normal Reference Laboratory Values. N Engl J Med. 1992; 327(10):718–24.

7. Tietz NW. Clinical Guide to Laboratory Tests, 2nd ed. Philadelphia: W.B. Saunders Co.; 1990.

8. Tietz NW (ed). Fundamentals of Clinical Chemistry, 3rd ed. Philadelphia: W.B. Saunders Co.; 1987.

9. Tilkian SM. Clinical Implications of Laboratory Tests, 4th ed. St. Louis: C.V. Mosby Co.; 1992.

10. Wallach J. Interpretation of Diagnostic Tests, 5th ed. Boston: Little Brown & Co.; 1986.

11. Young DS. Implementation of SI Units for Clinical Laboratory Data. Ann Intern Med. 1987;106:114–129.

ACKNOWLEDGMENTS

The authors acknowledge Roderick C. Jorgenson, Lisa K. McDonald, Susan J. McVey, Debra A. Pluemer, and William D. Simmons for their helpful comments.

Diagnostic Procedures

Robert M. Breslow

Diagnostic procedures are an integral part of the clinical approach to patient care. The physical examination and patient history, clinical laboratory, and diagnostic procedures are key elements in confirming or making a diagnosis. All of these diagnostic building blocks potentially influence a patient's pharmaceutical care. For example, if a patient is admitted to the hospital after experiencing abdominal pain with coffee ground emesis and the clinical laboratory demonstrates a decreased hematocrit and hemoglobin with guaiac positive stools, there is a high suspicion of an upper gastrointestinal bleed. As confirmation, an endoscopic procedure would assist in determining this diagnosis and ultimately influencing the choice and duration of drug therapy. Further diagnostic procedures can guide the establishment of parameters to assess therapeutic outcomes.

This chapter provides a general overview of diagnostic procedures and the role of these diagnostic procedures in patient care, the pharmacotherapy treatment plan, and patient outcome. It is organized by organ systems, rather than diagnostic procedure classes. This format allows you to more quickly identify pertinent diagnostic procedures that apply to specific experiential settings. Each diagnostic procedure monograph consists of a description of the procedure, the procedure's intended purpose, normal and abnormal findings, and the procedure's pharmacy implications. These implications may be drug related or may prompt the monitoring of specific laboratory tests that may affect, or be affected by, the performance or outcome of a particular diagnostic procedure.

GENERAL PROCEDURES

Biopsy[1,2]

Description

A biopsy is performed, depending on the tissue to be biopsied, by means of an aspiration or cutting needle, fine-needle, scalpel, or punch. Biopsies may be closed (i.e., not requiring a surgical incision) or open (i.e., requiring a surgical incision). Common biopsy sites include the bone marrow, breast, bone, cervix, liver, lung, lymph node, muscle, myocardium, nerve, pleura, prostate, renal, skin, small bowel, and thyroid. Anesthetic, either local or general, is administered before the procedure.

Purpose

To gather a small piece of tissue for microscopic analysis (either histologic or cytologic).

Findings

Normal and abnormal findings are dependent upon the histology or cytology of the specific tissue being biopsied.

Pharmacy Implications

- Patients may require sedation with a parenteral benzodiazepine such as midazolam or diazepam. Patients should be monitored for over-sedation and/or respiratory depression.

- A local anesthetic such as lidocaine or bupivacaine may be necessary. Be sure to check for a potential history of allergic reactions.

- Patients may require general anesthesia. An anticholinergic such as parenteral atropine or glycopyrrolate, a sedative such as diazepam or midazolam, and an analgesic such as morphine or meperidine may be required as premedication administered 15 to 30 minutes before anesthesia.

- It is recommended that antiplatelet agents be stopped before open and needle biopsies. Stop aspirin 7 to 10 days before the procedure. NSAIDs which reversibly inhibit the enzyme cyclooxygenase (e.g., ibuprofen, naproxen) require discontinuation 2 to 4 days before the procedure.

Computed Tomography(CT)[3-6]

Description

Computed tomography (CT) [also is known as computed axial tomography (CAT)] scanning, is a painless, noninvasive method for obtaining a three dimensional picture of body structures using cross sectional (transverse) slice x-rays. A complete scan consists of many pictures.

In a CT scan, an x-ray source or beam, together with a gamma ray detector, rotates around the patient in a 360° arc. The x-ray beam is very narrow, allowing little internal scatter of radiation. The detector simultaneously measures the intensity of radiation. A computer calculates the amount of radiation absorbed by each volume of tissue and assigns a Gray scale number to it. The computer analyzes the numbers and reconstructs a cross-sectional picture which can be displayed on a screen or produced as a hardcopy for a permanent record and later interpretation.

Contrast media may be injected intravenously to enhance the images of brain, abdominal structures, and vasculature. Oral contrast media (diatrizoate) as a 2% solution (4 mL/200 mL H_2O) is administered before abdominal CT scans to provide contrast enhancement of certain abdominal structures.

Purpose

CT scans can confirm the diagnosis of suspected malignancies, assist in determining the staging and extent of neoplastic disease, and determine the effectiveness of therapy. CT scans of the brain and skull (cranial CT) may be performed to define the nature of head trauma, hydrocephalus, increased intracra-

Computed Tomography(CT)[3-6] *(Continued)*

Purpose (Continued)

nial pressure, cerebrovascular lesions, degenerative brain diseases, and infections. CT scans of the body (body CT) which examine the neck, thorax, abdomen, and extremities may provide information on the cause of jaundice, inflammatory processes, pleural or chest wall abnormalities, and suspected abnormal collections of blood or fluid. A spinal CT is performed to evaluate disorders of the spine and spinal cord.

Findings

Normal and abnormal findings are dependent upon the organs being evaluated.

Pharmacy Implications

- As patients must lie completely still for an extended period of time, uncooperative patients are sedated with benzodiazepines (e.g., midazolam, diazepam, or lorazepam) or a sedative such as chloral hydrate. Typical dose of these agents are:

  ° *Midazolam.* Children: 0.05 to 0.1 mg/kg IV or 0.1 mg/kg IM. Adults: 0.1 to 0.2 mg/kg IV.

  ° *Diazepam.* Adults: 0.1 to 0.3 mg/kg IV.

  ° *Lorazepam.* Adults: 0.04 mg/kg IV or 0.5 mg/kg IM up to 4 mg.

  ° *Chloral Hydrate.* Children: 50 to 70 mg/kg up to 2.5 gm.

- Intravenous iodine contrast media should be used cautiously in patients with known or suspected hypersensitivity to iodine. Ionized contrast media are more likely to produce hypersensitivity reactions. Non-ionized products rarely produce reactions and are, therefore, used in patients with previously documented histories of iodine hypersensitivity.

Gallium Scan[4,6,7]

Description

Radioactive gallium citrate (Ga^{67}) is administered intravenously 24 to 48 hours before the scan. The Gallium scan is performed over the entire body by the use of a gamma scintillation camera or a rectilinear scanner. The scanning device measures the radiation emissions of Ga^{67} and shows the distribution or uptake patterns of Ga^{67} throughout the body. The degree of radioactivity Ga^{67} possesses is minimal and not harmful. A complete scan takes approximately 30 to 60 minutes.

Purpose

Gallium scans are used to detect or evaluate primary or metastatic neoplasms; inflammatory lesions of bacterial, autoimmune, or other origin; malignant lymphoma or recurrent tumors following chemotherapy or radiation therapy; and bronchogenic carcinoma. In addition, these scans aid in the diagnosis of focal defects in the liver.

Gallium Scan[4,6,7] *(Continued)*

Findings

Normal	Ga^{67} uptake is seen in the liver, spleen, bones, and large bowel.
Abnormal	Ga^{67} uptake is seen in abscesses, inflamed tissues, and some tumors.

Pharmacy Implications Ga^{67} is excreted into the feces. This could interfere with the detection of inflammatory or neoplastic diseases of the colon. Therefore, a cleansing enema should be administered before the scan. Patients do not need to restrict food or fluid intake before the scan.

Magnetic Resonance Imaging (MRI)[4,8,9]

Description   The patient is placed inside a large circular magnet. The magnetic field causes the protons inside the body's atoms to spin in the same direction. A radio frequency signal is then beamed into the magnetic field which causes the protons to move out of alignment. When the radio signal is terminated, the protons move back into the position produced by the magnetic field, releasing energy as this occurs. A receiver coil measures the energy released and the time it takes for the protons to return to the aligned position. This provides information about the type and condition of the tissue from which the energy emanates. A computer then processes all the information and constructs a 2- or 3-dimensional picture of the tissues examined which appears on a television screen. A permanent copy of this image is produced on film or magnetic tape.

MRI combines the advantage of anatomic imaging with excellent soft tissue characterization. It does not use ionizing radiation and does not require a contrast agent to identify vascular structures. However, a specialized contrast agent, gadolinium, is now being used in certain circumstances to enhance images through impaired contrast.

Purpose   MRI is especially useful for diagnosis of brain and nervous system disorders, cardiovascular disease, and cancer. MRI provides very precise and detailed images of internal organs.

Findings   Normal and abnormal findings are dependent upon the anatomy being evaluated.

Pharmacy Implications   • Successful imaging requires patients to lie very still. Uncooperative patients and children should be sedated. (See CT Scan recommendations on page 6–3.) No contrast media is required.

Magnetic Resonance Imaging (MRI)[4,8,9] *(Continued)*

Pharmacy Implications
(Continued)

• MRI is contraindicated in patients with cardiac pace-makers, metal hardware of any kind inserted surgically, and recently inserted prostheses.

Ultrasonography[4,10]

Description

Ultrasound is a noninvasive, non toxic (without dyes) diagnostic procedure that examines internal structures utilizing high frequency sound waves. As sound travels through the body tissues, it is modified (weakened as it goes through tissues) and travels at different speeds depending upon the density and elasticity of the tissues. This is referred to as the acoustic impedance of the tissue.

In ultrasonography, a probe produces short pulses of sound. When the sound wave produced by the probe encounters an interface (the border between two adjacent structures) some of the waves are reflected (echoed) back to a transducer and an electric current is produced. The current is amplified and the resultant image is displayed on a cathode ray tube (CRT).

Ultrasound produces a good image when there are small differences in tissue density of the adjacent structures. However, when there are large differences, as between bone and soft tissue or air-filled spaces and soft tissue, the image is unintelligible because most of the sound waves are reflected back.

Although ultrasound cannot be used to evaluate bone or air-filled spaces, ultrasound can measure sound frequency shifts due to motion. Consequently, ultrasound can be used to evaluate blood flow, free fluid, and amniotic fluid.

Purpose

• Ultrasound is used to

  ° *Examine* internal soft tissue organs and structures including the eye, thyroid, breast, heart, liver, spleen, gallbladder, bile ducts, pancreas, uterus, ovary, bladder, and kidneys.

  ° *Detect and Evaluate* masses, abscesses, stones, motion, fluid, and other reasons for obstruction.

  ° *Determine* size, shape, and position of the organ under study.

  ° *Differentiate* solid, cystic, and complex masses.

Several enhancement techniques are now used to provide better contrast and visualization of various body structures and to provide more recognizable images with greater detail.

Ultrasonography[4,10] *(Continued)*

Findings

Normal
Absence of masses, obstructions, and abscesses. Normal shape, size, and position of organs.

Abnormal
Presence of masses, obstructions, or abscesses. Abnormal size, shape, or location of organs.

Pharmacy Implications
None.

ALLERGY/IMMUNOLOGY

Candida, Histoplasmin, and Mumps Skin Test[4,11,12]

Description
Skin testing is a method of detecting an individual's sensitivity to certain allergens or microorganisms responsible for disease. Skin testing may also be used to assess the integrity of a person's cell-mediated immune system. Three types of skin tests are generally used: scratch, patch, and intradermal tests. Reaction to a skin test demonstrates a hypersensitivity to the tested antigen. This indicates immunity to a disease or product or can indicate the presence of the active or inactive disease being studied.

An antigen is made from serum in which the organism responsible for the respective infection is present. The antigen is injected (0.1 mL) intradermally as a bleb on the volar surface of the forearm by use of a tuberculin syringe and a small (25- or 27-gauge) needle. All tests are read at 24 to 48 hours.

Purpose
Although each test can be used by itself to determine whether the patient under study has had the respective infection, the primary purpose of these recall antigens (those to which a patient has had, or may have had, previous exposure or sensitization) is to evaluate the competence of the cell-mediated immune system. These antigens are common and will usually provoke an immune response in patients with a competent cell-mediated immune system. These skin tests are referred to as "controls" because they are used to determine whether a negative response to a skin test (e.g., tuberculin) is the result of negative exposure to the antigen or to incompetent cell-mediated immunity.

Findings

Normal
A positive reaction indicates previous exposure and resistance to the respective antigen. A positive test is observed when an induration larger than 10 mm in diameter appears after injection of the respective antigen.

Candida, Histoplasmin, and Mumps Skin Test[4,11,12] *(Continued)*

Findings (Continued)

Abnormal   A negative reaction indicates that the patient has not been previously exposed to the respective antigen or is suggestive (more likely) of a compromised immune system (anergy). No erythema and a lesion <10 mm in diameter indicates a negative test.

Pharmacy Implications   Skin tests are refrigerated before use. Concurrent or recent use of corticosteroids can produce a false negative result due to suppression of the cell-mediated (delayed hypersensitivity) immune response. Antihistamines and H_2-blockers interfere with the cutaneous histamine response of the IgE-mediated immediate hypersensitivity reaction and can produce false negative results.

Tuberculin Skin Test (PPD)[4,11]

Description   Tuberculin is a protein fraction (purified protein derivative) of the soluble growth product of *Mycobacterium tuberculosis* or *Mycobacterium bovis*. The antigen is administered intradermally (0.1 mL) creating a bleb at the intradermal injection site (usually the volar or dorsal aspect of the forearm). The antigen is available in three concentrations described as tuberculin units (TU); 1 TU, 5 TU, and 250 TU. The test is evaluated within 48 to 72 hours.

Purpose   The tuberculin antigen is administered to determine if the patient has active or dormant tuberculosis. The skin test cannot distinguish between active or dormant infections.

Findings

Normal   Absence of redness or induration. Referred to as a negative skin test.

Abnormal   Induration of the skin, erythema, edema, and central necrosis. The larger the wheal diameter in millimeters around the injection site, the more positive is the result (negative <5 mm, doubtful or probable 5 to 10 mm, positive >10 mm). A positive skin test indicates prior exposure to the tubercle bacilli (TB) or previous BCG vaccination.

Pharmacy Implications   PPD is refrigerated and must be drawn up just before use. The 5-TU concentration is used most frequently; however, the 1-TU concentration is sometimes used as initial screening in patients with suspected TB to lessen the severity of the reaction. The 250-TU concentration, while rarely used, can be employed when TB is suspected and a state of anergy may be present.

Tuberculin Skin Test (PPD)[4,11] *(Continued)*

Pharmacy Implications
(Continued)

Concurrent or recent use of corticosteroids can produce false negative results due to suppression of the cell mediated (delayed hypersensitivity) immune system. Antihistamines and H_2-blockers interfere with the cutaneous histamine response of the IgE-mediated immediate hypersensitivity reaction and can produce false negative results. Lymphoid disease can produce a false positive result. Viral and certain bacterial infections can cause false negative results due to suppression of the delayed hypersensitivity reaction. Prior administration of BCG vaccine can also result in a false positive reaction.

CARDIOLOGY

Echocardiography[4,10,13,14]

Description

A transducer, placed on the chest where there is no bone or lung tissue, directs high frequency sound waves to the heart which reflects these waves (echoes) back to a transducer. These sound waves are then converted to electrical impulses and relayed to an echocardiography machine which creates a diagram on an oscilloscope.

Purpose

- Echocardiography is used to:

  ° *Diagnose or Rule Out* valvular abnormalities or pericardial effusion

  ° *Measure* the size of heart chambers

  ° *Evaluate* chambers and valves of the heart

  ° *Detect* atrial tumors and cardiac thrombi, and

  ° *Evaluate* cardiac function or wall motion after a myocardial infarction (MI).

Findings

Abnormal

Abnormal motion, pattern, and structure of the four cardiac valves, left ventricular dysfunction, valve abnormalities, wall thickening, tumors or thrombi in the heart, abnormal size of the heart or chamber size, or pericardial effusion.

Pharmacy Implications

None.

Electrocardiography (ECG)[4,11,15]

Description

ECG is a graphic recording of the electrical impulses of the heart that tracks the cardiac cycle from depolarization through repolarization. The electrical current generated by myocardial depolarization is natu-

Electrocardiography (ECG)[4,11,15] *(Continued)*

Description
(Continued)
rally conducted to the surface of the body where it is detected by electrodes placed on the patient's limbs and chest. The waves produced by this electrical activity are amplified for greater visibility before being printed on a moving graph paper strip. In order to capture the multidirectional electrical activity, 12 ECG leads are used simultaneously to achieve a comprehensive view of the electrical activity of the heart. Leads I, II, III, AVF, AVL, and AVR are attached to the limbs and provide an electrical view of the frontal plane of the heart; leads V1, V2, V3, V4, V5, and V6 are attached to the chest and produce a horizontal view of the heart's electrical activity. The tracing produced by the ECG shows the voltage of the waves, the time duration of waves, and the interval between them.

Purpose
ECG is used in the diagnosis of coronary artery disease, myocardial infarction (MI), pericardial effusion, pericarditis, rhythm disturbances as a result of ischemia or electrolyte abnormalities, and disorders of impulse formation and conduction. It is also helpful for evaluation of the effect of drugs on the heart.

Findings

Normal
See Table 6–1.

Abnormal
Abnormal heart rate, rhythm, axis or position of the heart; myocardial hypertrophy; or myocardial infarction. Conclusions can be reached about heart function after comparing the waves and intervals of the particular tracing against a normal tracing. However, this information cannot be used to depict the actual mechanical state of the heart or integrity of heart valves.

Pharmacy Implications
Cardioactive drugs (e.g., digoxin, quinidine, beta blockers) have various specific effects on the ECG tracing.

Electrophysiology Study (EPS)[11,13,16]

Description
Solid electrode catheters are most commonly inserted into the venous system and advanced into the right atrium, across the septal leaflet of the tricuspid valve and into the right ventricle in a fashion similar to cardiac catheterization. Discrete conduction intervals are measured by recording electrical conduction during the slow withdrawal of a bipolar or tripolar electrode catheter from the right ventricle through the HIS bundle to the sinoatrial (SA) node. As part of the study, ECG leads are attached to the patient's chest. After base line values have been determined, pacing (electrical stimulation of the heart) is used to induce

TABLE 6–1: Description of ECG Wave and Normal Findings

Wave/Interval	Explanation	Normal Finding
P wave	Impulse from SA node to atria. (Atrial depolarization)	Normal size, shape, and deflection
PR interval	P wave to QRS complex	0.1–0.2 sec
QRS complex	Depolarization of the ventricle	<0.12 sec
ST segment	Interval between depolarization and repolarization	No elevation or depression
T wave	Recovery phase after contraction. (Ventricular polarization)	No inversion

Electrophysiology Study (EPS)[11,13,16] *(Continued)*

Description (Continued)

arrhythmias. When an ectopic site takes over as pacemaker, EPS can help pinpoint its origin. If a sustained arrhythmia is induced, an attempt will usually be made to capture the heart by pacing to terminate the arrhythmia. If the patient's cardiovascular system cannot compensate for the arrhythmia, the patient may require cardioversion back into a normal sinus rhythm (NSR).

Purpose

- EPS aids in:

  ° *Diagnosis* of disorders of the heart's conduction system and provides insight into the etiology and mechanism of ventricular arrhythmias and other disturbances within the AV conduction system.

  ° *Selection* of an antiarrhythmic drug and/or evaluation of the effectiveness of antiarrhythmic drug therapy.

- EPS is used to:

  ° *Assess* the need for an implanted pacemaker in some patients.

  ° *Work-up* patients with syncope and sick sinus syndrome.

Findings

Normal

Normal conduction intervals, refractory periods, recovery times, and absence of arrhythmias. Normal conduction intervals in adults are: H–V interval 35 to 55 msec; A–H interval 45 to 150 msec; P–A interval 20 to 40 msec.

Electrophysiology Study (EPS)[11,13,16] *(Continued)*

Findings (Continued)

Abnormal	Prolonged conduction intervals (see Table 6–2), abnormal refractory periods, abnormal recovery times, and induced arrhythmias.
Pharmacy Implications	• No food or fluids at least six hours before the study.
	• EPS is contraindicated in patients with severe coagulopathy, recent thrombophlebitis, and acute pulmonary embolism.

Exercise Electrocardiography (Stress Test)[4,13]

Description	Electrical cardiac principles are the same as for the ECG; however, the exercise stress test requires more preparation and patient participation. The electrode sites are shaved if necessary and the skin is cleansed to remove the superficial epidermal skin layer and excess skin oil. The chest electrodes are placed according to the lead system selected to provide the desired tracing. Electrodes are held in place by adhesive or a rubber belt. The lead wire cable is draped over the patient's shoulder, with the lead wires connected to the previously placed electrodes. A baseline rhythm strip is run and checked for dysrhythmias. The blood pressure is checked and a stethoscope is used to listen for the presence of S_3 and S_4 gallops or chest rales. The patient then steps onto a treadmill moving at a slow speed. A monitor is continuously observed for any changes in cardiac electrical activity and a rhythm strip is checked at preset intervals for any abnormalities as the treadmill speed is increased. Blood pressure is monitored at predetermined intervals and changes in systolic blood pressure are recorded. Testing stops when the target heart rate is reached or if unstable changes occur pertaining to the ECG, blood pressure, heart rate, or patient status (i.e., exhaustion or angina).

TABLE 6–2: Conduction Intervals and Potential Causes

Interval Prolonged[a]	Possible Cause
H-V	Acute or chronic disease
A-H	Atrial pacing, chronic conduction system disease, carotid sinus pressure, recent MI, and drugs
P-A	Acquired, surgically-induced, congenital atrial disease, and atrial pacing

[a] H-V = Time from the onset of Bundle of His deflection to ventricular activation; A-H = Time from atrial activation to onset of His deflection; P-A = Time from onset of the p wave on the ECG to atrial deflection.

Exercise Electrocardiography (Stress Test)[4,13] *(Continued)*

Purpose

- The stress test is used to:
  - ° *Test* cardiac reaction to increased demands for oxygen.
  - ° *Help Diagnose* the source of chest pain or other cardiac pain.
  - ° *Help Determine* the functional capacity of the heart after cardiac surgery or myocardial infarction.
  - ° *Screen* for coronary artery disease.
  - ° *Establish* the limits of an exercise program.
  - ° *Identify* dysrhythmias.
  - ° *Evaluate* the effectiveness of antiarrhythmic or antianginal drug therapy.

Findings

Normal

A normal ECG tracing with expected wave forms and intervals. (See ECG on page 6–9.)

Abnormal

Most prominent abnormal findings are a flat or down sloping ST segment depression and an up sloping, but depressed ST segment.

Pharmacy Implications

- Use of beta blockers may make the stress test difficult to interpret because the heart will be prevented from reaching the maximal target rate.

Holter Monitoring[3]

Description

Holter monitoring records heart rate and rhythm for a period of time (24 to 72 hours). Although a Holter monitor is usually used in ambulatory patients, it also can be used in patients restricted to bed. Three to five electrodes are placed on the chest and heart rate and rhythm are recorded on magnetic tape. The tape is then analyzed for evidence of cardiac arrhythmias that would normally not have been present during a routine ECG test.

Purpose

- Holter monitoring is used to:
  - ° *Diagnosis* cardiac arrhythmias.
  - ° *Evaluate* therapy for cardiac arrhythmias.
  - ° *Identify* asymptomatic patients at high risk for sudden cardiac death.
  - ° *Evaluate* syncopal episodes in which arrhythmias are not evident.

Findings

Holter monitoring can demonstrate the relationship between symptoms such as syncope, palpitations, or shortness of breath and a cardiac arrhythmia. Unfor-

Holter Monitoring[3] (Continued)

Findings (Continued)	tunately, symptom(s) and the Holter monitor abnormality must occur during the same testing period.
Pharmacy Implications	Patients keep a diary of all activities and symptoms during the period tested. All medications are recorded at the exact time taken.

Magnetic Resonance Imaging (MRI) of the Heart

See General Procedures: MRI on page 6–4.

Multiple Gated Acquisition Scan (MUGA)[4,16–18]

Description

Human serum albumin or erythrocytes labeled with a radioactive isotope (technetium 99-m pertechnetate) are injected into the patient. As the isotope labeled albumin or erythrocyte passes through the ventricle of the heart, a scintillation camera, triggered by the patient's ECG signals, records 14 to 64 points of a single cardiac cycle. This produces sequential images that can be viewed like a motion picture film. A MUGA scan allows evaluation of ventricular performance including wall motion, ejection fraction (EF), and other indices of cardiac function. The MUGA scan can also be performed after exercise. When compared to the results at rest, changes in ejection fraction and cardiac output (CO) can be assessed. The test is also known as cardiac blood pool scanning, because the blood, not the heart itself, is imaged.

Purpose

- MUGA is used to:

  ° *Evaluate* left ventricular function in order to assess prognosis in patients after an acute MI.

  ° *Evaluate* the efficacy of coronary artery disease therapies.

  ° *Differentiate* ventricular hypokinesis from left ventricular aneurysms.

  ° *Detect* intracardiac shunting in patients with congenital heart disease or septal rupture after a myocardial infarction.

  ° *Detect* right ventricular failure.

  ° *Provide* useful information in patients with aortic regurgitation.

Findings

Normal

The left ventricle contracts symmetrically and the isotope appears evenly distributed in the scans. Ejection fraction (EF) is approximately 50% to 65%.

Multiple Gated Acquisition Scan (MUGA)[4,16–18] *(Continued)*

Findings (Continued)

Abnormal	Asymmetric blood distribution in the myocardium, the presence of coronary artery disease as seen by segmental abnormalities of ventricular motion; the presence of cardiomyopathies as seen by globally reduced ejection fractions; right to left shunting seen by early arrival of activity in the left ventricle or aorta; and the presence of aneurysms in the left ventricle.
Pharmacy Implications	None.

Myocardial Biopsy[19]

Description	A catheter is inserted into the heart through an artery or vein and a cutting instrument attached to the catheter is used to remove tissue samples.
Purpose	Myocardial biopsy is used to diagnose cardiac disease (including cardiomyopathy) and assess suspected rejection of a transplanted heart.
Findings	
Normal	Normal pathology and histology.
Abnormal	Signs of rejection in a transplanted heart. Graded 0 through 4 based upon degree of interstitial lymphocytic infiltration.
Pharmacy Implications	Discontinue antiplatelet agents before the procedure. Aspirin should be stopped 7 to 10 days before and other NSAIDs should be stopped 2 to 4 days before the procedure.

Thallium Stress Test/Scan[20, 21]

Description	This nuclear medicine study can be performed with the patient at rest or exercising on a tread mill. Thallium-201 with biologic properties similar to potassium being taken up intracellularly, is administered intravenously. Blood flow then distributes the radionuclide to the myocardium and other organs. A gamma camera is used to measure the radioactivity throughout the myocardium. Healthy myocardium rapidly takes up the thallium whereas areas of infarcted myocardium show little or no radioactivity.
	The stress test is performed using a multi-stage treadmill test and ECG monitoring with thallium-201 being administered at the time of peak exercise. The myocardium is reimaged 3 hours later and myocardial perfusion again assessed following redistribution of the thallium. For those patients unable to exercise, adenosine or dipyridamole is administered intravenously along with the thallium to simulate the change in cardiac blood flow that occurs with exercise.

Thallium Stress Test/Scan[20, 21] *(Continued)*

Purpose

- The thallium stress test is used to:

  ° *Evaluate* regional myocardial perfusion.

  ° *Detect* evidence of recent or remote myocardial infarction.

  ° *Identify* viable myocardium in a previously infarcted portion of the myocardium.

Findings

Normal

Homogeneous distribution of thallium throughout the myocardium.

Abnormal

A thallium defect demonstrates a region of decreased myocardial blood flow. Infarcted areas can be demonstrated on the images immediately after injection and at the time of delayed imaging. Ischemic areas are detected on the early images as defects, but disappear with delayed imaging due to thallium redistribution.

Pharmacy Implications

- Patients should not eat for several hours before the test to prevent increased distribution of the thallium to the gut.

- Hold beta blockers for 48 hours before the test if exercise is to be performed to prevent a blunted response to exercise.

- Chest pain, headache, and dizziness occur frequently with dipyridamole. Chest pain, headache, and flushing are common with adenosine.

- Aminophylline can be administered IV (50 to 250 mg) to counteract the systemic adverse effects of IV dipyridamole.

ENDOCRINOLOGY

Adrenocorticotropic Hormone Stimulation Test (Cosyntropin)[4, 22-24]

Description

Cosyntropin (a synthetic derivative of ACTH) 250 μg IM or IV (preferred route) is administered to the patient after a blood sample is drawn to measure the base line cortisol level. Blood samples are then drawn at 30 and 60 minutes after the cosyntropin has been administered and serum cortisol concentrations are determined from these samples by radioimmunoassay technique.

Purpose

The adrenocorticotropic hormone stimulation test is a useful screening test to aid in the differentiation of primary and secondary adrenal failure and is used to diagnosis adrenal insufficiency.

Adrenocorticotropic Hormone Stimulation Test (Cosyntropin)[4, 22–24] (Continued)

Findings

Normal	Serum cortisol will rise at least 10 µg/dL above the baseline determination. Generally, a doubling of the baseline level is a normal response. Baseline determinations are affected by time-of-day due to diurnal variation.
Abnormal	Baseline cortisol level will be low and will display an inadequate response by rising <10 µg/dL over the baseline. This does not fully differentiate primary (adrenal) failure from secondary (pituitary) failure. Further testing is necessary.

Pharmacy Implications

- Patient may fast overnight, but this is not always done.

- If cosyntropin is to be given IV, inject IV push at a rate not to exceed 2 minutes.

- Estrogens, spironolactone, cortisone and its analogues, and lithium can interfere with the test.

- Dexamethasone does not affect the test due to its noninterference with the assay technique.

- Smoking, obesity, and alcohol can produce increased cortisol levels.

Dexamethasone Suppression Test (DST)[4, 22–26]

Description

The low dose dexamethasone suppression test involves the administration of 1 mg of dexamethasone at midnight, and on the following morning at 0800 hr a plasma cortisol level is drawn. Variants of this low dose study include dexamethasone 500 µg Q 6 hr for 2 days or 2 mg Q 6 hr for 2 days. In both cases, the plasma cortisol is measured on the second day. The RIA method of measuring the plasma cortisol concentration is generally preferred. For use in evaluating depression, 1 mg of dexamethasone is administered at 2300 hr and cortisol levels are measured at 1600 hr and 2300 hr the following day.

Purpose

- The DST is a screening test for the presence of Cushing's syndrome. It is most useful for ruling out Cushing's as the diagnosis. The overnight test does not easily differentiate between pituitary, adrenal, or ectopic etiologies. The two-day test provides more information and may be more diagnostic with respect to the etiology, but is less frequently performed due the time required.

- The DST also aids in the diagnosis of major endogenous depression.

Dexamethasone Suppression Test (DST)[4, 22–26] *(Continued)*

Findings

Normal	Plasma cortisol <5 μg/dL.
Abnormal	• Failure to suppress (cortisol >5 μg/dL) suggests that the pituitary-adrenal axis is not suppressible and Cushing's disease may be present.
	• Only about 50% of patients with major depression fail to suppress. Consequently, the usefulness of the DST as a screening test for depression is limited.
	• Patients with significant psychiatric disorders, thyrotoxicosis, obesity, acromegaly, pregnant females, and alcoholics often have elevated plasma cortisol levels and may confound the screening test. Diurnal rhythm (time of day) can also influence the result.

Pharmacy Implications

• Patient must fast overnight.

• ACTH, cortisone, estrogens, hydrocortisone, oral contraceptives, ethanol, lithium, or methadone taken 2 weeks before testing increases plasma test results. Phenytoin and androgens may decrease plasma cortisol levels.

Oral Glucose Tolerance Test (OGTT)[4,27,28]

Description

A blood sample to determine the fasting (baseline) blood glucose for the patient is drawn first. Then, the patient drinks a highly concentrated glucose solution (75 gm/300 mL for nonpregnant adults and 100 gm/400 mL for pregnant women). Subsequently, a timed series of blood glucose tests is performed at 30, 60, 90, and 120 minutes for nonpregnant adults and 1, 2, and 3 hours for pregnant women to determine the rate of removal of glucose from the bloodstream. This test is not performed if the fasting blood sugar is >140 mg/dL since virtually all patients will have blood glucose determinations that meet or exceed the diagnostic criteria for diabetes mellitus.

Purpose

OGTT is used to diagnose [or rule out (R/O)] overt diabetes, glucose intolerance, Cushing's syndrome, and acromegaly.

Findings

Normal

Adult, Non-pregnant	Fasting blood glucose	115 < mg/dL
	After 75 gm of oral glucose	30 min < 200 mg/dL
		60 min < 200 mg/dL
		90 min < 200 mg/dL
		120 min < 140 mg/dL

Oral Glucose Tolerance Test (OGTT)[4,27,28] *(Continued)*

Findings (Continued)

Abnormal

Adult

- **Diabetes Mellitus**
    - ° Sustained elevated blood glucose levels during at least 2 OGTTs.
    - ° The 2 hour sample and at least one other between 0 and 2 hr >200 mg/dL.

- **Impaired Glucose Tolerance**
    - ° 2 hr OGTT blood glucose level of 140 to 200 mg/dL.
    - ° 0 to 2 hr OGTT blood glucose level >200 mg/dL.

- **Gestational Diabetes**
    - ° This diagnosis may be made if 2 blood glucose values equal or exceed:

Fasting	105 mg/dL
1 hr	190 mg/dL
2 hr	165 mg/dL
3 hr	145 mg/dL

Pharmacy Implications

- Patient should be instructed to fast overnight (12 hr).

- 75 gm glucose (Glucola) is given to nonpregnant adults and 100 gm to pregnant women on morning of the test.

- Insulin or oral hypoglycemics should not be given until after test is completed.

- The following drugs should be discontinued at least 3 days before the test: hormones (including oral contraceptives), alcohol, salicylates, indomethacin, diuretics (especially thiazide), guanethidine, hypoglycemic agents, propranolol, corticosteroids, MAOIs, lithium, nicotinic acid, phenothiazines, and ascorbic acid.

Thyrotropin Releasing Hormone Test (Protirelin)[29,30]

Description

The test is performed by administering protirelin (TRH) 500 µg IV over 15 to 30 sec following the drawing of a blood sample from the patient to determine a baseline thyroid stimulating hormone (TSH). Plasma TSH levels are drawn 30 and 60 min after TRH is administered.

Thyrotropin Releasing Hormone Test (Protirelin)[29,30] (*Continued*)

Purpose	• Protirelin is used to:

    ° *Diagnose* suspected hyperthyroidism in individuals whose routine thyroid function tests are not fully diagnostic.

    ° *Assess* the integrity of the pituitary thyrotropes to aid in differentiating hypothyroidism due to intrinsic pituitary disease from hypothalamic dysfunction.

    ° *Aid* in the diagnosis of mild hypothyroidism.

Findings

Normal — TSH rise >5 μU above the baseline TSH excludes the diagnosis of hyperthyroidism.

Abnormal

• **Hyperthyroidism.** No TSH rise or <5 μU rise.

• **Primary Hypothyroidism.** Initially high baseline levels of TSH (exaggerated response).

• **Secondary Hypothyroidism.** Little or no response when pituitary failure present.

• **Hypothalamic Hypothyroidism.** TSH will rise at 45 or 60 min after TSH.

Pharmacy Implications

• Results can be affected by patients on thyroid supplementation.

• A 14-hour overnight fast is recommended.

GASTROENTEROLOGY

Abdominal X-Ray (KUB)[4, 31, 32]

Description

A KUB x-ray is also called a "scout film." The patient lies on his or her back and an x-ray is taken of the kidneys, ureters, and bladder (KUB). No contrast media are used for this study.

Purpose

• KUB is used to:

    ° *Diagnose* intra-abdominal abnormalities such as nephrolithiasis, intestinal obstruction, tissue masses, abnormal accumulation of gas, free air in the abdomen, or enlargement or perforation of the tissues.

    ° *Evaluate* size, shape, and position of the liver, spleen, and kidneys.

Abdominal X-Ray (KUB)[4, 31, 32] *(Continued)*

Findings

Normal

No masses, smooth peritoneal space, and normal size and position of organs. Right kidney is slightly lower than the left.

Abnormal

Foreign bodies are present, abnormal fluid, ascites, abnormal kidney location or shape, urinary calculi, calcification of blood vessels, cysts, or tumors.

Pharmacy Implications

- Normally, there is no patient preparation.

- The presence of feces or gas can obscure the film which may necessitate the administration of a laxative (milk of magnesia) at bedtime the night before the exam or 75 mL of senna fruit concentrate at 1600 hr on the day before the film. However, this is not frequently done.

- The presence of barium obscures the clarity of the film. The KUB should be scheduled before exams requiring administration of oral contrast media.

Barium Enema[33,34]

Description

Barium contrast is instilled through the rectum by means of a rectal tube up to the ileocecal valve and is retained while films are taken. Examination of the large intestine is performed using x-ray and fluoroscopy. These show position, filling, and movement of the colon. The barium contrast opacifies the bowel mucosa and outlines folds of the large intestine.

Purpose

- Barium enemas are used to:

  ° *Diagnose* colorectal cancer and inflammatory bowel diseases such as ulcerative colitis.

  ° *Detect* the presence of polyps or diverticula.

  ° *Evaluate* the structure of the large intestine.

Findings

Normal

Normal position, contour, filling, rate of passage of barium, movement, and patency of colon.

Abnormal

Presence of tumors, diverticula, obstructions, inflammation, or other abnormal findings.

Pharmacy Implications

- A typical procedure protocol includes:

  ° A liquid diet two days before procedure.

  ° Drinking 32 oz of water the day before exam from Noon to 2300 hr.

  ° Drinking 300 mL magnesium citrate at 1700 hr. [If severe renal disease is present, the patient should drink 1 bottle (75 mL) senna fruit concentrate.]

Barium Enema[33,34] *(Continued)*

Pharmacy Implications
(Continued)

• A typical procedure protocol includes:

   ° Taking four 5 mg bisacodyl tablets at 1900 hr. (Swallow the tablets whole. Do not administer within one hour of antacids or milk.)

   ° No food or drink after midnight.

   ° A 2,000 mL cleansing enema before the procedure.

   ° Taking 30 mL Milk of Magnesia orally as a cathartic after procedure. In a renal patient with compromised renal status, administer 30 mL of sorbitol 70% orally after procedure.

Barium Enema With Air Contrast[4,33,34]

Description

This test is often referred to as double contrast barium enema or pneumocolon. It involves the same principles as a standard barium enema, but includes the instillation of air into the bowel in addition to contrast medium. This method improves detection of subtle changes in the colon, but is not as thorough an exam as a colonoscopy.

Purpose

See Barium Enema.

Findings

See Barium Enema.

Pharmacy Implications

See Barium Enema.

Enterocylsis[35,36]

Description

Enterocylsis is a radiographic examination of the small bowel by delivering barium directly into the jejunum by way of an orogastric or nasogastric tube, followed by a radiolucent methylcellulose solution. Enterolysis provides an improved and more detailed view of the entire small bowel as compared to the standard small bowel series.

Purpose

Enterolysis is used to evaluate malabsorption, inflammatory bowel disease, and the presence of a small bowel obstruction.

Findings

Normal

The presence of normal appearing bowel mucosa, small bowel wall thickness, normal fluid transit time, and the absence of lesions, obstructions, or fistulas.

Abnormal

Inflamed mucosa, accelerated transit time, and presence of masses, obstruction, narrowed lumen, and fistulas.

Pharmacy Implications

• See Barium Enema.

• Metoclopramide 10 mg IV may be administered 20 to 30 minutes before the procedure to aid in intubation of the small bowel.

Barium Swallow (Upper GI with Small Bowel Follow Through-UGI/SBFT)[4,35,36]

Description

A fluoroscopic x-ray examination of the pharynx, esophagus, stomach, duodenum, and upper jejunum comprise the upper GI portion of the exam. An oral contrast medium (barium) is swallowed permitting visualization of the lumen in these areas. To evaluate the remainder of the jejunum and the ileum (small bowel follow through), a series of hourly films may be required to track the contrast medium through the small bowel. This portion of the exam is complete when the ileocecal valve has filled with the contrast material.

Purpose

- A barium swallow is used to:

  - *Detect* congenital abnormalities of the bowel.

  - *Diagnose* the presence of tumors, pyloric stenosis, and varices.

  - *Aid* in the diagnosis of diverticula, ulcers, polyps, hiatal hernia, gastritis, regional enteritis, malabsorption, and motility disorders.

Findings

Normal

Normal size, contour, motility, and peristalsis.

Abnormal

Deformed contour from intrinsic tumor, filling defects, and/or stenosis with dilation. May also see ulcers and other irregularities.

Pharmacy Implications

- Barium sulfate or diatrizoate meglumine (Gastrografin) must be given during procedure.

- No oral ingestion (including medications, antacids) after 2200 hr the day before the exam.

- Administer 30 mL Milk of Magnesia 30 mL after the procedure as a cathartic. In a renal patient with compromised renal status, administer 30 mL of sorbitol 70% after the procedure.

Cholangiography (Percutaneous Transhepatic)[37,38,39]

Description

A 22-gauge, 6-inch long needle is used to puncture the skin and is passed into the intrahepatic biliary tree. Contrast material is then administered via this needle into the biliary tree. A fluoroscopic examination is performed and individual radiographs are taken.

Purpose

- Cholangiography is used to:

  - *Aid* in the diagnosis of obstructive jaundice (differentiate intrahepatic and extrahepatic causes of cholestasis).

Cholangiography (Percutaneous Transhepatic)[37,38,39] *(Continued)*

Purpose (Continued)

- Cholangiography is used to:
  - *Outline* the detail of the intra- and extrahepatic ducts and the biliary tree.
  - *Identify* the presence of stones, tumors, lesions, strictures, and biliary duct fistula.

Findings

Normal

Normal sized ducts and duct anatomy. Absence of stones or lesions.

Abnormal

Extrahepatic obstructive jaundice is associated with dilated ducts and a cause of the obstruction is identified (stones, biliary carcinoma, or pancreatic carcinoma impinging on the common bile duct). Non-obstructive jaundice is associated with normal sized ducts and leads to a diagnosis of intrahepatic cholestasis.

Pharmacy Implications

- Patient NPO 4 hours before the procedure.

- Contrast dye may produce a hypersensitivity reaction.

- The patient may receive a parenteral anxiolytic like diazepam before the procedure.

- Prophylactic antibiotics may be administered (e.g., ampicillin, an aminoglycoside, cefoxitin or cefotetan, cefoperazone or ceftriaxone) before and after the procedure.

- Discontinue aspirin 7 to 10 days before the procedure and NSAIDs 2 to 4 days before the procedure.

- Evaluate patients for non-drug related impaired coagulopathy.

- If coagulation studies (PT) are abnormal, oral or parenteral (IM, IV) vitamin K may be given daily before the procedure or fresh frozen plasma (FFP).

Cholangiography (T-Tube)[4]

Description

An iodine contrast dye is injected into a T-tube (a self-retaining drainage tube attached to the common bile duct during gall bladder surgery), and a fluoroscopic examination is made. The T-tube is then unclamped and the contrast material drains out. This test is often referred to as postoperative cholangiography.

Purpose

The T-tube cholangiography is used to evaluate the patency of the common bile duct following gall bladder surgery and evaluate the presence of an extrahepatic obstruction.

Cholangiography (T-Tube)[4] *(Continued)*

Findings

Normal	Patent common bile duct with no obstructions.
Abnormal	Extrahepatic obstruction noted.
Pharmacy Implications	Contrast dye may produce a hypersensitivity reaction.

Computed Tomography (CT) of the Abdomen

See General Procedures: Computed Tomography on page 6–2.

Endoscopy[4, 40]

Endoscopy is visual examination of various internal body structures using a fiber optic instrument. The fiber optic instrument is made up of a flexible tube and a lighted
mirror lens system. Depending upon the orifice into which the endoscope is inserted,
the diameter of the endoscope will vary. Endoscopy can be used for diagnostic pur-
poses since this device allows direct visualization. Endoscopy can be used to perform
therapeutic procedures and tissue biopsies.

Colonoscopy

Description   Colonoscopy is examination of the colon and termi-
nal ileum by use of a flexible fiber optic endoscope.

Purpose   • Colonoscopy is used to:

° *Further Evaluate* an abnormal barium enema.

° *Help Determine* the cause of a lower GI bleed.

° *Screen* for the presence of cancer.

° *Evaluate* patients with colonic cancer or inflammatory bowel disease.

° *Determine* the cause of unexplained diarrhea.

° *Perform* polypectomy.

° *Arrest* the bleeding from lesions.

° *Decompress* a dilated colon, reduce an intestinal volvulus, or dilate strictures.

° *Remove* foreign objects from the large bowel.

° *Perform* tissue biopsies to aid in the diagnosis
of suspected disease.

Findings

Normal	Absence of inflammation, normal mucosa, and nor-mal anatomy.
Abnormal	Presence of polyps or tumors, areas of inflammation, signs of bleeding, presence of foreign objects, and abnormal anatomy.

Endoscopy[4, 40] *(Continued)*

Pharmacy Implications

- **Standard Prep for a typical procedure protocol** includes:

  ° A clear liquid diet 2 days before the procedure.

  ° *On evening before the procedure:* administration of magnesium citrate 300 mL PO at 1700 hr (Use senna concentrate 75 mL instead of magnesium citrate in patients with renal disease); administration of a bisacodyl tablet 10 mg PO at 1900 hr; encouragement of oral fluids; and NPO after midnight.

  ° *On morning of procedure:* administration of 1500 mL of a normal saline solution enema times two and meperidine IM ordered for on call or 30 minutes before procedure.

- **Preparation for colonoscopy with lavage** (either evening before or morning of colonoscopy) includes:

  ° Metoclopramide 10 mg (IM, IV, or PO) 30 min before GI lavage solution.

  ° GI lavage solution (polyethylene glycol-electrolyte solution) 1.2 to 1.8 L/hr until diarrhea clears (usually ≈4 L). Stop lavage if patient develops vomiting or severe abdominal pain. If the patient is unable to tolerate PO, an NG tube may need to be placed.

  ° If biopsy or surgical procedure is performed, prophylaxis of bacterial endocarditis for susceptible individuals (e.g., prosthetic heart valves, congenital cardiac malformations, valvular disease, and history of endocarditis) should be administered before the procedure. Ampicillin 2 gm + gentamicin 1.5 mg/kg (Max: 80 mg per AHA guidelines) (substitute vancomycin for ampicillin if penicillin allergic) is the recommended regimen. This may be repeated 8 hr after the initial dose.

Endoscopic Retrograde Cholangiopancreatography (ERCP)[4,41]

Description

A special sideviewing endoscope is passed into the duodenum and then cannulation is performed at the point of junction of the pancreatic duct and the common bile duct just before the two ducts enter into the duodenum (Ampulla of Vater). A tube is then placed in each duct and a radiographic contrast medium is injected. Radiographs are taken of the ducts. Areas visualized include the common bile duct, intrahepatic ducts, gallbladder, and pancreatic ducts.

Endoscopic Retrograde Cholangiopancreatography (ERCP)[4,41] (Continued)

Purpose

- ERCP is used to:

  ○ *Aid* in the diagnosis and treatment of certain biliary tree and pancreatic diseases.

  ○ *Evaluate* patients with suspected obstructive jaundice, disease of the biliary system, pancreatic cancer, recurrent pancreatitis, and the anatomy of the pancreas and ductal system before intervention.

  ○ *Place* biliary stents (devices used to keep the biliary or pancreatic duct open).

  ○ *Perform* sphincterotomy, remove common duct gallstones, and perform other minor surgical procedures related to the pancreatic and common bile duct.

Findings

Normal

Normal ductal anatomy (pancreatic duct and common bile duct) and the absence of lesions, stones, and other causes of obstruction.

Abnormal

Ductal dilation and/or strictures, and presence of stones or tumors.

Pharmacy Implications

- Administer atropine IM 30 minutes before the procedure to decrease secretions.

- Administer meperidine IM 30 minutes before the procedure to reduce pain perception. Meperidine is preferred due to less effect on Sphincter of Oddi as compared to other narcotic analgesics.

- IV benzodiazepines are sometimes used to alleviate anxiety and provide an amnesic effect (diazepam, midazolam, or lorazepam).

- If minor surgery is anticipated, ampicillin 2 gm (vancomycin 1 gm if penicillin allergic) and gentamicin 1.5 mg/kg (Max: 80 mg per AHA guidelines) are administered just before the procedure as a prophylactic measure to prevent infection from enterococci and gram-negative rods. These agents may be continued after the procedure if necessary. This regimen is also used as prophylaxis of bacterial endocarditis in susceptible individuals.

- Contrast dye may produce a hypersensitivity reaction.

Esophogogastroduodenoscopy (upper endoscopy)[4,42]

Description

Esophogogastroduodenoscopy is examination of the esophagus (esophagoscopy), stomach (gastroscopy), and duodenum (duodenoscopy) using an endoscope. The endoscope is placed through the mouth and

Description (Continued) throat and passed along the esophagus into the stomach and duodenum. Air is placed into the esophagus and stomach for better visualization.

Purpose
- Esophogogastroduodenoscopy is used to:

  ° *Directly Visualize, Examine, and Photograph* the inside of the esophagus, stomach, and duodenum.

  ° *Identify* the site of an upper GI bleed.

  ° *Visualize* abnormalities seen with an UGI series.

  ° *Evaluate* the healing of ulcers and gastric emptying and swallowing abnormalities.

  ° *Perform* polypectomy, sclerotherapy of esophageal varices, esophageal and gastric dilation, and tissue biopsies.

  ° *Remove* foreign objects.

  ° *Coagulate* bleeding sites.

  ° *Place* feeding tubes and percutaneous gastrostomy tubes.

Findings

Normal — Absence of inflammation, lesions, and bleeding. Mucosa and anatomy appear normal.

Abnormal — Inflammation (reddened mucosa) of the examined structures; identified area of bleeding (hemorrhage); hiatal hernia; lesions (benign or malignant); or visible ulcers.

Pharmacy Implications
- Patient is NPO for at least 6 hours before the examination.

- No antacids after 2200 on the day before the exam, or before the exam if being performed on an urgent basis.

- Administer atropine IM 30 minutes before the procedure to decrease secretions and prevent reflex bradycardia secondary to vagal stimulation from insertion of the scope. (Exercise caution with IM use in patients with a low platelet count, bleeding disorder, or being treated with anticoagulants.)

- Narcotics (e.g. meperidine) and benzodiazepines (e.g. midazolam) may be administered just before the exam to produce sedation, reduce anxiety, and decrease the perception of discomfort. The patient must be alert enough to assist in swallowing.

Pharmacy Implications (Continued)

- Local anesthetics may be used to anesthetize the throat. If used, the patient should be NPO for 1 to 2 hours after the procedure to reduce the risk of aspiration when swallowing. Initially, clear liquids are administered and the patient is closely observed for swallowing difficulties.

- If a biopsy is to be performed, parenteral antibiotic prophylaxis for bacterial endocarditis, in susceptible individuals, should be administered 30 minutes before the procedure. Ampicillin 2 gm IV (vancomycin 1 gm IV if penicillin allergic) plus gentamicin 1.5 mg/kg IV (Max: 80 mg per AHA guidelines). This may be repeated 8 hr after the initial dose.

Proctoscopy[4,43]

Description

Proctoscopy is an instrumental examination of a 12 inch area of the rectum using a proctoscope. (A proctoscope is a rigid tube with a lighted mirror and lens at the end.)

Purpose

- Proctoscopy is used to:

   ° *Confirm* or rule out ulcerative, pseudomembranous, or granulomatous colitis.

   ° *Examine* the rectosigmoid area for the presence of tumors, polyps, or hemorrhoids.

   ° *Aid* in the diagnosis of irritable bowel syndrome and Crohn's disease.

Findings

Normal

No tumors or inflammation. Rectal mucosa is smooth and pink. The rectum has normal anatomy.

Abnormal

Edematous, red, or denuded mucosa. Presence of grainy-like minute masses. The tissue is easily broken or pulverized. Visible ulcers or pseudomembranes. Spontaneous bleeding upon examination.

Pharmacy Implications

- Give laxatives and enema (tap water or phosphate) the evening before the procedure.

- One or two phosphate enemas or a suppository (bisacodyl) may be given one hour before the procedure.

- Barium within past week could interfere with the examination.

- Patient should be NPO two hours before the exam.

Proctoscopy[4,43] *(Continued)*

Pharmacy Implications
(Continued)

- If a biopsy is planned, parenteral antibiotic prophylaxis for bacterial endocarditis, in susceptible individuals, should be administered 30 minutes before the procedure. Ampicillin 2 gm (vancomycin 1 gm if penicillin allergic) plus gentamicin 1.5 mg/kg (Max: 80 mg per AHA guidelines). May be repeated 8 hr after initial dose.

Sigmoidoscopy (Flexible)[4,44]

Description

Sigmoidoscopy is direct visual examination of the distal 60 cm (24 inches) of the rectum and sigmoid colon using a flexible fiber optic scope.

Purpose

- Sigmoidoscopy is used to:
  - *Directly Visualize and Biopsy* abnormalities in the rectosigmoid area.
  - *Directly Evaluate* lesions seen on xray.
  - *Evaluate* patients who have undergone bowel resection and the cause of bloody diarrhea or rectal bleeding.
  - *Diagnose and Monitor* inflammatory bowel disease and the effectiveness of therapy.
  - *Reduce* a sigmoid volvulus.
  - *Screen* for colon cancers and follow patients with a known history of colon cancer.

Findings

Normal

Absence of inflammation, bleeding, and lesions. Normal anatomy.

Abnormal

Reddened or bleeding mucosa, presence of neoplastic disease.

Pharmacy Implications

- No preparation for patients who present with a primary complaint of diarrhea, who are suspected of having inflammatory bowel disease, or have a history of acute bright red rectal bleeding.

- Usual preparation includes withholding of breakfast on the morning of the procedure and the administration of phosphate enemas 130 mL PR twice given 30 minutes before the procedure.

- If a biopsy is planned, antibiotic prophylaxis of bacterial endocarditis, in susceptible individuals, is recommended. Administer ampicillin 2 gm (vancomycin 1 gm if penicillin allergic) IV plus gentamicin 1.5 mg/kg (Max: 80 mg per AHA guidelines) IV 30 minutes before the procedure. May be repeated 8 hr after initial dose.

Hepatobiliary Scintigraphy (HIDA, PAPIDA, or DISIDA SCAN)[4,45]

Description

A radionuclide tracer, 99mTcIDA (technetium labeled iminodiacetic acid derivatives), is injected intravenously and taken up by the liver and excreted into the biliary tree. A scintillation camera, by means of serial imaging (an image every 5 minutes for 1 hour), shows the radioactivity in the liver, bile ducts, gall bladder, and duodenum.

Purpose

- Hepatobiliary scintigraphy is used to:

  ° *Aid Diagnosis* of cholecystitis, biliary tract stones, tumors, cancer, obstruction, leaks, and anatomical anomalies of the biliary tree.

  ° *Evaluate* the biliary ducts for patency after surgical intervention.

  ° *Evaluate* liver function and to determine liver rejection after transplantation.

Findings

Normal

The gallbladder, bile ducts, liver, and portion of the small bowel are visualized within 1 hour showing normal size, shape, and function of the biliary system.

Abnormal

Radioactivity in the liver, but little or none in the gallbladder and duodenum indicates biliary obstruction. Decreased or absent radioactivity in the gallbladder, bile ducts, and duodenum or delayed uptake by the liver indicates hepatocellular disease.

Pharmacy Implications

None.

Liver Biopsy[4,40,46]

Description

The procedure employs a percutaneous needle aspiration of a core of tissue from the liver utilizing the Menghini needle (a long large bore needle). The biopsied tissue is then sent for histologic analysis.

Purpose

- Liver biopsy is used to:

  ° *Diagnose and Assess* the course of and response to therapy of hepatic cellular disease, such as cirrhosis or hepatitis.

  ° *Assist* in the diagnosis and staging of lymphomas and other malignancies.

  ° *Assist* in the diagnosis of metabolic disease, multisystem disease, and granulomatous infections.

  ° *Assess* the effect of hepatotoxic drugs (e.g., methotrexate).

  ° *Evaluate* suspected rejection of a transplanted liver.

Liver Biopsy[4,40,46] *(Continued)*

Findings

Normal

In all cases, presence of normal pathology and histology.

Abnormal

Presence of tumors or cysts; hepatic cellular changes consistent with cirrhosis or hepatitis; signs of organ rejection; signs of drug toxicity.

Pharmacy Implications

- It is recommended that antiplatelet agents be stopped before open and needle biopsies. Stop aspirin 7 to 10 days before the procedure. Discontinue NSAIDs which reversibly inhibit the enzyme cyclooxygenase (e.g., ibuprofen, naproxen) 2 to 4 days before the procedure.

- Preprocedure medications such as parenteral analgesics (e.g., meperidine, morphine) and parenteral sedatives/anxiolytics (e.g., lorazepam, diazepam, midazolam) may be administered.

- A local anesthetic (e.g., lidocaine) may be necessary. Check the patient's history of allergic reactions.

MRI of the Abdomen

See General Procedures: MRI on page 6–4.

Paracentesis[4,47]

Description

Paracentesis is the puncture of any cavity for the aspiration of fluid; however, the withdrawal of fluid from the abdomen (abdominal paracentesis) probably is the most commonly encountered. First, the area between the umbilicus and the pubis is cleaned and anesthetized. Then, a long 18-gauge needle is inserted through the abdominal wall into the peritoneum 1 to 2 inches below the umbilicus. Fluid is aspirated and sent to the laboratory for analysis.

Purpose

- Paracentesis is used to:

  - *Aid Diagnosis* of a suspected infection (peritonitis) or malignancy.

  - *Assess* the electrolyte and protein make-up of the fluid.

  - *Therapeutically Remove* ascitic fluid from the abdomen of patients with cirrhosis or abdominal malignancy.

  - *Determine* the presence of abdominal bleeding.

Findings

Normal (Peritoneal fluid). See Table 6–3.

TABLE 6–3: Normal Paracentesis Findings

Appearance	Clear and yellowish
Volume	<50 mL
Protein Content	0.3–4.1 gm/dL
Glucose	70–100 mg/dL
RBCs	None
WBCs	<300/mL
Bacteria and Fungi	None
Cytology	No malignant cells

Paracentesis[4,47] *(Continued)*

Findings (Continued)

Abnormal	Cloudy or turbid appearance; elevated protein content; elevated glucose; presence of RBCs or bloody fluid; WBCs >300/mL; and cytology positive for malignant cells.
Pharmacy Implications	None.

Small Bowel Series

See Barium Swallow on page 6–22.

Small Bowel Biopsy[4,40,48]

Description	Small bowel biopsy is usually performed using an apparatus called the Rubin-Quinton multipurpose tube. It is passed orally into the small bowel and a piece of jejunal tissue is harvested or duodenal fluid aspirated. Alternatively, a Carey capsule may be used to perform the biopsy. The specimen obtained with this device is more broad and less deep than the samples obtained with the Rubin-Quinton device. Fluoroscopy is used to check the position of the tube. Histologic and/or fluid analysis is performed on the samples.
Purpose	• Small bowel biopsy is used to:

  ○ *Determine* the cause of malabsorption or diarrhea.

  ○ *Assess* response to drug or other non-drug therapies.

  ○ *Verify* a suspected malignancy.

  ○ *Diagnose* and assess inflammatory bowel disease.

Small Bowel Biopsy[4,40,48] *(Continued)*

Purpose (Continued)	• Small bowel biopsy is used to:
	○ *Collect* pancreatic fluid for analysis and bile fluid for analysis to assess gallbladder disease.
	○ *Diagnose* bacterial overgrowth or giardiasis.

Findings

Normal	In all cases, presence of normal pathology, histology, and fluid composition.
Abnormal	Presence of histologic changes characteristic of inflammatory bowel disease or malignancy, the presence of giardia or bacterial overgrowth, or the presence of cholesterol crystals and white blood cells in bile fluid.

Pharmacy Implications

• The patient should be NPO.

• Spray the patient's throat with a local anesthetic (e.g., benzocaine, cetacaine, or lidocaine) to reduce the likelihood of gagging when the tube is passed.

• Preprocedure medications such as parenteral analgesics (e.g. meperidine) and parenteral sedatives/anxiolytics (e.g. lorazepam, diazepam, or midazolam) may be administered. However, the patient needs to be cooperative and somewhat alert to be able to swallow the tube.

• Current use of antiplatelet agents such as aspirin and other NSAIDs or anticoagulants such as warfarin is a contraindication to this test.

• An elevated PT or aPTT for a nondrug-related reason is a contraindication to performance of this procedure.

Ultrasonography of Abdomen

See General Procedures: Ultrasonography on page 6–5.

GYNECOLOGY

Breast Biopsy (Needle and Open)[4,49]

Description

• **Needle.** A needle is introduced into the breast mass where fluid (if present) is aspirated. Tissue obtained from the biopsy is sent for cytology. Diagnostically, this procedure is limited by the small tissue sample obtained from a needle biopsy; it may not be representative of the entire breast mass. There is also an increased risk of "seeding" the needle tract with potentially malignant cells causing further spread of the disease. Therefore, a needle biopsy is generally reserved for a fluid-filled cyst or an advanced malignant lesion.

Breast Biopsy (Needle and Open)[4,49] *(Continued)*

Description
(Continued)

- **Open.** In an open biopsy of the breast, an incision is made to expose the breast mass. If the mass is small enough (<2 cm) and looks benign, the mass is excised. If the mass is larger or looks malignant, a representative amount of tissue is incised from the mass and sent for receptor assay analysis and frozen section. Frozen section involves quick freezing of the tissue sample so it can be cut into microscopic sections and examined by the pathologist to determine if the tissue is malignant and if the tissue margins indicate adequate excision. This entire process takes 10 to 15 minutes and provides valuable information on whether more malignant tissue needs to be excised or if the wound can be closed.

Purpose

Needle and open breast biopsies are performed to determine if breast tumors are benign or malignant. Receptor assays are done on malignant tissues to determine if the tumor is estrogen-receptor (ER) and/or progesterone-receptor (PR) positive or negative. ER(+) and PR(+) tumors will respond best to hormonal chemotherapy like tamoxifen.

Findings

Normal

Results from a breast biopsy will reveal adequate amounts of cellular and noncellular connective tissue with proper development of tissue.

Abnormal

Presence of a benign tumor such as adenofibroma or the presence of a malignant tumor like adenocarcinoma, inflammatory carcinoma, sarcoma, and others. Plasma cell mastitis or the presence of intraductal papilloma and others.

Pharmacy Implications

- Local anesthetics are administered before needle and some open breast biopsies. Some open biopsies require the use of a general anesthetic in which case the patient is to remain NPO after midnight on the day before the procedure.

- A penicillinase-resistant antibiotic (e.g. dicloxacillin, cephradine, cefazolin, ampicillin/sulbactam) is sometimes used after an open breast biopsy as prophylaxis against penicillinase-producing staphylococcal infections.

Colposcopy[4]

Description

Colposcopy is a visual examination of the cervix and vagina using a colposcope, an instrument containing a magnifying lens and a light.

Colposcopy[4] *(Continued)*

Purpose
- Colposcopy is used to:
  - *Directly Observe* the cervix and vagina.
  - *Perform* a tissue biopsy of the cervix and vagina.
  - *Confirm* intraepithelial neoplasia or invasive carcinoma.
  - *Evaluate* other vaginal or cervical lesions.
  - *Monitor* antineoplastic therapy.

Findings

Normal	Vaginal and cervical mucosa and epithelium of normal color and appearance.
Abnormal	Presence of color tissue changes, or lesions.
Pharmacy Implications	None.

Hysterosalpingography[4]

Description
Hysterosalpingography is an x-ray examination to visualize the uterine cavity, fallopian tubes, and peritubal area by means of a contrast medium injected through a cannula inserted into the cervix. The uterus and fallopian tubes are viewed under fluoroscopy and x-ray films are taken.

Purpose
Hysterosalpingography is used to evaluate tubal patency as part of an infertility workup.

Findings

Normal	Normal anatomy with no tubal or uterine abnormalities.
Abnormal	Tubal adhesions or occlusions. Uterine abnormalities including foreign bodies, fibroid tumors, congenital malformations, or fistulas.
Pharmacy Implications	A sedative may be administered before the procedure.

Laparoscopy[4,7]

Description
A laparoscopy is the visual examination of the peritoneal cavity with an endoscope (laparoscope) through the anterior abdominal wall. A small incision is made at the level of the umbilicus with the patient under general anesthesia. A needle is inserted and approximately 2 to 3 L of CO_2 or NO_2 is instilled into the abdominal cavity to distend the abdominal wall and provide organ free-space to aid in visualization. If fallopian tube patency is being evaluated, a dye is injected through the cervix and observed. The laparoscope is inserted through the same incision at the umbilicus and the examination performed. The gas is removed after the exam is completed.

Laparoscopy[4,7] *(Continued)*

Purpose	• Laparoscopy is used to:
	○ *Detect* abnormalities or *Perform* procedures such as lysis of adhesions, ovarian biopsy, tubal ligation, and removal of foreign bodies.
	○ *Detect* ectopic pregnancy, endometriosis, or pelvic inflammatory disease.
	○ *Evaluate* pelvic masses.
	○ *Examine* the fallopian tubes of infertile women.
	○ *Harvest* eggs (ovum) for *in vitro* fertilization.

Findings

Normal	Uterus, ovaries, and fallopian tubes are of normal size and shape without adhesions, cysts, or presence of endometriosis.
Abnormal	Presence of cysts, adhesions, fibroids, endometriosis, ectopic pregnancy, infection, or abscess.

Pharmacy Implications

- Patient is NPO after midnight the night before the procedure.
- Pelvic or abdominal discomfort postoperatively may require analgesics.

Mammography[4]

Descriptions	A mammogram is an x-ray of the breast; a low energy x-ray beam (0.1 to 0.8 rads) delineates the breast on mammograms. Two radiographs are taken: 1) frontal view and 2) lateral view.
Purpose	• Mammography is used to:
	○ *Screen* for breast cancer and investigate or detect masses missed during physical examination of the breast.
	○ *Help* differentiate benign and malignant masses which have previously been located.

Findings

Normal	No calcification, no abnormal mass, normal duct contrast with narrowing of ductal branches.
Abnormal	Poorly outlined, irregular shape and opaque lesion suggest malignancy. Malignant cysts are usually solitary and unilateral, and contain an increased number of blood vessels. Benign cysts are usually round and smooth with definable edges.
Pharmacy Implications	• No medications/preparations are needed.

Mammography[4] *(Continued)*

Pharmacy Implications
(Continued)

• The American Cancer Society recommends a base line mammogram for all women between 35 and 40 years of age, an annual or biannual mammogram for ages 40 to 49, and a yearly mammogram after 50. Routine breast self-examination is recommended.

Ultrasonography of Pelvis, Uterus, and Ovaries

See General Procedures: Ultrasound on page 6–5.

HEMATOLOGY

Bone Marrow Biopsy[4,7]

Description

A biopsy of the bone marrow is most commonly obtained from one of four sites in the body: the posterior superior iliac spine (preferred site), the sternum, the spinous process, or the tibia. The area where the biopsy is to be performed is first injected with a local anesthetic. A needle is then inserted through the skin, subcutaneous fatty tissues, and into the cortex of the bone being sampled. Through this large bore needle, tissue plugs of bone marrow are removed for microscopic examination.

Purpose

• Bone marrow biopsy is used to:

  ° *Diagnose* disorders such as anemias, thrombocytopenia, leukemias, and granulomas.

  ° *Distinguish* between primary and metastatic tumors.

  ° *Determine* the cause of bone infection.

  ° *Aid* in the staging of neoplastic disease.

  ° *Evaluate* the effectiveness of chemotherapy and monitor myelosuppression.

Findings

Normal

Normal hematologic analysis with differential count. Normal relative amounts of fat and hemopoietic cells and normal number of megakaryocytes, immature platelets, plasma, and mast cells present.

Abnormal

Detection of osteoclasts or osteoblasts; groups of malignant cells found in the marrow; granulomas present; and cells seen with indistinct margins indicating marrow necrosis.

Pharmacy Implications

Patients may require sedation before the bone marrow biopsy with an IM or IV narcotic analgesic and/or an IM or IV benzodiazepine.

INFECTIOUS DISEASE

Gram's Stain[50]

Description	Gram's stain is a procedure whereby a specimen or sample of a body fluid (e.g. blood, sputum, urine, or wound aspirate) is fixed to a slide stained with a crystal violet solution; rinsed, then flooded with Gram's Iodine Solution; rinsed, decolorized with a mixture of ethanol and/or acetone; rinsed, then counter stained with safranin; rinsed, and then allowed to dry. This is a relatively quick screening method for identifying infecting bacteria. The composition of the cell wall appears to be the key element in the staining and differentiation of organisms.
Purpose	A Gram's stain is performed to classify bacterial organisms into gram-positive or gram-negative cocci or rods.
Findings	**Gram-positive** organisms retain the primary dye and appear dark purple.
	Gram-negative organisms will, after decolorization and counter staining, appear pinkish-red.
Pharmacy Implications	Knowledge of which organisms are gram-positive and gram-negative organisms and antibiotic sensitivity patterns to various antibiotics aids in the selection of appropriate empiric antibiotic therapy until final identification of organism is known.

Indium Labeled WBC Scan
(Indium-111 Leukocyte Total Body Scan)[4,11]

Description	Approximately 40 mL of blood is taken from the patient for labeling of the white blood cells (WBC) with radioactive Indium-111. The labeled WBCs are intravenously reinjected into the patient. At 24 and 48 hours after reinjection, imaging studies are performed on the patient. It takes approximately one hour for each imaging study. The radiation from this test is equivalent to one abdominal x-ray.
Purpose	Indium labeled WBC scans are used to diagnose infectious and inflammatory processes.
Findings	
Normal	Results will show high concentrations of the labeled WBCs in the liver, spleen, and bone marrow.
Abnormal	Results will show high concentrations of the labeled WBCs outside the liver, spleen, and bone marrow, such as in an abscess formation, acute and chronic osteomyelitis, orthopedic prosthesis, infection, and active inflammatory bowel disease.

Indium Labeled WBC Scan
(Indium-111 Leukocyte Total Body Scan)[4,11] *(Continued)*

Pharmacy Implications   Hyperalimentation, steroid therapy, and long-term antibiotic therapy can produce false-negative results because of their ability to change the chemotactic response of WBCs.

NEPHROLOGY
Renal Biopsy[3,4]

Description   The safest method is percutaneous needle biopsy employing a 7 inch, 20 gauge needle inserted through the skin and into the kidney capsule. However, if a tissue sample from a solid lesion is necessary, an open biopsy may need to be performed.

Purpose
- Renal biopsy is used to:
  - *Diagnose* diseases that alter the structure of the glomerulus.
  - *Determine* the nature of a renal mass identified by other diagnostic techniques.
  - *Monitor* the course of chronic renal disease.
  - *Evaluate* suspected rejection of a transplanted kidney.

Findings

Normal   Normal pathology and histology.

Abnormal   Presence of a tumor, clot, or renal stone. Presence of histologic changes characteristic of lupus erythematosus, amyloid infiltration, glomerulonephritis, renal vein thrombosis, pyelonephritis, and renal transplant rejection.

Pharmacy Implications   It is recommended that antiplatelet agents be stopped before open and needle biopsies. Stop aspirin 7 to 10 days before the procedure. NSAIDs which inhibit the enzyme cyclooxygenase (e.g. ibuprofen, naproxen) should be stopped 2 to 4 days before the procedure.

Renal Scan[4]

Description   A radioactive tracer, technetium-99m is injected intravenously. A scanning camera then takes images of the blood flow to and through the kidneys.

Purpose
- Renal scan is used to:
  - *Detect* or rule out masses.
  - *Investigate* kidney function.
  - *Evaluate* kidney transplant viability and renal blood flow.

Renal Scan[4] *(Continued)*

Findings

Normal	Normal size, shape, position, and function of the kidneys.
Abnormal	Tumors (irregular masses) within the kidney, obstructions, decreased renal perfusion, abnormal kidneys (shape or size), and presence of rejection.

Pharmacy Implications   None.

NEUROLOGY

Brainstem Auditory Evoked Response (BAER)[51,52]

Description

Electrodes are placed on the scalp to obtain a baseline electrical activity. Then a large number of clicks (10 clicks/sec for about 1000 clicks) are delivered to one ear and then the other. The computer enhances the electrical activity resulting from the clicks and records them as wave activity.

Purpose

- BAER is used to:

  ○ *Diagnose* cerebral deficiencies of the eighth nerve (e.g., multiple sclerosis, posterior fossa tumors).

  ○ *Assess* coma and cerebral death.

Findings

It takes about 10 msec for a sound stimulus to reach the cerebral cortex. Lesions at different sites in a tract along the 8th cranial nerve through the brainstem and into the cerebral cortex will alter these waves in different ways, providing a method of locating a suspected brainstem lesion.

Pharmacy Implications   None.

CT of the Head

See General Procedures: CT on page 6–2.

Electroencephalography (EEG)[4,11,53,54]

Description

Electrodes are placed on the scalp in the form of small discs. They are fastened to the scalp after an electrical conduction paste has been applied to the scalp/electrodes. The electrodes are connected by wires to an amplifier and are arranged in one of several patterns on the scalp. Electrical impulses from the brain (alpha, beta, and delta waves) are recorded on a moving paper tape. This tape is then compared against a standardized normal tape and against tapes showing patterns for specific pathologies to make a diagnosis. A period of hyperventilation and light stimulation at different frequencies is used to stimulate the brain. The EEG may be done under normal

Electroencephalography (EEG)[4,11,53,54] *(Continued)*

Description
(Continued)

conditions in a sleep-induced state or in a sleep-deprived state. All of these states have characteristic electrical patterns.

Purpose

- EEG is used to:

  ○ *Measure and Record* electrical impulses in the brain to diagnose seizure disorders. An EEG should be performed while the patient is having a seizure or as soon after the seizure as possible. Simultaneous video monitoring and EEG monitoring may be necessary to classify the seizure.

  ○ *Aid* in identifying brain tumors, abscesses, and subdural hematomas.

  ○ *Ascertain* information about the possibility of other cerebrovascular diseases such as cerebral infarcts and intracranial hemorrhage, and cerebral diseases such as advanced cases of multiple sclerosis, narcolepsy, and acute delirium.

  ○ *Determine* brain death.

  ○ *Aid* in the diagnosis and characterization of sleep apnea.

Findings

Normal

The EEG tracing produces a tape that is consistent with normal electrical brain activity in the awake and sleep state.

Abnormal

Brain wave activity consistent with a seizure disorder or other cerebral disease or lesion. A flat EEG results from cerebral hypoxia or ischemia from which there is no neurological recovery.

Pharmacy Implications

- A sleep EEG patient receives chloral hydrate 1 to 2 gm PO before the test to promote rest and sleep.

- Withhold caffeine-containing drinks for 8 hours before the test.

- Drugs altering brain wave activity (e.g. anticonvulsants, sedatives, tranquilizers) will interfere with an accurate tracing.

Electromyography (EMG)[4,11,53,55]

Description

Skin surface electrodes (bipolar electrodes) or needle electrodes (monopolar electrodes) are attached to measure and record muscle nerve impulses. A needle electrode is inserted into the muscle to pick up the electrical activity. This electrical activity is amplified and displayed on a cathode-ray oscillograph and a permanent record is obtained by recording on a magnetic

Electromyography (EMG)[4,11,53,55] *(Continued)*

Description
(Continued)

tape. When the muscle is voluntarily or electrically stimulated, a muscle action potential is produced.

Purpose

The amplitude, duration, number, and configuration of the muscle action potentials aid in differentiating neurogenic pathology from myogenic involvement.

Findings

Normal

A normally relaxed muscle is electrically silent at rest. During voluntary contraction, electrical activity increases markedly.

Abnormal

Waveforms that are different from normal muscle are evaluated to differentiate a muscle disorder from a denervation disorder. These results can aid in the diagnosis of muscular dystrophies, amyotrophic lateral sclerosis, peripheral nerve disorders, and myasthenia gravis.

Pharmacy Implications

Drugs that affect the nerve-muscle junction (e.g., cholinergics, anticholinergics, skeletal muscle relaxants) can interfere with the test results.

Lumbar Puncture (LP)[11,56]

Description

The patient lies on his side at the edge of a firm surface with knees drawn up and head bent forward to put the spine in hyper-flexion. The usual site of puncture is between the 3rd and 4th (or 4th and 5th) lumbar vertebrae. The area is cleaned with an antiseptic and locally anesthetized. The lumbar puncture needle (3 to 4 inches in length) is inserted through the skin in the midline between the vertebra, perpendicular to the surface of the back and diverted slightly upward toward the patient's head. When the needle penetrates the dura and enters the spinal canal, a slight decrease in resistance can be felt. Once the spinal canal has been penetrated cerebrospinal fluid (CSF) is removed.

Purpose

• Lumbar puncture is used to:

  ° *Obtain* a CSF specimen for diagnostic study.

  ° *Aid* in the diagnosis of suspected meningitis, intracranial hemorrhage, and CNS involvement from malignant disease (e.g., leukemia, lymphoma).

  ° *Determine* the CSF pressure to document impairment of flow or to lessen pressure by removing a volume of fluid.

  ° *Diagnose* organic central nervous system disease (e.g., multiple sclerosis).

Lumbar Puncture (LP)[11,56] *(Continued)*

Purpose (Continued)	• Lumbar puncture is used to:
	° *Evaluate* certain electrolyte disturbances.
	° *Remove* blood or exudate from the subarachnoid space.
	° *Administer* x-ray contrast media (e.g., myelogram) or to give drugs intrathecally (e.g., antibiotics and antineoplastic agents).
Findings	
Normal	Normal appearance, consistency, expected cell composition, absence of bacteria, normal chemistry of the fluid, and normal pressure. (See Chapter 5: Laboratory Tests for normal CSF composition).
Abnormal	See Table 6–4.
Pharmacy Implications	• Patients may experience a headache following removal of CSF, requiring treatment with an analgesic.
	• Patients should lie flat for up to 8 hr after the procedure.

MRI of the Head

See General Procedures: MRI on page 6–4.

Myelography[4]

Description	Myelography is a fluoroscopic and radiographic study using an iodine contrast (iophendylate, metrizamide, or iohexol) which is introduced by lumbar puncture into the spinal subarachnoid space to outline the spinal cord, nerve roots, and detect any distortion of dura mater. If a water soluble contrast medium (metrizamide or iohexol) is used it does not have to be removed from the spinal column after the study is complete. However, if an oil contrast medium (iophendylate) is used, removal from the spinal column is necessary because it cannot be excreted. This test is sometimes followed or replaced by CT scanning which can improve visualization.

Table 6–4: Abnormal CSF Fluid

Appearance	Cloudy fluid
Protein Content	>50 mg/dL
Glucose Concentration	<30 mg/dL or >70 mg/dL
WBCs	>10/mm^3
pH of Fluid	< or >7.3
Bacteria or Virus	Present
RBCs	Present

Myelography[4] *(Continued)*

Purpose	• Myelograph is used to detect abnormalities of the spinal cord (e.g., neoplasms, ruptured disks, extraspinal pathology, spinal stenosis) and to confirm the need for surgery.
	• Candidates for the test are patients with unrelieved back pain, absent knee or ankle reflex, past history of cancer with loss of leg or bladder control, and muscle weakness.

Findings

Normal — Normal outline of spinal cord and normal nerve structures. No masses present. Contrast medium flows freely through subarachnoid space.

Abnormal — Tumors present in the subarachnoid space or spinal cord; compression and stenosis of the spinal cord; herniated intervertebral disks; or nerve root injury.

Pharmacy Implications

• Patients should not receive solid food after midnight.

• A sedative and anticholinergic may be administered before the procedure.

• If metrizamide is used as the contrast medium, phenothiazines should not be administered for 48 hours before or for 24 hours after the procedure. Metrizamide may increase the risk of seizures. Phenothiazines can exacerbate this risk. Use benzquinamide for nausea and vomiting postprocedure.

• Iohexol use does not require avoidance of phenothiazines.

• Analgesics may be needed after the procedure to treat headache, back pain, and neck stiffness resulting from the test.

Muscle Biopsy[57,58]

Description — A muscle biopsy involves surgical incision and excision of the desired muscle segment (open biopsy) or by a needle method (percutaneous).

Purpose

• Muscle biopsy is used to:

  ° *Investigate* the origin of muscle weakness (neurogenic or myogenic).

  ° *Diagnose* localized or diffuse inflammatory disease of the muscle, and suspected genetic diseases of the muscle.

  ° *Assist* in the diagnosis of diffuse vascular, connective tissue, and metabolic diseases.

  ° *Evaluate* suspected myopathy.

Muscle Biopsy[57,58] *(Continued)*

Findings

Normal   In all cases, presence of normal pathology and histology.

Abnormal   Presence of myogenic changes.

Pharmacy Implications
- It is recommended that antiplatelet agents be discontinued before open and needle biopsies. Stop aspirin 7 to 10 days before the procedure. Discontinue NSAIDs which reversibly inhibit the enzyme cyclooxygenase (e.g., ibuprofen, naproxen) 2 to 4 days before the procedure.

- Preprocedure medications such as parenteral analgesics (e.g. meperidine, morphine) and parenteral sedatives/anxiolytics (e.g., lorazepam, diazepam, midazolam) may be administered.

- A local anesthetic (e.g., lidocaine) may be necessary.

Nerve Biopsy[59]

Description   The sural nerve, situated in the lower leg near the achilles tendon, and the deep peroneal nerve, located in an area of the calf below the knee, are the two most commonly biopsied nerves. An incision is made, the nerve is exposed, and by sharp dissection a 3 to 4 cm length of nerve or nerve tissue is removed for evaluation. A nerve deficit may occur as a result of the biopsy.

Purpose   Nerve biopsies are performed to diagnose neuropathic disorders producing a clinical picture of mononeuropathy multiplex, sarcoidosis, vasculitis, amyloidosis, leprosy, or genetically determined pediatric neurological disorders.

Findings

Normal   Presence of normal pathology and histology.

Abnormal   Presence of polyarteritis nodosa, amyloidosis, sarcoidosis, neuropathy, leprosy, metachromatic leukodystrophy, Krabbe's disease, ataxia telangiectasia, giant axonal neuropathy, and infantile neuroaxonal dystrophy.

Pharmacy Implications It is recommended that antiplatelet agents be stopped before open and needle biopsies. Stop aspirin 7 to 10 days before the procedure. Discontinue NSAIDs which reversibility inhibit the enzyme cyclooxygenase (e.g., ibuprofen, naproxen) 2 to 4 days before the procedure.

Visual Evoked Response (VER)[51,52]

Description   EEG electrodes are placed on the scalp over the occipital or visual cortex area. Baseline electrical activity is recorded. The patient is instructed to fix on a

Visual Evoked Response (VER)[51,52] *(Continued)*

Description (Continued)	point. A visual stimulus such as flashes of light or a sudden change of a checkerboard pattern is administered. First one eye is stimulated, then the other. The time interval between the stimulus and the response is recorded and displayed.
Purpose	VERs aid in the diagnosis of lesions of the optic nerve (e.g., multiple sclerosis, retrobulbar neuritis, toxic and nutritional amblyopias, ischemic optic neuropathy, Liber hereditary optic neuropathy).
Findings	A difference in the responses between the left and right eye, with an increased latency and duration in one eye, indicates a lesion in that optic nerve. However, there may be lesions in both optic nerves.
Pharmacy Implications	None.

OPHTHALMOLOGY

Funduscopy[60,61]

Description	The inner eye is viewed via an ophthalmoscope, an instrument with a special illumination system. A strong light is directed into the patient's eye by reflection from a small mirror. The light is reflected from the fundus of the eye back through the ophthalmoscope to the examiner. The opening of the instrument is held as close as possible to the patient's and the examiner's eye.
Purpose	Funduscopy examines the fundus of the eye including the optic disk, macula, retina, retinal vessels, choroid, and sclera. Base line and follow up funduscopy is recommended when hypertension or diabetes is present or when certain drugs are being taken.
Findings	
Normal	Optic disk is normal size, color, and vascularity. Macula is devoid of blood vessels and darker than surrounding retina. Retina is attached and has normal vascularity and color. Choroid and sclera should not be visualized.
Abnormal	Two descriptive approaches for staging or grading of retinopathy are used. The choice of grading methods for retinal vascular changes is influenced by the underlying disease. (See Table 6–5.)
	Optic disk has abnormal vascularity, elevation (bulging), small hemorrhages, and abnormal color. The macula is edematous and ischemic with degeneration appearing as a round white mass. Choroid and sclera-visualization of vessels. Malignant melanoma appears as a pigmented elevated mass.

Funduscopy[60,61] *(Continued)*

Pharmacy Implications	Drugs affecting the retina include chloroquine, hydroxychloroquine, phenothiazines, penicillamine, isoniazid, ethambutol, and indomethacin.

Slit Lamp Examination[60,62]

Description	Slit lamp examination involves the combination of a light and microscopic examination of the eye. Dilation of the pupil using a mydriatic and cyclopegic agent facilitates viewing.
Purpose	The slit lamp allows for examination of the lids, cornea, anterior chamber of the eye, and transparent and nearly transparent ocular fluids and tissues.
Findings	
Normal	Clear, avascular vitreous fluid.
Abnormal	Vitreous disease including retraction, condensation, and shrinkage. Presence of blood and floaters. Presence of cataracts or corneal deposits.
Pharmacy Implications	Slit lamp examination may be needed to evaluate drug-induced ocular toxicity associated with indomethacin, clofazimine, allopurinol, corticosteroids, gold salts, chloroquine, hydroxychloroquine, griseofulvin, chlorambucil, cytosine arabinoside, mitotane, tamoxifen, amiodarone, quinidine, phenothiazines, phenytoin, and isotretinoin.

TABLE 6–5: Retinal Vascular Grading Systems

Hypertensive Retinopathy (Keith-Wagner Method)

Grade I	Constriction of retinal arterioles only
Grade II	Constriction and sclerosis of retinal arterioles
Grade III	Hemorrhages and exudates in addition to vascular changes
Grade IV	Papilledema (edema of the optic disk)

Diabetic Retinopathy (Retinal Changes Fall Into Two Categories)

Background Retinopathy

— Multiple microaneurysms appear

— Veins dilate, multiple dot and blot hemorrhages occur, and hard waxy white and yellow exudates may leak from the retinal vasculature in the area of the macula

— Cotton-wool patches (microinfarcts of the retinal nerve fiber layer) appear in the superficial retina. Hard exudates may form what is described as the macular star

Proliferative Retinopathy

— Neovascularization occurs

— Neovascularization of the optic disk occurs

— End-stage retinopathy with organized vitreous hemorrhage, fibrosis, and retinitis profilerans (detached retina) leading to blindness.

Tonometry (Applanation)[60,63]

Description	After first anesthetizing the eye with a topical anesthetic, fluorescein is dripped in the eye to outline the corneal rings (standard area of the cornea). The applanating prism mounted at the end of an arm projecting vertically from a black box is placed in contact with the patient's cornea. A knob on the black box actuates a spring loaded device which allows an examiner to increase or decrease the pressure necessary to flatten a standard area of cornea. The pressure needed for flattening to occur is read off a scale on the knob.
Purpose	Tonometry measures the eye's intraocular pressure.
Findings	
Normal	10 to 20 mm Hg (16 mm average).
Abnormal	>24 mm Hg diagnostic for glaucoma.
Pharmacy Implications	Drugs that may increase intraocular pressure include anticholinergics, corticosteroids, and sympathomimetics.

ORTHOPEDICS

Arthroscopy[4,7,11]

Description	Arthroscopy is visual examination of a joint (most commonly the knee) using a special fiber optic endoscope called an arthroscope. Arthroscopy is commonly performed using a local anesthetic. However, general or spinal anesthesia may be used if surgery is anticipated. Approximately, 75 to 100 mL of normal saline solution is injected into the joint to distend it. The arthroscope is then inserted close to the knee tendon and upper tibia. All parts of the knee are examined at various degrees of flexion and extension, and joint washings are examined.
Purpose	• Arthroscopy is used to:
	○ *Diagnose* athletic injuries and differentiate and diagnose acute and chronic disorders of the knee and other large joints.
	○ *Perform* joint surgery or monitor progression of disease and effectiveness of therapy.
Findings	
Normal	Normal joint vasculature, normal color of synovium, and normal ligaments, cartilage, and suprapatellar pouch.
Abnormal	Torn and displaced cartilage and meniscus, trapped synovium, loose fragments of bone or cartilage, torn ligaments, chronic inflammatory arthritis, chondromalacia of bone, secondary osteoarthritis, presence of cysts or foreign bodies.

Arthroscopy[4,7,11] *(Continued)*

Pharmacy Implications
- Patient should be NPO from midnight before the procedure.
- A sedative usually given before the exam.
- Analgesics may be given after the procedure as needed for pain. Anti-inflammatory agents (NSAIDs) are commonly used along with narcotic analgesics.

Arthrography[4,64]

Description
An arthrogram is an x-ray of a joint following injection of contrast media into the synovium. Joints most often examined in this manner are the knee, hip, and shoulders.

Purpose
Arthrography elucidates soft tissue injury in cartilage and ligaments surrounding the joint that cannot be seen with conventional x-ray techniques.

Findings

Normal
Normal anatomy and condition of the joint supportive tissues.

Abnormal
Ligamentous and cartilaginous tears or injuries.

Pharmacy Implications
Hypersensitivity reactions to the iodine dye are less likely to occur due to the small amount of iodine present in the synovial space.

Bone Scan

Description
A bone scan is an x-ray of the whole body after intravenous injection of a Tc-99m methylene diphosphate. The radionuclide has particular affinity for bone and collects in areas of abnormal metabolism. There is a 2 to 3 hour waiting period after injection of the tracer to allow for full concentration in the bone.

Purpose
- Bone scans are used to:
  - *Determine* site of bone and bone marrow biopsy.
  - *Diagnose* myeloproliferative disorders.
  - *Identify* focal defects in bone and bone marrow.
  - *Stage* lymphoma or Hodgkin's disease or find cancer metastases.
  - *Aid* in the diagnosis of bone pain and inflammatory processes (e.g., infection-osteomyletis).

Findings

Normal
The radioisotope is distributed evenly throughout the bone. No "hot spots" (concentrated areas of uptake) are noted.

Abnormal
Presence of "hot spots" indicating increased concentration of the radioactive compound at sites of abnor-

Bone Scan *(Continued)*

Findings (Continued)	mal metabolism (e.g. infection, fracture, degenerative bone disease, failing bone grafts). Bone marrow depression following radiation or chemotherapy. Nonvisualization in myelofibrosis. Sites of primary bone tumors and bone metastases from other malignancies.
Pharmacy Implications	None.

OTOLARYNGOLOGY

Laryngoscopy[65,66]

Description
- Three types of examination can be performed:
  - ° *Indirect* involving the placement of a laryngeal mirror in the mouth and a light source to visualize the back of the tongue, the epiglottis, valleculae, the pyriform fossae, and the structures of the larynx.
  - ° *Direct Involving the Use of a Flexible Fiber Optic Nasolaryngoscope.* The scope is passed through the locally anesthetized nasal cavity and then suspended above the larynx to provide a direct view of the nose, nasopharynx, larynx, and adjacent structures.
  - ° *Direct Involving the Use of a Rigid, Lighted Laryngoscope.* This technique requires the patient to undergo general anesthesia. The scope is inserted through the mouth and passed through the throat to expose the larynx and its structures.

Purpose
- Laryngoscopy is used to:
  - ° *Examine* the visible structures for disease, trauma, and strictures.
  - ° *Detect and Remove* foreign bodies.
  - ° *Perform* tissue biopsies of suspicious lesions to aid in the diagnosis of cancer.

Findings

Normal — Normal position, color, and anatomy of the examined area. Absence of lesions, strictures, inflammation, and foreign bodies.

Abnormal — Color changes of laryngeal and adjacent structures. Position changes, presence of lesions, strictures, or foreign bodies.

Laryngoscopy[65,66] *(Continued)*

Pharmacy Implications	• **Indirect Laryngoscopy.** None.
	• **Direct Fiber Optic Laryngoscopy.** A sedative/anxiolytic (e.g., midazolam, diazepam) may be administered before the procedure.
	• **Direct Rigid Laryngoscopy.** An anticholinergic (e.g., atropine or glycopyrrolate) IM and a sedative/anxiolytic (e.g., midazolam) IM may be administered 30 minutes before the procedure.

PULMONARY

Bronchial Alveolar Lavage (BAL)

See Bronchoscopy.

Bronchoscopy[67]

Description	Bronchoscopy is the examination of the inside of the tracheobronchial tree by direct visualization. After first anesthetizing the throat with a local anesthetic, a flexible fiber optic bronchoscope is inserted through an oral endotracheal tube and into the tracheobronchial tree. An eyepiece at the proximal end of the bronchoscope allows viewing. A camera can also be attached to the eye piece.
Purpose	• Bronchoscopy is used to:
	° *View* nasopharyngeal and laryngeal lesions, and visualize the source of hemoptysis.
	° *Further Evaluate* a patient with positive sputum cytology.
	° *Perform* transbronchial biopsy of the lung, and bronchial alveolar lavage (BAL).
	° *Assess* recurrent nerve paralysis.
Findings	
Normal	No tumors, lesions, or source of bleeding, infection, or cancer.
Abnormal	Presence of tumors, infections, or other abnormal findings as stated above.
Pharmacy Implications	• Patient should not receive food or drink after midnight the evening before the procedure.
	• Administer parenterally a skeletal muscle relaxant (e.g., a benzodiazepine) and an anticholinergic (e.g., atropine) to dry up secretions 30 to 60 minutes be-

Bronchoscopy[67] *(Continued)*

Description
(Continued)

fore the procedure. An analgesic such as meperidine may also be administered IM or IV before the procedure.

- The patient should be NPO for 1 to 2 hours after the procedure to reduce the risk of aspiration. Administer clear liquids initially and observe for swallowing difficulties.

Chest X-ray[4,11]

Description

A chest x-ray is an x-ray of the chest from the front, side, and sometimes back. It is best performed with the patient in the standing position.

Purpose

Chest x-rays are useful in the diagnosis of pulmonary, mediastinal, and bony thorax disease. The standing position demonstrates the presence of fluid levels.

Findings

Normal

Absence of fluids, masses, and infection. Air filled spaces appear black.

Abnormal

The film will have opacities (shadowy or white areas) suggestive of the presence of fluid, tumors and other lesions, infectious processes, unusual air in the lungs, or a collapsed lung. Spinal deformities, bone destruction, and trauma can be observed.

Pharmacy Implications

None.

CT of the Chest

See General Procedures: CT on page 6–2.

Pulmonary Function Tests (PFTs)[80, 81]

Description

Using spirometry a patient is instructed first to inhale and then exhale as rapidly as possible. As the patient exhales into the spirometer, he displaces a bell and the pen deflection records the volume of air entering or exiting the lung (see Figure 6–1).

The *tidal volume* or the volume of air being inhaled and exhaled during normal breathing can be recorded. The *vital capacity* (VC) is the amount of air being moved during maximal inhalation and exhalation. *Residual volume* (RV) reflects the volume of air left in the lung after maximal expiration. *Total lung capacity* (TLC) is the sum of the vital capacity and the residual volume. Patients with restrictive lung disease often display a decrease in all lung volumes, while those individuals with obstructive disease often have normal TLC but decreased VC and an increased RV.

FIGURE 6–1: Spirometric Graphics During Quiet Breathing and Maximal Breathing. Reprinted with permission. Applied Therapeutics: The Clinical Use of Drugs. 5th edition. Applied Therapeutics Inc., 1992.

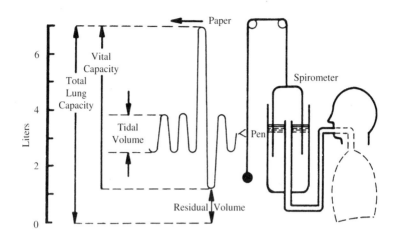

Pulmonary Function Tests (PFTs)[80, 81] *(Continued)*

Description
(Continued)

In evaluating the performance of the lung, forced expiration techniques together with a spirometer can measure lung volumes and air flow, providing useful information in graphic form (see Figures 6–2 and 6–3). The *forced expiratory volume* (FEV) measures the amount of air the patient can exhale after a maximal inhalation, often over a set period of time such as 1 sec (FEV_1). Together with the *forced vital capacity* (FVC), which measures the maximum volume of air exhaled with maximally forced effort after a maximal inhalation effort, these values can provide important performance measures of the lung. The *peak expiratory flow rate* (PEFR) measures the maximal flow that can be produced during the forced expiration. Generally, this measurement provides similar information as the FEV_1 but is less reproducible. Another measurement is the *forced expiratory flow* which occurs during the middle 50% of the expiratory curve [$FEF_{25\%-75\%}$, $FEF_{50\%}$ or maximal midexpiratory flow rate (MEFR)]. This measure is helpful for patients with emphysema since it represents the elastic recoil force of the lung and is less dependent on the patient's expiratory effort.

Spirometry can also be used to establish the reversibility of airway disease. The use of bronchodilators can be administered after baseline pulmonary function tests to

FIGURE 6–2: Reprinted with permission. Applied Therapeutics: The Clinical Use of Drugs. 5th edition. Applied Therapeutics Inc., 1992.

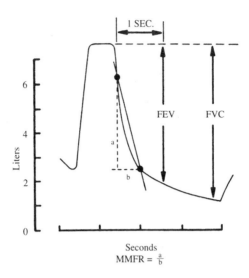

$$\text{MMFR} = \tfrac{a}{b}$$

FIGURE 6–3: Flow/Volume Curve Resulting from a Forced Expiratory Maneuver. Reprinted with permission. Applied Therapeutics: The Clinical Use of Drugs. 5th edition. Applied Therapeutics Inc., 1992.

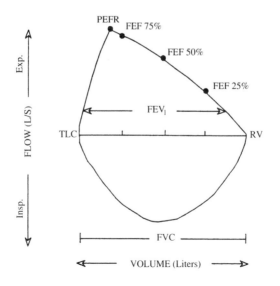

Pulmonary Function Tests (PFTs)[80, 81] *(Continued)*

Description *(Continued)*	determine the degree of reversibility. Generally a significant clinical reversibility is defined as a 15% to 20% improvement in the FEV_1 after administration of the bronchodilator.
	Arterial blood gases ($PaCO_2$, pH, PaO_2) are often performed at the same time as spirometry to assess the degree of blood oxygenation. The use of the carbon monoxide diffusing capacity (D_{co}) can help determine whether the ventilatory change is due to poor diffusion or ventilation. This test involves the inspiration of a small amount of carbon monoxide (CO) which is then held for 10 seconds while the blood CO test is measured. A reduction is seen in emphysema, pulmonary edema, and pulmonary fibrosis and is normal in asthma and pneumonia. For a more complete discussion the reader is referred to the Laboratory section.
Purpose	The respiratory system is responsible for the exchange of carbon dioxide (CO_2) and oxygen (O_2). Together with the circulatory system, body tissues can exchange CO_2 and receive adequate O_2. Occasionally, a variety of disease processes alter the exchanges of these gases between the alveoli and the blood stream. Thus, to provide an objective measurement of the respiratory system, pulmonary function tests can be performed.
	Pulmonary disorders are often classified as restrictive or obstructive. Typical air flow and volume curves can assist with classifying the disorder as shown in (see Figure 6–4).
Findings	
Normal	FEV_1/FVC 75% to 80%
Abnormal	In the obstructive pattern which reflects limitations to airflow during expiration, the expiratory flow rate is decreased. In later stages of the disease the FEV_1/FVC and $FEF_{25\%-75\%}$ are also reduced. The TLC may be normal or increased and the RV is elevated due to trapping of air during expiration. The ratio of RV/TLC is often increased.
	A restrictive pattern of lung disease which closely corresponds to impairment in inhalation (e.g., bronchitis, asthma) will present as a decrease in lung volumes, primarily TLC and VC.
Pharmacy Implications	• Administer bronchodilators before the procedure to evaluate degree of reversibility.
	• No preparation needed before or after the procedure, unless bronchodilators are used.

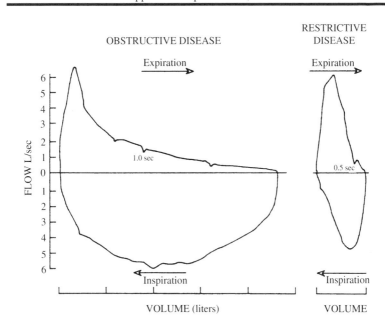

Sweat Test[4,68]

Description

Pilocarpine solution is applied topically to the forearm and 3 milliamps of current causes pilocarpine penetration into the skin and stimulates the sweat glands. The area is then washed with distilled water, and a preweighed filter paper is placed over the area for 30 to 60 minutes and covered to prevent evaporation. The filter paper is removed, weighed, and diluted in distilled water. A chloridometer is then used to determine the concentration of chloride. A minimum of 50 to 100 mg of sweat must be collected for an accurate result.

Purpose

Sweat tests are used to diagnose cystic fibrosis (CF) in conjunction with one or more other symptoms (i.e., documented exocrine pancreatic insufficiency, chronic obstructive airways disease, or a positive family history).

Findings

Normal

Chloride value in children is <40 mEq/L and in healthy adults may be up to 80 mEq/L.

Sweat Test[4,68] *(Continued)*

Findings *(Continued)*

Abnormal

- Chloride >60 mEq/L is diagnostic of CF if one or more of the above symptoms are present up to age of 20. Chloride levels of 40 to 60 mEq/L may be suggestive of CF in those patients who tend to have relatively normal pancreatic function.

- Other conditions which may cause elevations of sweat chloride include: untreated adrenal insufficiency; ectodermal dysplasia; glucose-6-phosphatase deficiency; hypothyroidism; hypoparathyroidism; familial cholestasis; pancreatic insufficiency; mucopolysaccharidosis; fucosidosis; and malnutrition.

Pharmacy Implications   None.

Thoracentesis[4,47,69]

Description

Thoracentesis involves the insertion of a needle into the pleural space. The patient may either straddle a straight backed chair or lay supine in bed with the affected side elevated. The patient's arm is extended at one side and a site at the 4th or 5th intercostal space along the posterior axillary line is selected. The skin is anesthetized and an infiltration needle is advanced over the upper boarder of the rib below the level of the fluid into the pleural space while anesthetic is being injected. The infiltration needle is withdrawn and a large gauge aspiration needle attached to a glass syringe with 3-way stopcock is introduced into the pleural cavity. Fluid is then withdrawn and via the stopcock the fluid is discharged through a side arm and tubing into a sterile heparinized flask. In the case of a large pleural effusion, an Intra Cath is used. This permits removal of the needle after the catheter has been diverted into the most dependent area of the pleural cavity and aspiration is then performed using a 3-way stopcock attached to the catheter. This catheter technique reduces the incidence of pneumothorax when the patient's position needs to be altered.

Purpose

- Thoracentesis is used to:
  - *Remove* pleural fluid for culture, cell count, specific gravity, chemical analysis, and cytology for characterization as either a transudate (due to abnormalities of hydrostatic or osmotic pressure) or an exudate (due to increased vascular permeability or trauma). Transudate fluid can be differentiated from exudate fluid by a protein content, the ratio of pleural to serum protein, the LDH content, and the ratio of pleural LDH to serum content.

Thoracentesis[4,47,69] *(Continued)*

Purpose *(Continued)*	° *Tap* pleural effusions to make the patient more comfortable.
	° *Inject* sclerosing agents such as antibiotics or cytotoxic agents into the pleural space to prevent further effusions.

Findings

Normal	No pleural fluid.
Abnormal	Blood in the pleural space (hemothorax) is generally a sign of a traumatic injury. Large volumes of pleural fluid due to inflammatory lung disease or neoplasms may be encountered. Cells may be found that will confirm the cell-type of a malignancy. Infectious organisms found in the pleural fluid.

Pharmacy Implications

- Drugs such as bleomycin (60 U in 50 mL normal saline solution) or doxycycline (500 mg in 30 mL normal saline solution) may be instilled into the pleural space as sclerosing agents.

- Patients may require a sedative and/or an analgesic 30 to 45 minutes before the procedure.

Ventilation-Perfusion Scintigraphy (V-Q Scan)[4,70–72]

Description	The perfusion portion of the study requires aggregates of albumin labeled with technetium (Tc-99m) to be injected intravenously into the patient. These particles lodge in capillaries and precapillaries of the lung. The lungs are viewed with a gamma camera immediately after injection for perfusion. The ventilation portion of the study involves the breathing of air mixed with radioactive gas. A nuclear scanner monitors the distribution of the gas in the lungs.
Purpose	V-Q scan is used to diagnose pulmonary embolism and to a lesser extent bronchiectasis, bronchial obstruction, and bronchopleural fistula.

Findings

Normal	Normal perfusion. No clinically significant pulmonary emboli.
Abnormal	Normal areas of ventilation combined with segmental perfusion defects indicating pulmonary embolus.
Pharmacy Implications	None.

UROLOGY

Cystometrography (CMG)[4,73]

Description

A catheter is placed through the urethra into the bladder. The catheter is connected to a cystometer which measures neuromuscular activity of the bladder. During the procedure the bladder is filled with sterile water, normal saline, carbon dioxide gas, or radiographic contrast. Throughout the procedure the patient is asked to report bladder sensory perceptions of hot and cold, fullness, and urge to void. Pressures and volumes are automatically recorded and plotted on a graph. The patient is also asked to report sensations associated with neurologic stimulation of the bladder and sphincter muscles (e.g., flushing, sweating, pain, nausea). Cholinergic and anticholinergic drugs may be instilled into the bladder to assess its function by altering neurostimulation to the bladder.

Purpose

CMG is used to assess the integrity of neuroanatomic connections between the spinal cord and the bladder. This exam is most useful in patients with known or suspected neurologic deficiencies (e.g., individuals who have sustained traumatic spinal cord injuries).

Findings

Normal

Bladder wall activity demonstrates appropriate motor and sensory function with a normal bladder filling pattern.

Abnormal

Findings reveal either an uninhibited, reflex or autonomous neurogenic bladder, or a sensory or motor paralytic bladder. Each dysfunction is associated with specific neurons from the spinal cord.

Pharmacy Implications

All drugs that can affect bladder function should be held before the procedure.

Cystoscopy[4,65]

Description

Direct visual examination of the entire surface of the urethra, prostate (in men only), and bladder by use of a rigid or flexible fiber optic scope. This examination is also known as cystourethroscopy.

Purpose

- Cystoscopy is used to:

  ° *Evaluate* patients with hematuria, voiding problems, history of bladder tumors, chronic urinary tract infections, or abnormalities revealed by other studies.

Cystoscopy[4,65] *(Continued)*

Purpose (Continued)
- Cystoscopy is used to:
  - *Perform* biopsies and extract stones from the lower ureters and from the bladder.
  - *Perform* bladder irrigation and to instill drugs.
  - *Perform* resection and fulguration of bladder tumors, and transurethral resection of the prostate.

Findings

Normal

Normal anatomy, absence of strictures, stones, and tumors.

Abnormal

Presence of stones, obstruction, stricture, tumors, signs of inflammation and infection, and sites of bleeding.

Pharmacy Implications
- Cystoscopy can be performed with local anesthetic (e.g., lidocaine gel instilled into the urethra).
- A benzodiazepine such as diazepam or midazolam may be administered before the procedure.
- Cystoscopy may be performed under general anesthetia in which case an analgesic such as morphine and an anticholinergic such as atropine may be administered preoperatively.

Intravenous Pyelography (IVP)[4,74]

Description

IVP is visualization of the kidneys and collecting system both intrarenal (renal calices) and extrarenal (ureter and bladder) by administration of an iodine contrast dye through a vein followed by x-rays taken at 5, 10, 15, and 20 minutes after the injection of dye. The term intravenous pyelography inaccurately describes the extent of this procedure since the term limits the anatomy studied to the renal pelvis and calyceal system. In actuality, the study examines anatomy beyond the scope of this term and should more appropriately be referred to as urography.

Purpose
- IVP is used to:
  - *Detect* congenital abnormalities, kidney obstruction, and changes in renal size.
  - *Determine* the presence of renal masses (tumors, cysts, abscesses, or stones).
  - *Assess* the extent of renal damage after traumatic injury.
  - *Evaluate* a unilateral non-functioning kidney.

Findings

Normal

No anatomical defects, no obstructions, no masses, and a functional collecting system.

Intravenous Pyelography (IVP)[4,74] *(Continued)*

Findings (Continued)

Abnormal	Presence of obstruction, masses, stones, signs of trauma to the kidney, or compromised function of the collecting system.

Pharmacy Implications

- Administer 75 mL senna fruit concentrate at 1600 the day before the procedure.

- The patient should only have clear liquids after the senna.

- Patients are NPO the morning of the exam.

- There is a potential for hypersensitivity reactions to the contrast dye.

- Do not perform IVPs in patients whose creatinine clearance is <25 mL/min.

- Maintain adequate hydration (IV or PO) after the procedure to prevent renal injury from the dye.

Kidneys, Ureters, Bladder (KUB)

See Abdominal X-Ray on page 6–19.

Retrograde Pyelography[4,11,75]

Description A ureter is catheterized through a cystoscope and dye is injected in a retrograde direction (opposite the normal flow of urine). An x-ray is then taken to visualize the ureters.

Purpose Retrograde pyelography allows visualization of the collecting structures of the kidney (renal pelvis) and ureters which together comprise the upper urinary tract. It is also used to confirm findings suspected on the IVP.

Findings

Normal	Normal anatomy of the ureters and kidney pelvis.
Abnormal	Intrinsic disease of ureters and pelvis of the kidneys. Also, diseases of the ureters including obstructive tumors or stones.

Pharmacy Implications See Cystoscopy.

Voiding Cystourethrography[4,76]

Description Contrast medium is instilled into the bladder via a Foley catheter. X-rays are taken as the bladder fills and when the patient voids.

Voiding Cystourethrography[4,76] *(Continued)*

Purpose
- A voiding cystourethrography is used to:
  - *Determine* potential causes of chronic urinary tract infections (UTIs), bladder emptying dysfunction, and incontinence.
  - *Evaluate* congenital abnormalities of the lower urinary tract, and evaluate and perform follow-up of patients with spinal cord injuries who have voiding difficulties.
  - *Evaluate* prostatic hypertrophy in males, suspected strictures of urethra, and a patient before renal transplantation.

Findings

Normal — Appropriate bladder and urethra structure and function.

Abnormal — Urethral strictures and diverticula, ureteroceles, prostatic enlargement, vesicoureteral reflux, or neurogenic bladder.

Pharmacy Implications — Iodine contrast medium may produce a hypersensitivity reaction. Special precautions should be taken in patients with known hypersensitivities to iodine compounds.

VASCULAR
Arteriography/Venography[47]

Description — An iodine contrast dye is injected into an artery (arteriogram) or a vein (venogram) by means of a needle or catheter in order to outline and view a portion of the arterial or venous system. The arteries or veins are then observed using fluoroscopy and x-rays.

Purpose — Arteriography is used to examine and evaluate the arterial or venous system of a particular organ or area of the body and to evaluate the flow into or out of that given area. This allows for the detection of lesions and abnormalities of flow and can allow for surgical correction if possible.

Findings

Normal — No flow abnormalities.

Abnormal — Presence of clots, strictures, obstructions, lesions, incompetent valves, or congenital abnormalities.

Pharmacy Implications
- Iodine contrast dye may produce hypersensitivity reactions or anaphylaxis. Special precautions should be taken in patients with known hypersensitivities to iodine compounds.

Arteriography/Venography[47] *(Continued)*

Pharmacy Implications
(Continued)

- When necessary, diphenhydramine, ranitidine, and prednisone may be started at least 12 hours before the procedure to prevent or reduce the severity of the hypersensitivity reaction.

- Adequate hydration should be provided to reduce the risk of renal injury from the contrast media.

Doppler Studies[4,53, 77]

Description

A doppler is an ultrasound blood flow detector which is sensitive to frequency shifts reflected from moving blood cells. The doppler is placed on the area for evaluation (e.g., peripheral artery, vein, or extracranial cerebrovascular vessel). A probe (transducer) directs high frequency sound waves through tissue and hits RBCs in the blood stream. The frequency of sound waves changes in proportion to the flow velocity of RBCs. The transducer then amplifies the sound waves which permits direct listening. A graphic recording of the blood flow can also be made from the sound waves. Systolic pressures using compression maneuvers are also measured. To evaluate arterial disease in the lower extremities, a pressure cuff is placed around the calf and inflated. A systolic pressure over the dorsalis pedis and posterior tibial arteries is obtained and waveforms are recorded. The cuff is then wrapped around the thigh and the procedure is repeated over the popliteal artery. The entire process allows segmental evaluation of the arterial tree in the lower extremities to aid in localizing the area of disease. An evaluation of the upper extremities can be performed in a similar fashion using forearm and upper arm compression taking ulnar, radial, and brachial artery readings. The pressures and waveforms from the ankle and brachial arteries are compared in the tested individual and an ankle-arm pressure index is calculated. Pulse volume recording (PVRs) can be done concurrently to quantitate blood volume or flow in an extremity. Because direct listening is subjective, it is desirable to have the same individual perform repeat studies on a given individual.

Purpose

Doppler studies allow the detection of arterial or venous obstruction or thrombi. They are also used to monitor patients who have had reconstructive or peripheral artery bypass surgery.

Findings

Normal

Multiphasic signal with prominent systolic sound and one or more diastolic sounds. Signals should

Doppler Studies[4,53, 77](Continued)

Findings (Continued)

Normal *(Continued)*	fluctuate with respiration, not heart beat. Ankle-arm pressure index (API) >1. Proximal thigh pressure is greater than arm pressure by 20 to 30 mm Hg. Increased flow velocity with compression of vessels. Flow should be spontaneous and phasic with respiration (venous).
Abnormal	Ankle-arm pressure index (API), the ratio between ankle systolic pressure and brachial systolic pressure, is <1. (See Table 6–6 for severity ranking.) Arm pressure is changed. Diminished or absent blood flow velocity signal. Calcified and non-compressible vessels produce unreliable measurements.

Pharmacy Implications   None.

Impedance Plethysmography (Occlusive Cuff)[4,78]

Description	Plethysmography is a non-invasive test that detects blood volume changes in the leg. A pneumatic cuff is placed around the mid thigh and inflated to occlude venous return. Occlusion is maintained for a minimum of 45 seconds and the cuff is then rapidly deflated. Electrodes placed around the calf detect changes in electrical resistance (impedance) due to alteration in blood volume distal to the cuff. The impedance changes occurring during inflation and deflation of the cuff are recorded on an ECG paperstrip. The changes in impedance during cuff inflation and deflation are compared against a discriminant line which separates normal from the abnormal graph.
Purpose	This procedure detects thrombi which produce obstruction to venous outflow. The test is sensitive and specific for occlusive thrombosis of the popliteal, femoral, or iliac veins. The test is relatively insensitive to calf vein thrombosis. Diagnostic accuracy of the test nears 90%. The test is unable to distinguish between thrombosis and non-thrombotic obstruction.

Table 6–6: Relationship of Ankle-Arm Pressure Index (API) and Disease Severity

API	Severity of Disease
1–0.7	Mild ischemia
0.75–0.5	Claudication
0.5–0.25	Pain at rest
0.25–0	Pregangrene

Impedance Plethysmography (Occlusive Cuff)[4,78] *(Continued)*

Findings

Normal	The graph for the patient will fall above the discriminant line (i.e., the test will be negative for proximal vein thrombi). However, false negatives can occur in patients with extensive collateral circulation which allows for adequate venous outflow and in patients where the proximal vein thrombosis is not occlusive.
Abnormal	The graph will fall below the discriminant line (i.e., positive for proximal vein thrombosis). False positives can occur when non-thrombotic occlusion (mechanical) is present and when arterial inflow disease limits the amount of venous filling, decreasing venous return.

Pharmacy Implications None.

Lymphangiography (Lymphography)[7,79]

Description Lymphography is the radiographic examination of the lymphatic system after radioactive material is injected into a lymphatic vessel in each foot (the hand, mastoid area, or spermatic cord is sometimes used). X-rays demonstrate the filling of lymphatic system with contrast media and, 24 hours later, the visualization of abdominal lymph nodes.

Purpose
- Lymphangiography is used to:
  - *Detect* obstruction, disease, or neoplasm in the lymphatic system.
  - *Stage* lymphoma.
  - *Distinguish* between primary and secondary lymph edema.
  - *Evaluate* the need for surgical treatment.
  - *Assess* the results of previous chemotherapy or radiation therapy.

Findings

Normal	Homogeneous and complete filling of the lymphatic system with the radioactive contrast material on the initial films.
Abnormal	Presence of enlarged, foamy looking nodes indicate lymphoma. Filling defects or lack of opacification of vessels indicate metastatic involvement of nodes by neoplasm. The number of nodes and their unilateral versus bilateral location and the extent of extranodal involvement determines staging of neoplastic disease.

Pharmacy Implications Check for hypersensitivity to iodine or other contrast media.

REFERENCES

1. Kline TS, ed. Handbook of Fine Needle Aspiration Biopsy Cytology. 2nd ed. New York:Churchill Livingstone, Inc;1988:9–16.

2. Teplick SK, Haskin PK. Imaging modalities. In: Handbook of Fine Needle Aspiration Biopsy Cytology. Kline TS, ed. 2nd ed. New York:Churchill Livingstone, Inc;1988:17–48.

3. Michaels D, ed. Procedures requiring the use of contrast media. In: Diagnostic Procedures: The Patient and the Health Care Team. New York: John Wiley and Sons; 1983:274–79.

4. Ford RD, ed. Diagnostic Tests Handbook. Springhouse: Springhouse Corporation; 1987.

5. Taub WH. Relative strengths and limitations of diagnostic imaging studies. In: Straub WH, ed. Manual of Diagnostic Imaging. Boston: Little, Brown and Company; 1989: 13–15.

6. Grossman ZD, et al, eds. The Clinicians Guide to Diagnostic Imaging Cost Effective Pathways. 2nd ed. New York: Raven Press; 1987.

7. Hamilton HK, Cahill M, eds. Diagnostics. Springhouse: Springhouse Corporation; 1986.

8. Edelman RR et al. Basic principles of magnetic resonance imaging. In: Edelman RR, Hesselink Jr, eds. Clinical Magnetic Resonance Imaging. Philadelphia: WB Saunders Company;1990:3–38.

9. Lufkin, RB. The MRI Manual. Chicago: Yearbook Medical Publishers, Inc;1990:21–41.

10. Hagen–Ansert SL. Textbook of Diagnostic Ultrasonography. 3rd ed. St. Louis: CV Mosby Company;1989:594–624.

11. Fischbach FT. A Manual of Laboratory Diagnostic Tests. 4th ed. Philadelphia, PA: JB Lippincott; 1992.

12. Webb DR. Diagnostic methods in allergy. In: Altman LC, ed. Clinical Allergy and Immunology. Boston:GK Hall Medical Publishers; 1984:149–68.

13. Timmis A. Essentials of Cardiology. Oxford: Blackwell Scientific Publications; 1988:40–45.

14. Gazes PC. Clinical Cardiology. 3rd ed. Philadelphia: Lea and Febiger; 1990.

15. Conover MB. Understanding Electrocardiography. 3rd ed. St. Louis: CV Mosby Co.; 1980.

16. DaCunha JP, ed. Diagnostics: Patient Preparation Interpretation Sources of Error, Post Test Care 2nd ed. Springhouse, PA: Springhouse; 1986:947–48.

17. Michaels D, Willis K. Noninvasive cardiovascular procedures. In: Michaels D, ed. Diagnostic Procedures: The Patient and The Health Care Team. New York: John Wiley & Sons; 1983: 441–442.

18. Alpert JS, Rippe JM, eds. Manual of Cardiovascular Diagnosis and Therapy. 2nd ed. Boston: Little, Brown and Co.; 1985:21.

19. Tilkian AG, Daily EK. Endomyocardial biopsy. In: Cardiovascular Procedures: Diagnostic Techniques and Therapeutic Procedures. St. Louis: CV Mosby Company; 1986:180–203.

20. Howard PA. Intravenous Dipyridamole: Use in Thallous Chloride TL 201 Stress Imaging. Annal Pharmacotherapy 1991;25:1085–91.

21. Anon. Persantine IV Hosp Pharm. 1991;26:356, 361–6.

22. Carpenter PC. Diagnosis of Adrenocortical Disease. In: Mendelsohn G, ed. Diagnosis and Pathology of Endocrine Diseases. Philadelphia: JB Lippincott; 1988:179–197.

23. Stern N, Griffon D. Protocols for stimulation and suppression tests commonly used in clinical endocrinology. In: Lavin N, ed. Manual of Endocrinology and Metabolism. 1st ed. Boston: Little, Brown; 1986:703–20.

24. Merkle WA. Secretion and metabolism of the corticosteroids and adrenal function and testing. In: Degroot LJ, ed. Endocrinology, Vol. 2. Philadelphia: WB Saunders; 1989:1610–1632.

25. Fitzgerald PA. Pituitary disorders. In: Fitzgerald PA, ed. Handbook of Clinical Endocrinology. Greenbrae: Jones Medical Publications; 1986:1–63; 450.

26. Carpenter PC. Cushing's syndrome: update of diagnosis and management. Mayo Clin Proc. 1986; 61:49–58.

27. Larenzi M. Diabetes mellitus. In: Fitzgerald PA. Handbook of Clinical Endocrinology. Greenbrae: Jones Medical Publications; 1986:337–406.

28. Stern N, Griffin D. Protocols for stimulation and suppression tests commonly used in clinical endocrinology. In: Lavin N, ed. Manual of Endocrinology and Metabolism. Boston: Little, Brown and Co.; 1986:703–19.

29. Singer PA. Thyroid function tests and effects of drugs on thyroid function. In: Manual of Endocrinology and Metabolism. 1st ed. Boston: Little, Brown, 1986:341–354.

30. Safrit HF. Thyroid disorders. In: Fitzgerald PA, ed. Handbook of Clinical Endocrinology. Greenbrae: Jones Medical Publications; 1986:122–169.

31. Field S. The acute abdomen-the plain radiograph. In: Grainger RG, Allison DJ, eds. Diagnostic Radiology: An Anglo-American Textbook of Imaging, Vol.2. Edinburgh: Churchill Livingstone; 1986:719–742.

32. Rice RP. The plain film of the abdomen. In: Taveras JM, Ferrucci JT, eds. Radiology: Diagnosis-Imaging-Intervention, Vol.4. Philadelphia: JB Lippincott; 1990:1–21.

33. Bartram CI. The large bowel. In: Grainger RG, Allison DJ, eds. Diagnostic Radiology: An Anglo-American Textbook of Imaging, Vol 2. Edinburgh: Churchill Livingstone; 1986:859–895.

34. Kressel HY, Laufer I. Double contrast examination of the gastrointestinal tract. In: Taveras JM, Ferrucci JT, eds. Radiology: Diagnosis-Imaging-Intervention, Vol.4. Philadelphia: JB Lippincott; 1990:1–21.

35. Nolan DJ. The small intestine. In: Grainger RG, Allison DJ, eds. Diagnostic Radiology: An Anglo-American Textbook of Imaging, Vol. 2. Edinburgh: Churchill Livingstone; 1986:833–858.

36. Maglinte DDT. The small bowel: anatomy and examination techniques. In: Taveras JM, Ferrucci JT, eds. Radiology: Diagnosis-Imaging-Intervention, Vol. 4. Philadelphia: JB Lippincott; 1990:1–7.

37. Levinson SC. Percutaneous transhepatic cholangiography. In: Drossman DA, ed. Manual of Gastroenterologic Procedures, 2nd ed. New York: Raven Press; 1987:162–168.

38. Bowley NB. The biliary tract. In: Grainger RG, Allison DJ, eds. Diagnostic Radiology: An Anglo-American Textbook of Imaging, Vol 2. Edinburgh: Churchill Livingstone; 1986:955–987.

39. Simeone JF. The biliary ducts: anatomy and examination technique. In: Taveras JM, Ferrucci JT, eds. Radiology: Diagnosis-Imaging-Intervention, Vol.4. Philadelphia: JB Lippincott; 1990:1–11.

40. Drossman DA. Colonoscopy. In: Drossman, DA, ed. Manual of Gastroenterologic Procedures, 2nd. ed. New York: Raven Press; 1987:110–118.

41. Bozynski EM. Endoscopic retrograde cholangio pancreatography. In: Drossman DA, ed. Manual of Gastroenterologic Procedures. 2nd ed. New York: Raven Press; 1987:103–109.

42. Sartar RB. Upper gastrointestinal endoscopy. In: Drossman DA, ed. Manual of Gastroenterologic Procedures, 2nd ed. New York: Raven Press; 1987:90–97.

43. Powell DW. Anoscopy and rigid sigmoidoscopy. In: Drossman DA, ed. Manual of Gastroenterologic Procedures, 2nd ed. New York: Raven Press; 1987:125–132.

44. Sandler RS. Flexible sigmoidoscopy. In: Drossman DA, ed. Manual of Gastroenterologic Procedures, 2nd ed. New York: Raven Press; 1987:119–124.

45. Drane WE. Radionuclide imaging of the liver, biliary system, and gastrointestinal tract. In: Chobanian SJ, Van Ness MM, eds. Manual of Clinical Problems in Gastroenterology. Boston: Little, Brown, and Company; 1988:290–296.

46. Tao LC, Kline TS. In: Kline TS, ed. Handbook of Fine Needle Aspiration Biopsy Cytology, 2nd. ed. New York: Churchill Livingstone; 1988:343–63.

47. Corbett JV. Diagnostic Procedures in Nursing Practice. Norwalk, CT: Appleton and Lange; 1987.

48. Weinstein WM, Hill TA. Gastrointestinal mucosal biopsy. In: Berk JE, ed. Gastroenterology, 4th ed. Vol. 1. Philadelphia: WB Saunders; 1985:626–44.

49. Paulfrey ME. Histology: breast biopsy. In: Hamilton HK, Cahill M, eds. Diagnostics. Springhouse: Springhouse Corporation; 1986:467–473.

50. Larson E. Clinical Microbiology and Infection Control. Boston, MA: Blackwell Scientific Publications; 1984:527–77.

51. Adams RD, Victor M. Principles of Neurology. 3rd ed. New York: McGraw-Hill; 1985:27–28.

52. Pryse-Phillips W, Murray TJ. Essential Neurology. 3rd ed. New York: Medical Examination Publishing Co.; 1986:103–104.

53. Berkow R, ed. The Merck Manual of Diagnosis and Therapy. 14th ed. Rahway: Merck Sharp & Dohme Research Laboratories, 1982.

54. Coniglio AA, Garnett WR. Status epilepticus. In: Dipiro JT et al, eds. Pharmacotherapy: A Pathophysiologic Approach. New York: Elsevier Science Publishing Company; 1989:599–610.

55. Vander AJ, et al, eds. Human Physiology: the Mechanisms of Body Function. 4th ed. New York: McGraw-Hill; 1985:690–91.

56. Rotschafer JC, Humphrey ZZ, Steinberg I. Central nervous system infection. In: Dipiro JT, et al, eds. Pharmacotherapy: A Pathophysiologic Approach. New York: Elsevier Science Publishing Co; 1989:1074–1088.

57. Kakulas BA, Adams RD, eds. Diseases of Muscle. Philadelphia: Harper and Row; 1985:771–86.

58. Anderson JR. Atlas of Skeletal Muscle Pathology. Lancaster: MTP Press Limited; 1985:11–17.

59. Connolly ES. Techniques of diagnostic nerve and muscle biopsies. In: Neurosurgery, Vol. 2. Wilkins RA, ed. New York: McGrawHill; 1985:1907–8.

60. Vaughn D, Asbury T. General Ophthalmology. 10th ed. Los Altos, CA: Lange Medical Publications, 1983.

61. Peters HB, Bartlett JD. Optical fundus in diagnosis. In: Physifax: Physicians Pocket Compendium of Normal Values, Tests, Diagnostic Criteria, Drug Therapy, and Other Useful Data. Montclair: Medication International, Ltd; 1984:97–120.

62. Lesar TS. Drug-induced ear and eye toxicity. In: DiPiro JT et al, eds. Pharmacotherapy: A Pathophysiologic Approach. New York: Elsevier; 1989:919–931.

63. Phillips CI. Basic Clinical Ophthalmology. London: Pitman Publishing, 1984:5586.

64. Stoker DJ. Arthrography. In: Harris NH, ed. Postgraduate Textbook of Clinical Orthopaedics. Bristol: Wright-PSG; 1983:882–90.

65. Karmody CS. Textbook of Otolaryngology. Philadelphia: Lea and Febiger; 1983.

66. Barton RP. Endoscopy. In: Keer Ag, Stell PM, eds. Scott-Brown's Otolaryngology: Laryngology. 5th ed. London: Butterworth's; 1987:31–41.

67. Ebadort AM. Branchoscopy. In: Michaels D, ed. Diagnostic Procedures: The Patient and the Health Care Team. New York: John Wiley and Sons; 1983: 493–506.

68. Behrman RE, Vaughn VC. Nelson Textbook of Pediatrics. 13th ed. Philadelphia: WB Saunders Co; 1987:928–29.

69. Lim RC. Surgical diagnosis and therapeutic procedures. In: Dunphy JE, Way LW, eds. Current Surgical Diagnosis and Treatment. Los Altos: Lange Medical Publications; 1981:1085–1097.

70. Sullivan D. Radionuclide imaging in lung disease. In: Putman C ed. Pulmonary Diagnosis: Imaging and Other Techniques. New York: Prentice-Hall; 1981: 67–78.

71. Bell WR, Simon TL. Current status of pulmonary thromboembolic disease: pathophysiology, diagnosis, prevention, and treatment. Am Heart J. 1982; 103:239–262.

72. Hull DR et al. Pulmonary angiography, ventilation lung scanning, and venography for clinically suspected pulmonary embolism with abnormal perfusion lung scan. Ann Intern Med. 1983; 98:891–899.

73. Blavis JG. Cystometry. In: deVere RW, Palmer JM, eds. New Techniques in Urology. New York: Futura Publishing Corporation; 1987:193–219.

74. Friedenberg RM. Excretory urography in the adult. In: Pollack HM, ed. Clinical Urography. Philadelphia: WB Saunders; 1990:101–243.

75. Imray TJ, Lieberman RP. Retrograde pyelography. In: Pollack HM, ed. Clinical Urography. Philadelphia:WB Saunders; 1990:244–55.

76. Hertz M. Cystourethrogaphy. In: Pollack HM, ed. Clinical Urography. Philadelphia: WB Saunders; 1990:256–295.

77. Bastarche MM, et al. Assessing peripheral vascular disease: noninvasive testing. AJN. 1983; 85:1552–1556.

78. Hirsch J. Natural history and diagnosis of venous thrombosis. Paper presented at a symposium sponsored by the Page and William Black Post-Graduate School of Medicine of the Mount Sinai School of Medicine, New York, NY; 1981 Oct 30.

79. Bryan GT. Diagnostic Radiography: A Concise Practical Manual. 4th ed. Edinburgh: Churchill Livingstone; 1987:289–96.

80. Menendez R, Kelly HW. Pulmonary-function testing in the evaluation of bronchodilator agents. Clin Pharm. 1983;2:120–128.

81. Kelly HW. Asthma. In: Koda-Kimble MA, Young LY eds. Applied Therapeutics: The Clinical Use of Drugs. 5th Ed. Vancouver: Applied Therapeutics; 1992:15-1-15–4.

Drug Administration

Dave Wegner
Mary Swandby

BACKGROUND

In recent years, parenteral routes of drug administration have been more widely used than in previous years. The development of more readily usable IV access devices, as well as marketing of an increasing percentage of parenterally administered medications, makes a working knowledge of parenteral administration techniques imperative. This chapter explores the routes of parenteral administration, available access devices, and delivery systems for many clinical situations.

ROUTES OF PARENTERAL DRUG ADMINISTRATION

Intramuscular (IM) Route

Intramuscular injections are administered through the skin and subcutaneous tissue and into the underlying muscle. The gluteal and deltoid muscles are the major sites for IM injections. The gluteal muscle is preferred when large volumes (i.e., 2–3 mL adults; 1–1.5 mL children) or when irritating drugs (e.g., Phenytoin) need to be given intramuscularly. When administering an IM injection, care must be taken to prevent accidental intravenous injection of the drug. This is accomplished by drawing back the plunger of the syringe to check for a blood return. If no blood appears, the medication can be administered; the presence of blood indicates the needle must be moved before administration. Common needle sizes for IM injections are 21 to 23 gauge. The gauge reflects needle diameter: the larger the number, the smaller the diameter. Needles are generally between 1 to $1^1/2$ inches long.

Drugs in solution or suspension (aqueous or oil) can be injected intramuscularly. Drugs in solution provide a prompt effect, whereas suspensions provide a delayed onset and a prolonged effect.

Subcutaneous (SC or SQ) Route

Subcutaneous injections place a small amount of fluid, usually <1 mL, through the skin and into the underlying subcutaneous tissue. Sites for these injections are often the front part of the thigh and the outer surface of the upper arm. A 25 gauge, 5/8" long needle is commonly used for these injections. Most drugs injected subcutaneously are solutions, with insulin suspensions being notable exceptions. Drugs known to cause local irritation should not be administered subcutaneously to avoid the potential for inflammation or abscess formation.

INTRAVENOUS (IV) ADMINISTRATION OF DRUGS

Many factors impact the decision to inject drugs intravenously, but none so much as the type of IV access available. As access devices have evolved over the last several years, the intravenous route has emerged as a major avenue for drug delivery, accounting for up to 40% of all drugs given in hospitals. With the advent of semipermanent centrally implanted catheters, considerations of pH, osmolality, and local irritation of peripheral veins have decreased in importance. Nevertheless, these factors are still significant when dealing with peripheral access devices.

Peripheral Venous Access

Butterfly. The butterfly needle is a steel needle of small diameter (about 22 gauge) attached to two wing like plastic stabilizers (see Figure 7–1). These devices are relatively inexpensive and provide patients requiring peripheral venous access greater mobility; however, infiltration is common. The delivery of the IV solution can be compromised when the patient moves the limb to which the butterfly is attached into an inappropriate position. Therefore, butterfly needles work well for infusions of medications on an intermittent basis. It is difficult to maintain a well functioning butterfly when giving medications known to irritate veins (e.g., nafcillin).

Heparin Well. Heparin wells are similar to butterfly needles, but have an injection port attached to the needle. Medications can be administered through the injection port, then flushed through the port with either saline or heparinized saline to prevent clot occlusion. The concentration of heparin is relatively low, usually 10 to 100 U/mL. Heparin wells are also inexpensive, but have the same limitations as butterfly needles.

FIGURE 7–1: Butterfly Infusion Set

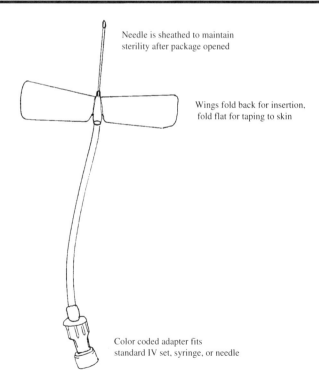

Needle is sheathed to maintain sterility after package opened

Wings fold back for insertion, fold flat for taping to skin

Color coded adapter fits standard IV set, syringe, or needle

Angiocatheters. This product consists of a polypropylene catheter fitted over a needle, which is withdrawn after insertion, leaving only the catheter in the vein. Angiocatheters are less irritating and less likely to infiltrate than a metal needle.

Central Catheters. Similar in construction to angiocatheters, central venous catheters are placed into the subclavian vein or into another of the large central vessels close to the heart. The high flow of blood in the central vasculature provides immediate dilution of fluids and medication. Consequently, hypertonic solutions such as parenteral nutrition can be delivered via the central route, where peripheral administration would be far too irritating to the vein. Placement of central lines is difficult, and insertion can result in a pneumothorax.

Infection is another serious risk when dealing with central lines. To overcome this problem, Hickman and other semipermanent implanted catheters were developed to minimize the infectious complications and the useful life of the catheter. Placement of a Hickman catheter is a surgical procedure. The silastic catheters are placed in the subclavian vein or other central vessel, then tunneled subcutaneously for several inches, before exiting somewhere on the chest wall. A small dacron cuff is located an inch or two from the exit site in the subcutaneous tissue. As the tissue heals postoperatively, scar tissue forms around the cuff, anchoring the catheter into place. While organisms may migrate from the outside around the exit site to the cuff area, the long subcutaneous tunnel prevents the organism from reaching the actual site where the catheter enters the central vein. There are many types of implanted catheters available, including Hickman, Raaf, Broviac, and Groshong. Groshong catheters are unique in that the tip is not open, but is closed with slit valves that open when under either forward or backward pressure. These unique catheters are expensive, and the cost of the surgical procedure adds to the overall expense.

Central Implanted Ports. Central implanted ports are another type of semipermanent central access device. As with central catheters, implantation of ports is also a surgical procedure. Ports are commonly made of steel or some type of plastic. The catheter itself is inserted into the subclavian or other central vein and then tunneled to the site several inches away where the port device is secured under the skin. Ports have a small reservoir and a central septum that is accessed by puncturing the skin with a right angle needle. Medication is infused through the needle. When the medication administration is complete, the needle is removed and the patient's device has no opening to the outside, being located entirely in the subcutaneous tissue. Ports work well for patients with intermittent needs for medication administration, such as chemotherapy or antibiotic therapy in cystic fibrosis. Continuous use of a port can lead to infection, and sterilization of a port device is difficult to accomplish with IV antibiotics.

Peripherally Inserted Central Catheters. Peripherally inserted central catheters, such as the Percucath or Landmark catheter, are inserted into the brachial vein and threaded upward over the clavicle until the tip is located in the central vasculature. They consist of an introducer needle, and a long pliable catheter (Percucath) or biologically reactive plastic (Landmark catheter). The biomer material in the Landmark softens and expands as it dwells in the vein, making initial insertion of the catheter easier, and securing the catheter in the vein as the material expands. These catheters work well for patients requiring home IV therapy, as they last much longer than butterfly needles or angiocaths. Due to the central administration of medication using this approach, some of the problems with administration of irritant drugs can be avoided as well.

Maintenance of Access Devices (Flushing)

All IV access devices used on an intermittent basis must be flushed periodically to maintain device patency. Heparinized saline, in concentrations of 10 to 100 U/mL every four hours to every day, is commonly used to flush heparin wells as well as Hickman or other central catheters. Sodium chloride 0.9% may be as effective as heparinized solutions for maintaining catheter patency. Hickman catheters should be flushed daily when not in use and after every infusion of medication. Groshong catheters, because of their closed tip, need only be flushed weekly with saline. Ports are flushed even less often, using 1000 U/mL heparin on a monthly basis. After medication is administered via a port, it can be flushed with saline or heparinized saline at least daily, and then "locked off" with more concentrated heparin when not in use.

METHODS FOR ADMINISTRATION OF IV MEDICATIONS

Intravenous medications can be administered in one of three ways. An intravenous push or "bolus" injection is the direct administration of the drug into the blood vessel. A small amount of blood should first be drawn back into the syringe to assure that the needle is in the vein. Suitability for this route of administration depends upon the pH or irritating potential of the drug, the sensitivity of the patient's vein, and the drug's therapeutic effect. Generally a bolus injection is administered over 3 to 5 minutes.

A *continuous infusion* of intravenous fluid is used to deliver a large volume of solution over several hours. Examples include:

>> Amphotericin B 30 mg in 250 mL 5% dextrose solution over 6 hr.

>> Dextrose 5% with potassium chloride 20 mEq/L Q 8 hr.

>> A total parenteral nutrition (TPN) solution infused on a continual basis.

Intermittent infusions are used to deliver a relatively small volume of fluid and drug over a short time at certain intervals. Examples include:

>> Vancomycin 1 gm in 100 mL of 5% dextrose over 1 hr BID (twice daily).

>> Penicillin G, 1,000,000 U in 50 mL of 0.9% sodium chloride over 30 minutes Q 6 hr.

Several different systems of intermittent intravenous infusion (see Figure 7–2) are described in Table 7–1 on page 7–6.

SELECTION OF IV ADMINISTRATION DEVICES

Many types of equipment are available to regulate flow during the administration of medications or solutions. These devices range in complexity from simple syringe pumps to programmable pumps with the capacity to simultaneously administer up to 10 different solutions at varying rates. The myriad of pumps, controllers, and devices available in the marketplace, requires a thorough understanding of the basic mechanisms of drug delivery, as well as the impact of these products on the preparation and stability of medications. Features such as size, alarms, disposability, computer programming, and multiple functions in a single device distinguish one piece of equipment from another. In selecting a particular device it is important to assess the equipment for ease of use, cost impact, drug stability, and appropriateness of the technology

FIGURE 7–2: Intravenous Delivery Systems.

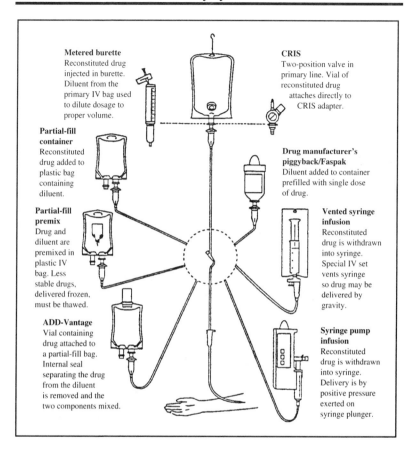

Metered burette
Reconstituted drug injected in burette. Diluent from the primary IV bag used to dilute dosage to proper volume.

Partial-fill container
Reconstituted drug added to plastic bag containing diluent.

Partial-fill premix
Drug and diluent are premixed in plastic IV bag. Less stable drugs, delivered frozen, must be thawed.

ADD-Vantage
Vial containing drug attached to a partial-fill bag. Internal seal separating the drug from the diluent is removed and the two components mixed.

CRIS
Two-position valve in primary line. Vial of reconstituted drug attaches directly to CRIS adapter.

Drug manufacturer's piggyback/Faspak
Diluent added to container prefilled with single dose of drug.

Vented syringe infusion
Reconstituted drug is withdrawn into syringe. Special IV set vents syringe so drug may be delivered by gravity.

Syringe pump infusion
Reconstituted drug is withdrawn into syringe. Delivery is by positive pressure exerted on syringe plunger.

for specific patient populations. A brief description of administration controllers, pumps, and other types of devices used to administer medications follows.

Controllers

Controllers are IV infusion devices that do not use pressure to regulate fluid flow rates. Controllers often use drop sensors to detect the movement of fluid and gravity to propel the fluid. Pumps, on the other hand, force fluid with positive pressure. Very few medications require a pump for dosing accuracy, most fluids and drugs are quite accurately administered with a controller. When medications infiltrate out of the vascular space, extravasation injury is less extensive when a controller is used due to the lack of pressure during administration.

Pumps

Pumps should be used for administration of medications at very slow flow rates and when dosing requires extreme accuracy. Although the use of pumps has expanded

TABLE 7–1: Intermittent Intravenous Infusion Systems

System	Advantages	Disadvantages
Metered burette	Accurate measure of diluent volume. Good for pediatric and fluid restricted patients when standard 50 or 100 mL minibags could cause fluid overload.	System is open to room air via a vent. Difficult to rinse chamber between doses of incompatible drugs (i.e., ticarcillin and tobramycin).
Partial fill containers	Drug is diluted and ready for administration.	Stability of most drugs is shortened when diluted. Fluid status must be watched closely in patients with multiple medications.
Partial fill container (drug only, no diluent)	Longer expiration dating for most drugs than with diluted partial fill containers. Require less storage space.	Drug must be diluted from primary IV solution before administration.
Partial fill premix	Saves time in IV admixture area. May reduce waste.	Need to thaw and label with expiration date before use. Diluent type and volume is determined by manufacturer. Available only in limited dosages.
ADDvantage system	Saves time in IV admixture area. Drug is reconstituted immediately before use, so waste is minimal.	End user must rupture seal to mix drug and diluent. Possibility that only this diluent may be administered. Drugs must be in special vials, limiting availability.
CRIS system	Possible cost savings depending upon cost of sets and empty vials.	Drug vial top must be 20 mm to attach to the system. Difficult to tell if drug has be administered unless drug is colored.
Manufacturer's piggyback/ FASPAK	FASPAK bags may be diluted by the end user with primary IV solution to save pharmacy preparation time.	Piggyback bottles are large and use a large amount of storage space. Doses may not fit in standard medication cart systems.
Vented syringe infusion	Cost of syringe is usually less than cost of other containers. No electronic device is required.	Requires a two step dilution process in the pharmacy. Required special sets add to the cost.

TABLE 7–1: Intermittent Intravenous Infusion Systems *(Continued)*

System	Advantages	Disadvantages
Syringe pump infusion	Very accurate at delivering desired volume over the time desired. Cost of syringe is usually less than the cost of other containers.	Costs associated with rental or purchase of pumps. This level of accuracy is not needed for most drugs. It requires a two step dilution process in pharmacy. Pump maintenance is a problem. Positive pressure may increase severity of infiltration injury.

significantly in recent years, pumps are often used unnecessarily. Pumps commonly employ one of three mechanisms to propel fluid: linear peristalsis, rotary peristalsis, or piston drive. Pumps have been developed for many clinical settings, including patient controlled analgesia, multiple channel machines for ICU settings, subcutaneous implanted pumps for insulin or analgesics, ambulatory pumps with multiple functions for use in the home, and circadian rhythm pumps for the administration of chemotherapy. Caution must be exercised to assure that these very expensive devices are selected appropriately to serve a given patient population and used only when indicated.

Disposable Infusion Devices

With the advent of home IV therapy, the search for an easy-to-use, disposable infusion device has led to the development of many such systems (e.g., Homepump, Intermate). Home antibiotic therapy and home chemotherapy are the two common applications of these devices. These devices have an elastomeric reservoir that is filled with a single dose of drug to be infused. When activated, the balloon-like reservoir deflates, forcing the fluid through a rate-controlling one way valve. While the single use systems are simple for patients to use, they are extremely expensive when compared to the price of syringes, bags, pumps, and tubing.

Fluid and Electrolyte Therapy

Linda M. Calkins
Bill R. Check

Fluid and electrolyte therapy is complicated and presents even the most experienced practitioner with challenges. This chapter provides an overview of fluid and electrolyte balance (including recommended daily requirements), reviews the appropriate use of common IV solutions, and gives guidelines for monitoring IV therapy. For a more comprehensive presentation of fluid and electrolyte disorders, see the reference listing at the end of this chapter.

INTRACELLULAR AND EXTRACELLULAR ELECTROLYTES

In a healthy individual, body fluid and electrolytes are maintained in a delicate balance by normal homeostatic physiological mechanisms and vary little on a daily basis. The kidneys are primarily responsible for maintaining fluid and electrolyte balance; and cell membranes maintain the intracellular composition of the electrolytes. The electrolyte content in intracellular fluid (ICF) differs significantly from that in extracellular fluid (ECF). (See Table 8–1.)

Na^+ and K^+ diffuse passively across cell membranes along concentration gradients. The Na^+-K^+-ATPase pump is responsible for actively retaining K^+ intracellularly and Na^+

TABLE 8–1: Concentrations of Electrolytes in ICF and ECF[a]

Electrolyte	Concentration (mEq/L)
ICF	
Na^+	10
K^+	140
Cl^-	2
HCO_3^-	8
Mg^{++}	35
Ca^{++}	3
$P(HPO_4)$	95
ECF	
Na^+	142
K^+	4
Cl^-	103
HCO_3^-	25
Mg^{++}	3
Ca^{++}	5
$P(HPO_4)$	2

[a] ICF = Intracellular Fluid; ECF = Extracellular Fluid.

extracellularly, thus maintaining an intracellular K^+ concentration of 140 mEq/L with an extracellular K^+ concentration of 4 mEq/L (i.e., against the concentration gradient).

OSMOLALITY

Despite the significant differences in the electrolyte composition of the ICF and ECF, the osmolality of the ICF is equal to that of the ECF and varies little in a healthy individual. Cell membranes are freely permeable to water. Water will move from an area of lower solute concentration to an area of higher solute concentration to re-establish equilibrium and eliminate osmotic gradients. When measured, plasma osmolality usually is 280 to 295 mOsm/L.

Plasma osmolality (Posm) can be estimated by the following formula:

$$\text{Posm in mOsm/L} = 2 \times \text{Plasma [Na+] in mEq/L} + \frac{\text{BUN in mg/dL}}{2.8} + \frac{\text{Blood Glucose in mg/dL}}{18}$$

$$e.g., \text{Posm} = 2(140) + (15/2.8) + (100/18)$$
$$= 291 \text{ mOsm/L}$$

The osmolality of intravenous (IV) solutions can be calculated as follows:

$$\text{mOsm/L} = \left(\frac{\text{mg/L}}{\text{MW}} \right) (\text{Number of Particles})$$

$Where:$ MW = Molecular Weight
Number of Particles = Number of Particles Produced by Dissociation of the Substance

For example, the osmolality (in mOsm/L) of normal saline and for 5% dextrose in water (D_5W) can be calculated as follows:

$$0.9\% \text{ NaCl}: \left(\frac{9000 \text{ mg/dL}}{58.5 \text{ mg/mM}} \right) (2) = 308 \text{ mOsm/L}$$

$$5\% \text{ D}_5\text{W}: \left(\frac{50000 \text{ mg/L}}{180 \text{ mg/mM}} \right) (1) = 278 \text{ mOsm/L}$$

TOTAL BODY WATER (TBW)

Normally, total body water (TBW) in adult males is approximately 60% of total body weight. Fat cells contain little or no water. In adult females, TBW is approximately 50% of total weight. These percentages vary with age (higher in the term infant, decreasing in infancy and childhood, and further decreasing in adolescence) and degree of obesity. TBW is subdivided into intracellular fluid and extracellular fluid. Approximately two-thirds of TBW is ICF, the remaining one-third is ECF. The extracellular fluid is further subdivided into intravascular and interstitial fluid. The intravascular component consists of plasma and comprises approximately 25% of the ECF. The interstitial compartment consists of fluid between cells or tissues [e.g., lymph, cerebrospinal fluid (CSF), GI secretions, ocular fluid, synovial fluid] and comprises approximately 75% of the ECF (see Figure 8–1).

FIGURE 8–1: Total Body Water (TBW).

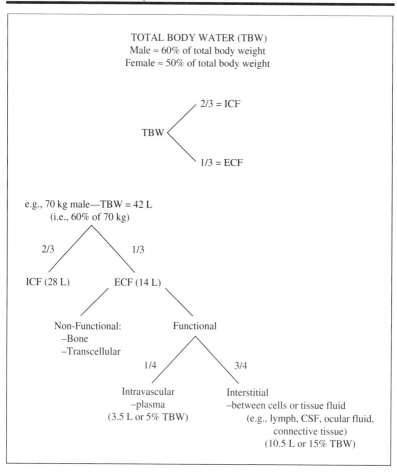

ESTIMATION OF TOTAL BODY ELECTROLYTES

The following examples illustrate how to estimate total body electrolyte content:

Example. Estimation of total normal body K^+.

$$K^+ \text{ in ECF} = 4 \text{ mEq/L}$$
$$\text{ECF } K^+ = (4 \text{ mEq/L}) (14 \text{ L})$$
$$= 56 \text{ mEq}$$

$$\textit{Whereas } K^+ \text{ in ICF} = 140 \text{ mEq/L}$$
$$\text{ICF } K^+ = (140 \text{ mEq/L}) (28 \text{ L})$$
$$= 3920 \text{ mEq}$$

Example. Estimation of sodium deficit in a 70 kg male patient with true hyponatremia (serum sodium 110 mEq/L).

$$Normal\ Serum\ Na^+ = 140\ mEq/L$$

$$\begin{aligned} TBW &= (Weight\ in\ kg)\ (0.6) \\ &= (70\ kg)\ (0.6) \\ &= 42\ L \end{aligned}$$

Calculate the sodium deficit of a 70 kg patient with a serum Na+ = 110 mEq/L.

$$\begin{aligned} Desired\ Change\ in\ Serum\ Na^+ &= 140 - 110 \\ &= 30\ mEq/L \end{aligned}$$

$$\begin{aligned} \textit{Thus},\ Na\ Deficit &= (30\ mEq/L)\ (42\ L) \\ &= 1260\ mEq\ Na^+ \end{aligned}$$

In general, fluid and electrolyte requirements can be determined by the following formula:

$$Requirement = Baseline\ Needs + Abnormal\ Losses + Deficits - Excesses$$

NORMAL FLUID AND ELECTROLYTE REQUIREMENTS

Consumed calories provide energy, and utilization of this energy results in heat production and water loss to the environment. For every 100 kcal expended, 100 mL of water are lost (i.e., obligatory losses) and must be replaced for the body to maintain normal functions of elimination and temperature regulation. Daily water and electrolyte requirements must be reduced for patients with organ failures.

Water

The average adult requirement of 30 to 40 mL/kg/day is needed to maintain normal body functions of elimination and temperature regulation. (See Table 8–2.) The intake and output of fluids must be monitored and recorded (see Appendix 8–1) when fluids are provided to patients who are unable to regulate their own intake of fluid.

Sodium (Na+)

Normal intake should generally supply at least 70 mEq Na+/day; however, after several days on a sodium-free diet, sodium essentially disappears from the urine. Therefore, the absolute minimum requirement is unknown, but "enough sodium" must be provided in relation to water to prevent hyponatremia.

Potassium (K+)

The minimum requirement of potassium is 25 mEq/day to replace normal losses via the urine and stool. Patients with normal renal function generally require 40 to 60 mEq/day of potassium. (See Appendix 8–2 for recommended guidelines for the administration of intravenous potassium.)

Calcium (Ca++)

The usual daily calcium requirement is 0.2 to 0.3 mEq/kg/day.

TABLE 8–2: Daily Water Balance in Adults

In		Out			
		Obligatory Loss		**Facultative Loss**	
Water consumed	1000 mL	Urine	900 mL	Kidney reserve	500 mL
Water in food	1200 mL				
Water of oxidation[a]	300 mL	Fecal	100 mL	Insensible reserve	200 mL
	2500 mL	Insensible losses	800 mL		
			1800 mL		700 mL
			2500 mL		

[a] When carbohydrates or fat are oxidized, CO_2 and water are produced. Water of oxidation is produced at a rate of 12 mL/100 kcal metabolized.

Magnesium (Mg^{++})

The daily magnesium requirement varies: normal healthy patients require 0.08 mEq/kg/day. Depleted patients or patients with excessive losses require 0.3 to 0.4 mEq/kg/day of magnesium and patients with severe catabolic stress require 0.6 to 0.8 mEq/kg/day.

Chloride (Cl^-)

To avoid developing metabolic alkalosis and hyperchloremic acidosis, the Na:Cl intake ratio should be approximately 1:1.

Phosphate ($PO_4^=$)

As as anion, phosphorous dissociates into various forms and therefore is reported and ordered on a millimolar concentration. The usual minimal daily requirement of phosphate is approximately 20 mmol/day or an average of 7 to 9 mmol/1000 kcal.

ABNORMAL LOSSES

Insensible Water Losses

Evaporative losses of water through skin and lungs are increased with hyperventilation, fever, hyperthyroidism, obesity, severe skin disease or injury, a hot environment, and burns. These "insensible" losses of water can be significant; for example, each degree (centigrade) above normal body temperature can increase "insensible" water loss by about 10% to 13%.

Third Space Fluid

Third space fluid results from an internal shift of fluid out of the vascular tree and into extravascular space (e.g., ascites or after abdominal surgery).

Body Fluid Loss

Excessive diarrhea, fistula losses, and nasogastric (NG) suction will increase daily water requirements (see Table 8–3). Measurement of fluid output and composition can aid in determining the necessary replacement needs.

Drugs

Drugs such as diuretics, semisynthetic penicillins, amphotericin, alcohol, and intravenous dantrolene (mannitol content) will increase water loss.

DEFICITS/EXCESSES

Deficits can be estimated from physical examination, patient history, serum electrolytes, urine electrolytes, and urine specific gravity (see Table 8–3).

A large amount of gastric fluid loss (e.g., NG-suction, vomiting) usually results in a loss of sodium that is less concentrated than in plasma (i.e., free-water is lost), more potassium, and no bicarbonate. Thus, the plasma sodium concentration usually increases, the plasma potassium concentration usually decreases, and the plasma bicarbonate usually rises (i.e., the patient becomes hypernatremic, hypokalemic, and alkalotic).

PEDIATRIC REQUIREMENTS

Caloric/Water Requirements (See Table 8–4.)

Example. Calculation of the caloric/water requirements for a 24 kg patient.

$$
\begin{array}{lll}
\text{1st 10 kg:} & 100 \times 10 = & 1000 \text{ kcal} \\
\text{10–20 kg:} & 50 \times 10 = & 500 \text{ kcal} \\
\text{Over 20 kg:} & 20 \times 4 = & \underline{80 \text{ kcal}} \\
& & 1580 \text{ kcal/24 hr}
\end{array}
$$

The normal water requirements for a hospitalized patient are 100 mL/100 kcal expended.

TABLE 8–3: Electrolyte Composition of Body Fluids

Fluid	Volume (mL/day)	Na+ (mEq/L)	K+ (mEq/L)	Cl− (mEq/L)	HCO3− (mEq/L)
Plasma		142	4.5	102	26
Gastric	2000–2500	60	9.0	84	0
Bile	600–800	149	4.9	101	45
Pancreatic	700–1000	141	4.6	77	92
Small bowel	300–1500	105	5.1	99	50
Ileal		129	11.2	116	29
Cecal		80	21	48	22
Sweat	400–500	45	4.5	58	0

[a] Adapted with permission. Maxwell MH, et al. In: Clinical Disorders of Fluid & Electrolyte Metabolism. New York: Mc Graw-Hill;1987:1183.

TABLE 8–4: Caloric/Water Requirements

Wt (kg)	kcal Requirement over 24 hr
First 10 kg	100 kcal/kg
10–20 kg	1000 kcal + 50 kcal/kg/24 hr for each kg over 10 kg
>20 kg	1500 kcal + 20 kcal/kg/24 hr for each kg over 20 kg

Distribution of Obligatory Water Losses Under Normal Conditions

Under normal conditions, the insensible (evaporative) water loss is as follows:

>> **Skin.** 30 mL/100 kcal expended.

>> **Lungs.** 15 mL/100 kcal expended.

>> **Urine.** 50 mL/100 kcal expended.

>> **Stool Water.** 5 mL/100 kcal expended.

Electrolyte Requirements

Remember: Maintenance fluid and electrolyte requirements in the newborn period are different from those of older children (see Table 8–6).

TABLE 8–5: Maintenance Electrolyte Requirements[a]

Electrolyte	Daily Requirements	Maximum
Na^+	3–4 mEq/kg/24 hr *or* 25–40 mEq/1000 kcal/24 hr	100–150 mEq/24 hr
K^+	2–3 mEq/kg/24 hr *or* 25–40 mEq/1000 kcal/24 hr	80–120 mEq/24 hr
Cl^-	2–4 mEq/kg/24 hr *or* 25–40 mEq/1000 kcal/24 hr	100–150 mEq/24 hr
Ca^{++}[b]	1–2.5 mEq/kg/24 hr *or* 10–35 mEq/1000 kcal/24 hr	9–35 mEq/24 hr
Mg^{++}[c]	0.2–0.5 mEq/kg/24 hr *or* 3–10 mEq/1000 kcal/24 hr	8–16 mEq/24 hr
PO_4[c]	2 mM/kg/24 hr *or* 35 mM/1000 kcal/24 hr	15–30 mM/24 hr

[a] Reprinted with permission. Benitz WE, Tatro DS. In: The Pediatric Drug Handbook, 2nd Ed. Chicago: Year Book Medical Publishers;1988:292.

[b] Provision of calcium is of practical importance primarily in the parenteral fluid management of infants and newborns. It is generally not necessary to give supplemental calcium to older children and adults, except as part of a program of total parenteral nutrition. These recommendations are equivalent to 200–500 mg of calcium gluconate/kg/24 hr, up to a maximum of 2 gm/24 hr in infants or 3–4 gm/24 hr in older children, adolescents, or adults.

c Supplementation of magnesium and phosphate is important primarily with total parenteral nutrition, but may also be important in some specific clinical situations. For example, magnesium may be essential in treatment of refractory hypocalcemia, and phosphate supplementation may be required in some patients with diabetic ketoacidosis.

TABLE 8-6: Maintenance Fluid and Electrolyte Requirements in the Newborn Period[a]

Age	Calories (kcal/kg/24 hr)	Water (mL/kg/24 hr)	Electrolytes		
			Na$^+$ (mEq/kg/24 hr)	K$^+$ (mEq/kg/24 hr)	Ca^{++}[b] (mg/kg/24 hr)
Premature	100–150	100–250	2–8	2–6	200–1000
Term					
0–24 hr	50–60	50–60	0–2	0–2	0–500
24–48 hr	75–80	75–80	0–2	1–2	200–500
48–72 hr	90–100	90–100	1–4	1–2	200–600
>3 days	100–120	100–180	1–4	1–2	200–800

[a] Reprinted with permission. Benitz WE, Tatro DS. In: The Pediatric Drug Handbook, 2nd Ed. Chicago: Yearbook Medical Publishers;1988:293.
[b] mg/kg/24 hr of the gluconate salt.

TABLE 8-7: Common IV Solutions

Solution Type	Dextrose (gm/L)	Na$^+$ (mEq/L)	K$^+$ (mEq/L)	Cl$^-$ (mEq/L)	Ca^{++} (mEq/L)	Lactate$^-$ (mEq/L)	mOsm/L
5% D/W[a]	50						253
10% D/W	100						505
5% D/0.9% NaCl	50	154		154			559
5% D/0.45% NaCl	50	77		77			406
5% D/0.2% NaCl	50	34		34			330
0.45% NaCl		77		77			154
0.9% NaCl		154		154			308
Ringers Lactate		130	4	109	3	28	274
D$_5$ 1/2 NS[b] + 20 mEq KCl/L	50	77	20	97			446
D$_5$ 1/4 NS + 20 mEq KCl/L	50	34	20	54			370
0.9% NaCl + 20 mEq KCl/L		154	20	174			348
3% NaCl		513		513			1026

[a] D/W = Dextrose in Water.
[b] NS = Normal Saline (NaCl).

COMMON IV SOLUTIONS

In general, do not infuse more than 500 mOsm/L into a peripheral vein because phlebitis, pain, and venous sclerosis can result. Do not infuse less than 150 mOsm/L (too hypotonic; can cause hemolysis and hematuria). When fluids are administered centrally, a wider range of tonicity is tolerated because the fluid is quickly diluted.

COMMON IV RATES

TABLE 8–8: Common IV Rates

Rate (mL/hr)	Duration of 1000 mL bag (hr)	Number of mL Administered per 24 hr
TKO (To Keep Open)		
5–50 mL/hr	Varies	120–1200
25	40	600
40	25	960
50	20	1200
75	13	1800
100	10	2400
125	8	3000
150	7	3600
200	5	4800

INDICATIONS FOR STANDARD INTRAVENOUS SOLUTIONS

TABLE 8–9: Indications for Standard Solutions

Solution[a]	Indications
D_5W	Free H_2O source Na-restricted patient Diluent for IV drug administration (e.g., drips)
$D_5$1/4 NS (D_5/0.2 %NaCl)	Maintenance therapy
$D_5$1/2 NS (D_5/0.45 %NaCl)	Provide both sodium and free water, maintenance therapy
NS	Approximately isotonic No free water Used to expand intravascular fluid volume No dextrose content and can be useful when blood sugar concentration is high
Ringers Lactate	Electrolyte composition/osmolality are similar to extracellular fluid Used to replace losses due to surgery or burns
1/2 NS	Provides free water without dextrose (e.g., diabetics)

[a] D_5W = 5% Dextrose in Water; $D_5$1/4 NS = 5% Dextrose in 1/4 Normal Saline; $D_5$1/2 NS = 5% Dextrose in 1/2 Normal Saline; NS = Normal Saline (0.9% NaCl); 1/2 NS = 1/2 Normal Saline (0.45% NaCl).

MONITORING FLUID STATUS

To assess and determine the magnitude of a patient's fluid disorder, the severity of a patient's clinical signs and symptoms provides useful information. Table 8–10 presents examples of various clinical monitoring parameters that assist in the assessment of a patient's fluid status.

TABLE 8–10: Monitoring Fluid Status[a]

Parameters	Signs and Symptoms
Total body water	Body weight changes Intake and output records (see page 8–16)
Extravascular extracellular fluid	Peripheral edema (sacral edema in supine position) Pulmonary congestion (crackles, x-ray, blood gases) Ascites or other third-space fluid
Intravascular fluid volume	Pulse and blood pressure; orthostatic changes in blood pressure Renal perfusion indicators: urine output, urine chemistry (sodium, specific gravity, osmolality), BUN:Cr ratio S_3 heart sound Central venous pressure (CVP) measurement, jugular venous distention (JVD), hepatojugular reflex (HJR) Peripheral circulation (color and temperature of extremities, rate of capillary refill) Hct and Hgb (assuming RBC mass constant)
Intracellular and free water volume	Serum osmolality and Na Thirst sensation Mental status changes Skin and mucous membranes Skin turgor

[a] See Chapter 5: Clinical Laboratory Tests for normal laboratory values and further discussion.

MANIFESTATIONS OF ABNORMAL SERUM ELECTROLYTES

TABLE 8–11: Manifestations of Abnormal Serum Electrolytes

Substance	Symptoms	Manifestations
Potassium[a]	Hyperkalemia	Weakness, flaccid paralysis, hyperactive deep tendon reflexes, confusion ECG changes: peaked T-waves, wide QRS, asystole K^+ 7–8 mEq/L is associated with ventricular fibrillation in 5% of patients K^+ 10 mEq/L is associated with ventricular fibrillation in 90% of patients

(Continued)

TABLE 8–11: Manifestations of Abnormal Serum Electrolytes *(Cont.)*

Substance	Symptoms	Manifestations
Potassium[a]	Hypokalemia	Muscle weakness, cramps, tetany, rhabdomyolysis, and myoglobinuria Nausea, vomiting, paralytic ileus, polyuria, polydypsia ECG changes: flattening of T-waves, U-wave becomes obvious, ST-depression, ectopy, and prolongation of PR-interval
	Policy and procedure for potassium administration	See page 8–18
Sodium	Hypernatremia	Confusion, stupor, coma Muscle tremors, seizures Pulmonary and peripheral edema Respiratory paralysis and death
	Hyponatremia	Headache, lethargy, confusion, seizures, coma Muscle twitches, irritability Nausea, vomiting, anorexia
Calcium[b]	Hypercalcemia	Anorexia, nausea, vomiting, polyuria, polydypsia, constipation Abdominal pains, renal stones Fatigue, hypotonia, lethargy, coma ECG changes: shortening of QT-interval Mental confusion, hyperactivity
	Hypocalcemia	Peripheral and perioral paresthesias Hyperactive deep tendon reflexes Abdominal pain and cramps Lethargy and irritability (in infants) Generalized seizures, tetany, laryngospasm ECG changes: prolonged QT-interval
Magnesium	Hypermagnesemia	3–5 mEq/L: nausea, vomiting, hypotension 7–10 mEq/L: hyporeflexia, weakness, drowsiness >12 mEq/L: coma, bradyarrhythmias, respiratory failure
	Hypomagnesemia	Anorexia, nausea, vomiting Weakness, muscle twitches, palpitations, asterixis Tremors, vertigo, convulsions, tachycardia, ventricular ectopy

TABLE 8–11: Manifestations of Abnormal Serum Electrolytes *(Cont.)*

Substance	Symptoms	Manifestations
Phosphate	Hyperphosphatemia	Usually no symptoms; symptoms can arise from coexistent hypocalcemia Increased risk of calcium-phosphate crystals (i.e., *in vivo* calcification) if concurrent hypercalcemia exists. Keep serum Ca PO_4 product ≤80 mg/dL
	Hypophosphatemia:	Anorexia, nausea, irritability Apprehension, confusion, paresthesias, seizures, coma, weakness, respiratory failure

[a] Serum potassium is influenced by the serum glucose. See Chapter 5: Clinical Laboratory Tests for further discussion.

[b] Serum calcium concentration is influenced by the serum albumin. See Chapter 5: Clinical Laboratory Tests for further discussion.

MISCELLANEOUS FLUID AND ELECTROLYTE EQUATIONS: GENERAL RELATIONSHIPS

>> For each 100 mg/dL above normal serum glucose, the serum Na^+ will be "falsely low" by about 1.6 mEq/L.

>> For each decrease in the plasma pH of 0.1 unit, the serum K^+ increases by about 0.6 mEq/L (as a very rough estimate).

>> A loss of 100 to 200 mEq of total body K^+ is required to decrease the serum K^+ by 1 mEq/L if the initial serum K^+ is >3 mEq/L.

>> When the initial serum K^+ is <3 mEq/L, a total body K^+ deficit of 200 to 400 mEq is needed to lower serum K^+ by 1 mEq/L.

$$\text{Anion Gap} = Na - (HCO_3 + Cl)$$
$$= 8 \text{ to } 12 \text{ mEq/L}$$

Or

$$\text{Anion Gap} = (Na + K) - (HCO_3 + Cl)$$
$$= 12 \text{ to } 16 \text{ mEq/L}$$

Significance: When metabolic acidosis occurs, it may not be associated with the accumulation of abnormal, unmeasured anions and an increased anion gap. For example, patients with hyperchloremic metabolic acidosis do not have an increased anion gap. Conditions that are associated with an increased anion gap include: diabetic ketoacidosis; azotemia and uremia; lactic acidosis; salicylate intoxication; alcoholic (ethyl alcohol) nondiabetic ketoacidosis; and intoxication due to the accumulation of other acids as in methanol, paraldehyde, and ethylene glycol intoxications.

> **"MULEPAK"** is a useful mnemonic for conditions
> associated with increased lactic acidosis.
>
> **M**ethanol or ethanol
>
> **U**remia
>
> **L**actic acidosis
>
> **E**thylene glycol
>
> **P**araldehyde
>
> **A**spirin
>
> **K**etoacidosis

Bilirubin

For every 3 mg/dL the bilirubin is above 10 mg/dL, the serum magnesium will be "falsely low" by 0.1 mg/dL. (See also Chapter 11: Common Pharmaceutical Calculations.)

$$\text{Corrected Mg}^{++} = \left(\frac{\text{Reported Bili} - 10}{3} \right) (0.1) + \text{Reported Mg}^{++}$$

Calcium

See also Chapter 11: Common Pharmaceutical Calculations. If serum albumin is low, the serum calcium will appear "falsely low" by the following relationship:

$$\text{Corrected Ca}^{++} = \text{Serum Calcium} + (4.0 - \text{Serum Albumin}) (0.8)$$

REFERENCES

1. Maxwell MH et al., eds. Clinical Disorders of Fluid & Electrolyte Metabolism. 4th ed. New York, NY: McGraw-Hill; 1987.

2. Saxton CR, Seldin DW. Clinical interpretation of laboratory values. In Kokko JP, Jannen RL, eds. Fluids and Electrolytes. Philadelphia, PA: W.B. Saunders; 1986:3;62.

3. Winters RW, ed. Principles of Pediatric Fluid Therapy. 2nd ed. Boston, MA: Little, Brown, & Co.; 1982: 1;22, 57;65, 94;101.

4. Benitz WE, Tatro DS, eds. The Pediatric Drug Handbook. 2nd ed. Chicago, IL: Year Book Medical Publishers; 1988: 289;338.

5. Dunagan WC, Ridner ML, eds. Manual of Medical Therapeutics. 25th ed. Boston, MA: Little, Brown & Co.; 1986.

6. Gomella LG et al., eds. Clinicians Pocket Reference. 6th ed. East Norwalk, CT: Appleton-Lange; 1986: 185;189.

7. Samiy AH et al., eds. Textbook of Diagnostic Medicine. Philadelphia, PA: Lea and Febiger; 1987: 302;324.

8. Schroeder SA et al., eds. Current Medical Diagnosis and Treatment. East Norwalk, CT: Appleton & Lange; 1988:31;39.

9. Finberg L et al., eds. Water & Electrolytes in Pediatrics: Physiology, Pathology, & Treatment. Philadelphia, PA: W.B. Saunders; 1982:17;22.

10. Aubier M et al. Effect of hypophosphatemia on diaphragmatic contractility in patients with acute respiratory failure. N Eng J Med. 1985;313:420;424.

11. Dubois GD, Ariess AC. Clinical Manifestations of Electrolyte Disorders. In: Fluid, Electrolyte & Acid Base Disorders. NY: Churchill Livingston Inc.; 1985:1087–1144.

INTAKE AND OUTPUT RECORD

INPUT

8 Hour Totals	IV	Colloid	Lipid	TPN	Oral	Free Water	Nasogastric			Total
2300-0700										
0700-1500										
1500-2300										
Total Intake										

OUTPUT

8 Hour Totals	Urine	Nasogastric[a]	Stool[a]	Emesis[a]	Wound			Total
2300-0700								
0700-1500								
1500-2300								
Total Loss								

Net I/O _____.

Daily Wt _____ Kg.   Wt. change _past 24 hrs_ _____.

Scale Number _____.

a.   When appropriate record ⊕ or ⊖ for guaiac.

APPENDIX 8–2: Guidelines for IV Potassium Salt Administration

Potassium is administered to replace chronic potassium losses or replenish an existing potassium deficit. Serum potassium concentrations should be monitored closely during therapy. Three modes of administration are available: dietary alterations; oral potassium supplements; and IV therapy.

In asymptomatic patients, the oral route of potassium administration is preferred whenever possible. IV therapy is appropriate in patients with severe hypokalemia and in those unable to take oral supplements. Bolus administration should be the last option. Special care should be exercised to ensure that no drugs or flush solutions are pushed through the line while the potassium salt is present in high concentrations. Sliding scale orders are inappropriate for general use and should be implemented only in special instances.

Arrhythmias are a potentially life-threatening complication when serum potassium concentrations rise quickly. Prominent manifestations are found on ECG with a potassium bolus and/or hyperkalemia. The earliest changes may be peaked, narrow T-waves and a shortened QT interval representing rapid depolarization. With increasing potassium concentrations, the QRS complex widens and merges with the T-wave to produce sine-wave patterns. This may be followed by ventricular fibrillation or standstill (potassium concentrations ≥ 8 mEq/L). In addition, potassium salts are extremely irritating to tissue. Therefore, extreme caution must be used to avoid extravasation (especially in patients with poor circulation or who are comatose).

The following guidelines were developed to emphasize prudent potassium administration, recognizing the potential life-threatening danger of inappropriate IV potassium administration. They are intended as only "guidelines" and do not preclude a practitioner from ordering or administering potassium in special instances, unique patient populations, or situations she deems medically necessary.

ADULTS

Table 8–A: Guidelines for Potassium Administration in Adults

Potassium Concentration	ECG	Rate for Peripheral Administration	Rate for Central Adminstration
≥ 2.5 mEq/L	Asymptomatic	10 mEq/hr	20 mEq/hr
<2.5 mEq/L	Symptomatic	40 mEq/hr	40 mEq/hr

Maximum Concentration of Potassium Salts Per Liter of IV Fluid

- Peripheral 40 mEq/L.

- Central 120 mEq/L.

(Continued)

ADULTS *(Continued)*

Recommended Dilutions

- Peripheral 10 mEq in at least 50 mL of IV fluid.

- Central 20 mEq in at least 50 mL of IV fluid.

PEDIATRICS ($\leq$40 kg)
Rate of Administration

- Administer doses of up to 1 mEq/kg over at least 1 hr to a maximum of 40 mEq/hr.

- For total doses of >1 mEq/kg, rate of administration must not exceed 0.5 mEq/kg/hr.

- Administration rates >0.2 mEq/kg/hr require cardiac monitoring.

Maximum Concentration of Maintenance IV Fluid

- Peripheral 40 mEq/L.

- Central 120 mEq/L.

Recommended Dilution

- Central and Peripheral 1 mEq in at least 5 mL of IV fluid.

Maximum Concentration

- 1 mEq in 1 mL of IV fluid on a syringe pump in an ICU setting only.

Enteral Nutrition

Timothy D. Wolf

9

Enteral nutrition is a method of providing nutritional support to patients with normal gastrointestinal (GI) function who are unable to eat to meet metabolic demands. With the development of enteral formulas appropriate for a variety of disease states, nutrition delivery can be provided to the GI tract via artificial means. As a means of nutritional support, enteral nutrition is preferred over parenteral nutrition because it is safe, effective, and economical for patients. It avoids the potential complications of parenteral therapy associated with central venous catheter insertion (e.g., catheter sepsis, pneumothorax, and catheter embolus). Administered by tube or by mouth, enteral products can serve as the sole source of nutritional support, as a dietary supplement to oral intake, or as an adjunct during transition from parenteral to oral feedings. When the enteral route for nutritional support is not viable, Chapter 10: Parenteral Nutrition should be reviewed. Calculations of adult nutritional requirements are presented in the Parenteral Nutrition chapter.

This chapter is aimed at providing a basic understanding and appreciation for the various types of enteral products and pediatric formulas available. Similarly, approaches for administering and monitoring the products to ensure efficacy and minimize toxicity or interactions are highlighted. (See Chapter 10: Parenteral Nutrition for a detailed discussion of nutritional calculations.)

NUTRITIONAL TERMS

A wide variety of dietary terms are used to describe nutritional plans for patients and some of the more common terms are listed below:

>> **Clear Liquid Diet.** A clear liquid diet may be used for pre- and post-operative procedures, before many diagnostic tests, and during acute illness. It should only be used for a brief period of time for conditions requiring easily digestible, easily consumable nourishment. Clear liquid diets are low in irritants and contain foods that are liquid at room and body temperature.

>> **General Diet.** A general diet provides various nutrients essential to the body for maintenance, repair, growth, and development. It is used for all patients not requiring restrictions, modifications, or special additions to their dietary regimen. A general diet includes milk and milk products, meat and meat substitutes, bread and cereal products, fruit and vegetables, saturated and unsaturated fats, and desserts.

>> **High Fiber Diet.** The high fiber diet is designed to decrease transit time through the intestine, increase stool volume, and decrease intraluminal pressure. It may be prescribed for patients with:

constipation, hemorrhoids, diverticulosis, or irritable bowel syndrome. A high fiber diet contains a minimum of 7 gm crude fiber. Adequate fluid intake is critical to prevent constipation and/or bowel obstruction.

>> **Low Cholesterol Diet.** This diet limits the cholesterol intake to ≤300 mg/day; total fat should not represent more than 30% of the total daily caloric intake. It contains equal amounts of saturated, monounsaturated, and polyunsaturated fats. The calories provided are aimed at maintaining an ideal weight.

>> **Low Sodium Diet.** A low sodium diet is indicated in congestive heart failure (CHF), hypertension, liver cirrhosis, some renal diseases, and following the administration of sodium-retaining hormones or drugs (e.g., adrenocortical steroids). The various amounts of sodium per day that often are representative of a low-sodium diet are: No added salt (NAS) (150 to 200 mEq); 90 mEq; 45 mEq; 22 mEq; and 11 mEq of salt per day.

>> **ADA Diet.** This is a diet based on the American Diabetes Association (ADA) guidelines which attempt to achieve control of blood glucose concentration and blood lipid levels. It provides adequate nutrition for growth and allows achievement and/or maintenance of reasonable weight to delay or prevent the complications associated with diabetes. Guidelines are available for insulin dependent diabetes mellitus (IDDM), non-insulin dependent diabetes mellitus (NIDDM), and diabetes during pregnancy.

>> **Low Carbohydrate, High Protein, High Fat Diet.** This diet is designed for patients recovering from a recent gastrectomy and/or who have developed a dumping syndrome. It is intended to prevent a hyperosmolar condition from developing in the proximal jejunum following gastrectomy. It is also used for patients who need to provide a gradual release of glucose into the blood stream, (e.g., in the treatment of hypoglycemia).

>> **Low to Moderate Protein Diets.** These diets minimize the accumulation of nitrogenous waste products (i.e., urea, uric acid, creatinine, organic acids, ammonia) when used in the treatment of hepatic disorders or in acute or chronic renal failure. Protein intake is approximately 0.4 to 1.2 gm/kg ideal body weight (IBW) or a total of 20 to 60 gm/day.

>> **High Protein Diets.** These diets are used during stress or trauma (e.g., surgery, burns, cirrhosis, infection, malnutrition, extreme heat or cold) or as replacement therapy for protein losses due to peritoneal dialysis or protein-losing enteropathy. These diets provide 1.5 to 2.0 gm/kg IBW or 90 to 150 gm/day of protein.

INDICATIONS/CONTRAINDICATIONS
FOR ENTERAL NUTRITION SUPPORT[1]

In general, enteral products are selected after a thorough and complete assessment of the patient's digestive/absorptive state and/or fluid and electrolyte demands. In addition, it is important to establish the delivery route (i.e., nasogastric, gastrostomy, or jejunostomy) which is dependent on the patient's clinical condition. Table 9–1 lists typical indications and contraindications for use of enteral nutrition.

TABLE 9–1: Typical Indications and Contraindications of Enteral Nutrition

Indications	Contraindications
Carcinoma of the head and neck	Paralytic ileus
Radical surgery to the upper GI tract, oral pharynx, and upper respiratory tract	Failure to meet nutritional needs on a properly managed trial of enteral nutrition
Endotracheal intubation	Peritonitis
Esophageal stricture	Small bowel or gastric obstruction
Depressed mental status, anorexia nervosa	Abdominal distention
Swallowing difficulties/dysphagia	Severe malabsorption
Paralysis	GI hemorrhage
Correction of malnutrition secondary to chronic disease	Enteral therapy associated with intractable diarrhea
When oral intake alone does not meet calorie and protein needs	
Hypermetabolic states, major body burns, and trauma	
Chemotherapy	
Radiotherapy	
Geriatric patients	

PROFILE: ENTERAL PRODUCTS

Commonly available enteral product formulas are described in Table 9–2. These products can further be categorized into the following groups:

>> **Standard Oral Supplements.** These products are most commonly used as tube feedings, are lactose-free, and generally well tolerated by most patients.

>> **Isotonic formulas** are indicated for patients with normal gut function or when the GI tract has been at rest for over 3 days. Fat calories are usually 50% of the formula as medium chain triglycerides with the remaining percentage composed of corn and soy oils. The electrolyte composition of isotonic formulas is moderate to enhance flexibility of use, especially in patients with electrolyte imbalances.

>> **High calorie/high protein formulas** are indicated for use in trauma, surgery, thermal injury, severe hypermetabolic states, multiple fractures, volume restrictions, and sensitivity. Like standard oral supplements, these formulations are lactose-free.

>> **Partially hydrolyzed peptide formulas** are indicated for patients with protein or fat maldigestion/malabsorption (e.g., Crohn's disease, cystic fibrosis, fistulas, short-bowel syndrome) or during transition from parenteral to enteral feedings. The protein source is comprised of essential amino acids that promote rapid and uniform nitrogen transport and absorption.

>> **High nitrogen, partially hydrolyzed formulas** are indicated for patients with extensive trauma, thermal injury, or with hypercatabolic states where digestive and absorptive capacity may be marginal.

>> **Elemental formulas** are indicated for maldigestion, malabsorption, protein restricted patients with liver or renal disease. These products are low in fat; therefore, supplementation with purified unsaturated fatty acids (PUFA) is necessary for long-term use to prevent essential fatty acid (EFA) deficiency.

>> **Elemental diet formulas** are indicated for maldigestion and malabsorption when protein restriction is unnecessary. These formulas have a high osmolarity and can cause diarrhea unless initiated slowly at a reduced concentration.

>> **Fiber-containing formulas** are indicated for patients requiring tube feeding, but not requiring a residue diet. The fiber may help normalize whole gut transit time.

>> **High fat/low carbohydrate formulas** are indicated for patients with compromised respiratory function and fluid restriction. These products provide concentrated nutrition and decrease carbon dioxide production and respiratory quotient.

>> **Modular components** contain a single source of calories as carbohydrates, protein, or fat. Polycose is composed of a glucose polymer and has a negligible electrolyte content. Medium Chain Triglyceride (MCT) provides calories as fat for fat malabsorption states that accompany short-bowel syndrome and pancreatic insufficiency. Propac provides protein and is indicated for disease states with high protein requirements (e.g., burn/trauma, sepsis). Lipomul is a source of EFA and increases non-protein calories without increasing the formula osmolality and carbohydrate load.

>> **Low calorie formula diets** are indicated for outpatient use as part of a specialized weight loss program under close medical supervision.

MONITORING THE TUBE-FED PATIENT

Once tube feedings are initiated, the patient must be monitored to ascertain efficacy of the nutritional support regimen and identify and correct intolerance problems, metabolic complications, or other adverse effects. Patients should be weighed daily or as appropriate. The patient's input and output should be accurately recorded: the volume of tube feeding (TF) and volume of free water administered to the patient should be recorded separately. Patients also should be observed for evidence of intolerance (e.g., bloating, nausea, emesis, diarrhea) and hydration status (e.g., edema, skin turgor, conditions of mucous membranes, rales).

Laboratory tests should be monitored as follows to assess efficacy or toxicity of the regimen:

>> **Initially** a chemistry panel, electrolytes (serum), and hematology panel are performed. The *chemistry panel* includes glucose, blood urea nitrogen (BUN), cholesterol, total bilirubin, alkaline phosphatase, gamma glutamyl transferase (GGT), aspartate aminotransferase (AST), lactate dehydrogenase (LD), creatinine, calcium, phosphorus, magnesium, uric acid, total protein, and albumin assessments. *Serum electrolytes:* sodium (Na^+), potassium(K^+), chloride (Cl^-), and total carbon dioxide are measured. The *hematology panel* includes white blood cell (WBC) count, red blood cell (RBC) count, hemoglobin (Hgb), hematocrit (Hct), mean cell volume (MCV), and mean corpuscular hemoglobin concentration (MCHC) assessments.

>> **Follow-up** includes electrolyte measurements daily for 5 days, and chemistry survey, electrolytes, and hematology survey weekly; 24-hour total urea nitrogen should be measured as appropriate.

PROPER ADMINISTRATION OF TUBE FEEDINGS

The proper administration of tube feeding products is important to achieve and assure patient tolerance. Consider the following points when administering a particular product.

Continuous drip given over a 24 hour period is the preferred method for administration of tube feedings. Potential complications associated with tube feedings

Table 9-2: Enteral Products Profile

Nutrients/1000 mL

Products	Na mmol/L (mg)	K mmol/L (mg)	Protein gm	Fat gm	Carbohydrate gm	Water mL	Non-Protein Calorie: N ratio	Osmolality mOsm/kg H₂0	Calories kcal/mL
Standard Oral Supplements									
Ensure	36.8 (845)	40 (1564)	37.2	37.2	145	800	153:1	450	1.06
Sustacal	40 (930)	54 (2100)	61	23	140	840	79:1	625	1
Resource Liquid Nutrition	36.7 (845)	40 (1561)	37.2	37.2	145	823	153:1	400	1.06
Carnation Instant Breakfast	45.3	—	62.4	37.5	142	—	89:1	700	1.06
Attain	35	41	40	35	135	—	134:1	300	1
Isotonic Formulas									
Osmolite	27.6 (634)	25.9 (1014)	37.2	38.5	145	841	153:1	300	1.06
Isocal	23 (530)	34 (1320)	34	44	133	840	167:1	300	1.06
Nutren	27.1	32	40	38	127	860	134:1	300	1
High-Calorie/High Protein Formulas									
Ensure Plus HN	51.3 (1180)	46.6 (1820)	62.6	50	200	769	125:1	650	1.5
Travasorb MCT Liquid	22.8 (524)	25.6 (1480)	73.8	48.5	185	—	100:1	450	1.5
Sustacal HC	36.7 (844)	37.6 (1477)	60.8	57.4	190	780	134:1	650	1.5
Partially Hydrolyzed Peptide Formulas									
Travasorb HN	40.1 (922)	30 (1171)	45	13.5	175	—	114:1	560	1
Vital HN	20.3 (467)	34.2 (1334)	41.7	10.8	185	867	125:1	460	1

(Continued)

Table 9–2: Enteral Products Profile (Continued)

Products	Nutrients/1000 mL									
	Na mmol/L (mg)	K mmol/L (mg)	Protein gm	Fat gm	Carbohydrate gm	Water mL	Non-Protein Calorie: N ratio	Osmolality mOsm/kg H₂0	Calories kcal/mL	
High Nitrogen–Partially Hydrolyzed Formula Isotein HN	27 (620)	27.4 (1070)	67.8	33.9	156	652	86:1	300	1.2	
Elemental Formula (Free Amino Acids) Tolerex	20.4 (468)	30 (1169)	20.6	1.4	231	—	284:1	550	1	
Elemental Diet Formula Vivonex T.E.N.	20 (460)	20 (782)	38.2	2.8	206	845	149:1	630	1	
Fiber Containing Formulas Jevity	40.4 (930)	40.3 (1570)	44.4	36.9	152	835	125:1	310	1.06	
High Fat, Low Carbohydrate Formula Pulmocare	57 (1310)	48.6 (1902)	62.6	92.1	106	785	92:1	545	1.5	
Modular Components Polycose									23 kcal/tbsp	
Medium Chain Triglyceride (MCT) Oil										
Propac			1 pkt = 15 gm					7.7	1 pkt = 78 kcal	
Lipomul									6	
Low Calorie Formula Diets Medifast 70			70 gm/ 500 cal							
Optifast 70			70 gm/ 500 cal							

(e.g., hyperglycemia, pulmonary aspiration, and diarrhea) can be reduced by continuous feedings. Bolus feedings are not recommended and should not be given unless the feeding tube is in the stomach and previous feedings have been well tolerated.

To initiate a **continuous tube feeding**:

1) Depending upon tube location, confirm placement of tube by irrigation with air or aspiration of stomach or small bowel contents.

2) Dilute the product to half strength; start administration at 50 mL/hr. This is especially important for high osmotic products.

3) If the feeding is tolerated, (i.e., absence of glucosuria, hyperglycemia, diarrhea, abdominal discomfort, residuals <150 mL), increase the *rate* of feeding by increments of 25 mL/hr each day until the desired rate of infusion is achieved.

4) Once the final rate (as determined by energy needs) is achieved, increase the *strength* in one-fourth increments every 24 hours.

5) If diarrhea or abdominal discomfort is present after the advancement of the feeding, return to the previous rate or strength for another 24 hour period.

Before initiation of tube feedings, check placement of the feeding tube to make sure it has been properly positioned. Place the patient in an upright position with the head elevated to a ≥30° angle during feeding. Before subsequent feedings, check gastric residuals. If residuals are >150 mL, feedings should be held.

Give adequate "free water" to replace insensible water loss (500 to 1200 mL/day). Total fluid requirements should include insensible losses which range from 1 to 2 mL/kcal with greater amounts for extrarenal losses (e.g., burns, fistulas, open wounds, fever). (See Chapter 8: Fluid and Electrolyte Therapy for a more detailed discussion). Adequate "free water" is especially important when administering high protein formulas or >1 gm/kg protein intake as these products can produce a solute diuresis leading to dehydration. Record input and output every 8 hours, with tube feeding volume recorded separately from water intake.

To prevent precipitating bacterial growth, refrigerate commercial tube feeding products after opening. If the formula is not used within 24 hours, it should be discarded. Further, no more than an 8-hour supply of feeding should be prepared and hung in the patient care area. Change the external tube and feeding bag daily. Irrigate the feeding tube with 120 mL of water if the feeding is stopped for any reason and at least every 6 to 8 hours to prevent clogging.

Finally, if a tube feeding product is given orally, chilling improves palatability. If this is unacceptable, consider flavored products.

TABLE 9–3: Tube Feeding Complications

Type/Complication	Causes	Management
Gastrointestinal		
Diarrhea (most common)	Bacterial contamination of formula; improper administration; use of antibiotics; lactose intolerance; impaction; malnutrition	Discard bags and tubing after 24 hr; use only 4–8 hr of feeding; use isotonic formula at tolerable rate by continuous delivery via pump; avoid or recognize drugs causing diarrhea; avoid lactose containing formulas; rule out impaction before treating diarrhea; use elemental formula or parenteral nutrition
Constipation	Low residue formula used in long-term, tube-fed patients	Provide additional fluids by mouth or tube feeding; increase ambulation or use a high-fiber, high-residue formula; administer bulking agents (psyllium)
Bloating	Presence of a mild ileus; intolerance to lipids in formula; swallowing excessive amounts of air (e.g., head and neck surgery)	Use elemental formulas requiring less digestion; increase ambulation; administer bisacodyl suppository
Inadequate gastric emptying	Gastric atony, prepyloric ulcers, bowel ileus	Verify tube placement; monitor stomach content residuals before bolus feedings or every 2–4 hr during continuous feedings
Vomiting	Psychological association with the illness; unpleasant odor of formulas containing free amino acids or the reinstilling of large amounts of aspirated gastric residuals	Reduce anxiety; use intact protein containing formulas or antiemetic when indicated; decrease the rate of delivery and feeding beyond the pylorus

(Continued)

9–9

TABLE 9–3: Tube Feeding Complications *(Continued)*

Type/Complication	Causes	Management
Gastrointestinal *(Continued)*		
Nausea	Delayed gastric emptying; gastric distention; formula too hot or too cold, or given too rapidly	Stop feedings and determine cause; check gastric residual to determine the progress of gastric emptying after 1–2 hr; restart feedings at slower rate and/or dilute
Gastrointestinal bleed (rare)	Some data suggest that enteral hyperalimentation may protect against GI bleeding while treating malnutrition	Discontinue enteral feeding and change to parenteral nutritional support
Mechanical		
Tube obstruction	Formula with a caloric density of 1.5 to 2.0 kcal/mL; inadequate crushing of medications or inadequate dilution/flushing of psyllium or antacids	Use feeding pumps for dense formulas and/or larger-bore feeding tubes; give medications as elixirs or mixed with water or formula; avoid mixing formulas with liquid medications with a pH $\leq$5; instill a few mL of Coca-Cola or meat tenderizer to help unclog tubes; use cranberry juice for psyllium administration
Displacement	Vomiting; cough; incorrect tube placement; detached tape holding tube to nose	Check tube placement by x-ray; listen for air being injected through the tube into the stomach with a stethoscope, followed by aspiration of a small amount of gastric contents
Irritation	Esophageal reflux; peptic esophagitis; pressure necrosis of esophageal and tracheal wall at cuff inflation site	Provide nose and mouth care; change tape; increase salivation in the mouth by allowing chewing gum, hard candy, or ice chips
Rupture (rare)	Continuous tube feeding in a closed system	Periodic disconnection of feeding tube from the infusion apparatus; assess for abdominal distention; pain in upper left quadrant or epigastric area may be a sign of gastric rupture

(Continued)

TABLE 9–3: Tube Feeding Complications *(Continued)*

Type/Complication	Causes	Management
Mechanical *(Continued)*		
Pneumonia	Gastric contents refluxing into bronchus secondary to delayed gastric emptying; improper placement of tube in tracheal or bronchus; incompetent lower esophageal sphincter	Place feeding tube beyond the pylorus; use small, soft feeding tube; keep maximum gastric content residuals to <150 mL.
Metabolic		
Hyperglycemia	Common in patients who are diabetic, hypermetabolic, or receiving corticosteroids or glucagon	Check blood glucose and urine acetone frequently with advancing enteral feedings; decrease rate of feeding; administer insulin if needed; hydrate patient or change to a lower carbohydrate content formula **Note:** Hyperglycemic-hyperosmolar coma may occur if glucose is infused faster than 0.5 gm/kg/hr, or if the patient is diabetic, a latent diabetic, or with hyperosmolar formulas causing intracellular dehydration
Tube feeding syndrome (develops 4–14 days after feedings initiated)	*Signs and Symptoms:* Lethargy, cardiovascular instability, fever, confusion, and decreased level of consciousness. *Results from:* Intake of excessive protein and inadequate fluids with subsequent dehydration, hypernatremia, hyperchloremia, and azotemia. Renal tubular dysfunction; primary water deficit; adrenal corticosteroid secretion producing sodium retention; advanced age and renal arteriosclerosis	Monitor electrolytes, BUN, Hct, and fluid intake and output. Reduce protein content of formula and/or provide more free water

(Continued)

TABLE 9–3: Tube Feeding Complications *(Continued)*

Type/Complication	Causes	Management
Metabolic *(Continued)*		
Hypernatremia	High sodium and low water intake	Monitor fluid intake and output, serum sodium, and BUN and rehydrate patient
Hyponatremia	Isotonic or hypotonic feedings; excessive antidiuretic hormone production; total body sodium deficiency or overhydration	Restrict fluids, administer diuretics, replace sodium losses
Hyperkalemia	Metabolic acidosis with or without renal insufficiency; anabolic metabolism; excessive potassium supplementation after tube feedings started	Monitor serum potassium and adjust formula
Hypokalemia	Diuretic use; GI losses; high doses of insulin; in combination with hypomagnesemia and hypophosphatemia in malnourished patients	Monitor serum potassium and adjust formula
Hyperphosphatemia	Renal insufficiency in tube-fed patients	Monitor serum phosphate and adjust formula
Hypophosphatemia	May occur in a malnourished patient placed on nutritional support who subsequently becomes anabolic	Monitor serum phosphate and adjust formula
Hypomagnesemia	Inadequate replacement of magnesium. May see: Increased reflexes, coarse tremors, muscle cramps, dysrhythmias, paresthesias, and positive Chvostek's and Trousseau's signs	Monitor serum magnesium and adjust formula
Hypozincemia	Sequestration of zinc in the liver resulting from systemic infection and decreased carrier protein levels in protein deficiencies	Monitor serum zinc and adjust formula

INDICATIONS AND GOALS
FOR PEDIATRIC ENTERAL NUTRITION

In infants, enteral nutrition is intended to provide adequate replacement for human breast milk. For those infants allergic or intolerant to various components of human breast milk or standard infant formulas, enteral nutrition should provide adequate substitute feeding.

Generally, caloric goals of pediatric enteral nutrition are calculated using the infant's weight as described by:[5]

>> **Low Birth Weight (LBW) Infants.** 120 kcal/kg/day.

>> **≤6 Months.** 100 to 200 kcal/kg/day.

>> **6 Months to 1 Year.** 100 to 105 kcal/kg/day.

>> **>1 Year.** 80 to 100 kcal/kg/day.

Protein requirements for infants during the first year of life are 2 to 3 gm/kg/day and should supply 7% to 16% of the total daily caloric intake. For low birth weight infants, protein intake should be greater, at approximately 3.5 to 4 gm/kg/day. The total daily caloric intake of carbohydrates and fats should be 35% to 65% and 30% to 55%, respectively.

HUMAN VERSUS COWS' MILK FORMULATION

Normal infant formulas are formulated from cows' milk. Table 9–4 provides a comparison of the differences and similarities between whole cows' milk and human milk.

Methods of Altering Cows' Milk
for Manufacture of Milk-Based Formulas[6]

To create milk-based formulas from cows' milk a variety of approaches have been used. First, the poorly absorbed butterfat is replaced by coconut and polyunsaturated vegetable oils to which Vitamin E has been added to change the fat composition. For infants with pancreatic insufficiency (cystic fibrosis), bile acid deficiency, prematurity, or other malabsorption problems, MCT has been used. MCT increases the absorption of calcium and phosphorus and may improve carbohydrate tolerance.

Next, the protein content is reduced by decreasing the total amount of calories from protein. In some instances, the lactalbumin:casein ratio is altered from 20:80 to 60:40 to more closely simulate breast milk. For infants allergic to milk protein, methionine has been added to the soy protein. Likewise, protein hydrolysates may also be used in formulas for infants with food allergies or digestive disorders such as cystic fibrosis. Finally, the cystine content is sometimes increased to more closely simulate breast milk.

To more closely simulate human milk, the carbohydrate caloric source in milk-based formulas is increased to 40%. The added carbohydrate may be lactose, corn syrup, tapioca, sucrose, or dextrose. For infants allergic to or intolerant of lactose, lactose may be totally replaced.

The renal solute load in cows' milk is too high for routine infant feeding and can lead to dehydration. Milk-based formulas are formulated with a lower percentage of protein calories and a lower mineral content, which brings the renal solute load closer to that of human milk.

Lastly, the mineral ratio of calcium to phosphorus in cows' milk may be altered to more closely resemble that of human breast milk.

TABLE 9–4: Comparison of Human Milk to Cows' Milk[6]

Component	Category	Cow's Milk	Human Milk
Fat	% of total calories	50%	55%
	Triglycerides	More difficult to absorb. Primarily short and long chain.[a] Primarily saturated	More medium chain and monounsaturated fatty acids that are easier to absorb. Contains lipoprotein lipase and bile salt stimulating pancreatic lipase
Protein	% of total calories	20% (3 times that of breast milk)	7% (7%–16% recommended)
	Lactalbumin:Casein[b]	20:80	60:40
	Taurine[c] and Cystine[d]	Almost none	High levels
Carbohydrate[e]	% of total calories	30%	38% (35%–65% recommended)
Form			
	Lactose	Lactose	Lactose
	Renal solute load	228 mOsm/L	79 mOsm/L
	Sodium	2.2 mmol/100 mL	0.7 mmol/100 mL
	Ca/PO$_4$ ratio	1.3:1	2–2.4:1

[a] Long chain triglycerides may form insoluble complexes with calcium.

[b] Casein is relatively insoluble and occurs in milk as a "tough curd," in contrast to lactalbumin which is highly soluble and occurs in milk as whey. The increased curd slows gastric emptying and may cause GI distress.

[c] Taurine is needed for maintenance of cellular structural and functional integrity.

[d] Increased cystine is needed because infants may not be able to convert methionine to cystine, which is necessary for somatic growth.

[e] Lactose is preferred as it increases the absorption of calcium and magnesium.

PROFILE: PEDIATRIC FORMULAS

Table 9–5 lists several examples of pediatric-based formulas. Product differences are described in Table 9–6.

ENTERAL FORMULAS AND DRUG COMPATIBILITY
Drug-Nutrient Incompatibilities

Potential interactions can occur when various medications are administered concurrently with an enteral product. (See Tables 9–7, 9–8, and 9–9.) To avoid potential drug-nutrient incompatibilities, tube feedings should be stopped and at least 60 mL of water instilled through the tube, before and after drug administration. The most frequent compatibility problems involve strongly acidic or buffered syrups with pH values ≤4. Incompatibilities between formulas and drugs can cause immediate dumping and increased viscosity and particle size resulting in clogged feeding tubes.[8] At pH values ≤5, *in vitro* clotting has occurred with Pulmocare, Ensure Plus, Osmolite, Enrich, Ensure, and Resource.[9]

TABLE 9–5: Pediatric Formulas Profile

Type	Product	Characteristics
Milk based formulas	Enfamil	Lower sodium, 60:40 lactalbumin:casein ratio
	Similac	Similac with whey available
	SMA	Lowest sodium, 60:40 lactalbumin:casein ratio
Soy formulas	Prosobee	No sucrose
	Nursoy	Lower sodium
	Isomil	Isomil SF is available which is sucrose free
	RCF	Carbohydrate free, must supplement with fructose or glucose polymers (e.g., Polycose)
Altered protein and/or fat	Nutramigen	Protein hydrolysate
	Pregestimil	Protein hydrolysate, MCT (40% of fat) and glucose polymers
	Portagen	Soy formula with MCT (low essential fatty acids)
	Lofenalac	Low phenylalanine
Low birth weight and premature formulas		Provide more calcium, protein, and sodium, an increased vitamin E to polyunsaturated fat ratio, altered carbohydrate consisting of lactose and corn syrup and part of the fat as MCT. Some have increased zinc and/or folic acid.
Renal formula	Similac PM 60/40	Low renal solute load, low sodium, low phosphorus

TABLE 9–6: Pediatric Formula Composition[5,7]

Formula	Calories kcal/30 mL	Na mmol/L	K mmol/L	Cl mmol/L	Ca:P Ratio	Renal Solute Load	Protein gm/L	Fat gm/L	CHO[a] gm/L
Standard Formulas									
Mature human milk	22	7	14	12	2.2:1	73	11	45	68
Enfamil	20	9	18	12	1.5:1	99	15	37	70
Similac 20	20	11	20	15	1.3:1	108	15	36	72
SMA 20	20	6	14	10	1.5:1	90	15	36	72
Therapeutic Formulas									
Milk Allergy									
Isomil	20	13	24	12	1.4:1	129	20	36	68
Nursoy	20	9	19	11	1.4:1	123	21	36	69
Nutramigen	20	14	16	14	1.5:1	107	22	26	88
Prosobee	20	11	21	16	1.3:1	128	20	36	69
Fat/Carbohydrate Restriction									
Portagen	20	14	22	16	1.3:1	147	24	32	78
Pregestimil	20	14	19	16	1.5:1	125	19	27	91
RCF (Ross Carbohydrate Free)	12	13	18	15	1.4:1	126	20	36	0

(Continued)

TABLE 9–6: Pediatric Formula Composition[5,7] (Continued)

Formula	Calories kcal/30 mL	Na mmol/L	K mmol/L	Cl mmol/L	Ca:P Ratio	Renal Solute Load	Protein gm/L	Fat gm/L	CHO[a] gm/L
Therapeutic Formulas (Continued)									
High Protein or Calorie Requirements (LBW Infant Formulas)									
Enfamil Premature	24	14	23	19	2:1	152	24	41	89
Similac Special Care	24	18	29	21	2:1	156	22	44	86
Premie SMA	24	14	19	15	1.9:1	224	44	86	—
Sodium Restriction									
Lonalac	20	1.7	49	22	1.1:1	289	34	35	48
Lofenalac	20	14	18	13	1.3:1	133	22	26	88
Renal Insufficiency									
Similac PM 60/40	20	7	15	11	2:1	96	15.8	37.6	68.8

[a] CHO = Carbohydrate.

TABLE 9–7: Enteral Formulas and Drug Compatibility[10]

Product	Compatibilities[a]		
	Osmolite HN	Vital	Osmolite
Aluminum hydroxide suspension (Amphojel)	C	C	I
Potassium gluconate (Kaon Liquid)	I	C	I
Potassium chloride powder (K-Lor)	C	C	C
Furosemide (Lasix)	C	C	C
Morphine sulfate	C	C	C
Magnesium and Aluminum hydroxide with simethicone 20 mg (Mylanta)	C	C	C
Magnesium and Aluminum hydroxide with simethicone 30 mg (Mylanta II)	I	C	I
Sodium phosphate (Phospho Soda)	I	C	I
Magaldrate (Riopan)	C	C	I
Cimetidine (Tagamet)	I	C	I

[a] I = Incompatible; C = Compatible

Pharmacokinetic Alterations[12, 13]

Alterations can result from the pharmacological actions of drugs which produce side effects such as nausea, vomiting, diarrhea, decreased appetite, and electrolyte and metabolic abnormalities. Likewise, medications' side effects must be considered in patients receiving enteral formulas and not be solely attributed to formula intolerance. Further, drug bioavailability and metabolism can be altered by the concomitant use of enteral formulas. (See Tables 9–9 and 9–10.)

TABLE 9–8: Enteral Formulas and Drug Compatibility[11]

Product	Compatibilities[i]	
	Enrich	Vivonex TEN
Cimetidine elixir	C	C
Prochlorperazine elixir (Compazine)	C	C
Docusate sodium elixir (Colace)	C	C
Diphenoxylate and atropine elixir (Lomotil)	C	C
Magnesium hydroxide (Milk of Magnesia)	C	C
Simethicone drops (Mylicon)	C	C
Metoclopramide syrup (Reglan)	I[a]	C
Diphenhydramine elixir (Benadryl)	C	C
Guaifenesin syrup (Robitussin)	I[b]	C
Pseudoephedrine (Sudafed)	I[c]	C
Acetaminophen elixir (Tylenol)	C	C
Ferrous sulfate elixir (Feosol)	I[d]	C
Potassium chloride elixir	C	C
Sodium phosphate (Fleets phosphosoda)	I[e]	C
Zinc sulfate capsules	I[f]	C
Amoxicillin suspension (Amoxil)	C	C
Nitrofurantoin suspension (Furadantin)	C	C
Cephalexin (Keflex)	C	C
Trimethoprim/Sulfamethoxazole suspension (Septra)	C	C
Chlorpromazine concentrate	I[g]	C
Thioridazine concentrate (Mellaril)	I[h]	C
Thiothixene (Navane)	C	C
Doxepin concentrate (Sinequan)	C	C
Phenobarbital elixir	C	C
Phenytoin suspension (Dilantin)	C	C
Digoxin elixir (Lanoxin)	C	C
Furosemide liquid	C	C

[a] Forms thin, granular formula.
[b] Separation particles.
[c] Thick, gelatinous mass.
[d] Large particles.
[e] Thin, granular.
[f] Soft, gelatinous mass.
[g] Soft, thick.
[h] Thin, large particles.
[i] I = Incompatible; C = Compatible.

TABLE 9–9: Interactions of Selected Formulas with Medications[12]

Product	Effect on Drug
Ensure	Theophylline: ↑ in osmolality Phenytoin susp.: ↓ drug concentration[a] Methyldopa: ↓ drug concentration
Ensure Plus	Theophylline: ↑ in osmolality Phenytoin susp.: ↓ drug concentration[a] Methyldopa: ↓ drug concentration
Osmolite	Theophylline: ↑ in osmolality Phenytoin susp.: ↓ drug concentration[a] Methyldopa: ↓ drug concentration

[a] No significant drug concentration changes with injectable phenytoin.

Table 9–10: Drugs That Undergo Altered Excretion and Absorption When Taken With Food[13]

Captopril	Nitrofurantoin
Carbamazepine	Penicillins
Dicumarol	Phenytoin suspension
Digoxin	Procainamide
Griseofulvin	Propranolol
Hydralazine	Rifampin
Hydrochlorothiazide	Tetracycline
Isoniazid	Theophylline
Metoprolol	

REFERENCES

1. ASPEN Board of Directors. Guidelines for the use of enteral nutrition in the adult patient. JPEN. 1987; 11(5): 435–439.

2. Breach CL, Saldanha LG. Tube feeding complications, Part I: gastrointestinal. Nutritional Support Services. 1988; 8(3):15–19.

3. Breach CL, Saldanha LG. Tube feeding complications, Part II: mechanical. Nutritional Support Services. 1988; 8(5):28–32.

4. Breach CL, Saldanha LG. Tube feeding complications, Part III: metabolic. Nutritional Support Services. 1988; 8(6):16–19.

5. Serrano Murphy VA, Bubica G. General pediatric therapy. In: Young LY, Koda-Kimble MA, eds. Applied Therapeutics: The Clinical Use of Drugs. 4th ed. Vancouver: Applied Therapeutics; 1988:1821.

6. McKenzie MW et al. Infant formulas. In: Feldmann EG, Blockstein WL, eds. Handbook of Nonprescription Drugs. 9th ed. Washington: American Pharmaceutical Association; 1990:529–561.

7. Benitz WE, Tatro DS. The Pediatric Drug Handbook. 2nd ed. Chicago: Year Book Medical Publishers, Inc.; 1988:339–347.

8. Cutie AJ et al. Compatibility of enteral products with commonly employed drug additives. JPEN 1983; 7:186–191.

9. Marcuard SP, Perkins AM. Clogging of feeding tubes. JPEN. 1988; 12(4): 403–405.

10. Fagerman KE, Ballou AE. Drug compatibilities with enteral feeding solutions coadministered by tube. Nutritional Support Services. 1988; 8(5); 31–32.

11. Burns PE et al. Physical compatibility of enteral formulas with various common medications. J Am Diet Assoc. 1988; 88(9):1094–1096.

12. Holtz L et al . Compatibility of medications with enteral feedings. JPEN. 1987; 11(2):183–186.

13. Egging P. Enteral nutrition from a pharmacist's perspective. Nutritional Support Services. 1987; 7(4):17.

Parenteral Nutrition

Cheryl A. Ray

10

The clinical applications of total parenteral nutrition (TPN) have greatly expanded over the past decade. Undernutrition which results from lack of nutrients and/or abnormal assimilation of nutrients, clinically affects the visceral protein mass, plasma proteins (albumin, globulins, transferrin, and other transport proteins), immunoglobulins, clotting factors, red and white blood cells, and lymphocytes. Without these factors, it is impossible to maintain circulating plasma volume, hematologic integrity, and defense against injury and infection.

The goal of parenteral nutrition is to maintain nutritional balance and/or replenish needed nutrients. To determine nutritional requirements, assessment of the patient is essential. This includes determining the patient's energy reserves, somatic and visceral protein mass, and degree of catabolism. This chapter discusses nutritional calculations, indications for TPN, and techniques for administering and monitoring outcome measures of TPN efficacy and toxicity.

INDICATIONS FOR PARENTERAL SUPPORT

Intravenous parenteral support is indicated when enteral access is unavailable or inadequate for more than seven days. The absence or failure of the gastrointestinal (GI) tract usually requires TPN therapy. TPN should be considered in the following examples:

>> Short-bowel syndrome. Adequate nutrient absorption requires more than 40 cm of intestine; more is required in the elderly.

>> Malabsorption syndromes (e.g., celiac disease, inflammatory bowel disease).

>> Motility disorders (e.g., intestinal pseudo-obstruction, prolonged postoperative ileus).

>> Sepsis with multi-system organ failure.

>> Radiation enteritis/chemotherapy.

>> Unremediable bowel obstruction with prolonged projected survival.

>> Severe malnutrition.

>> Chronic intractable diarrhea of infancy.

>> Severe pancreatitis.

>> Enterocutaneous fistula.

>> Hypermetabolic states such as severe burns.

>> Transplantation (bone marrow, liver, pancreas).

>> Necrotizing enterocolitis prevention and treatment in premature or low birth weight infants.

FLUID REQUIREMENTS

Maintenance fluid requirements depend upon the state of hydration, body size (surface area), environment (e.g., phototherapy, radiant warmers), and underlying disease. Because dehydration, hypernatremia, and hyperosmolarity may occur with inadequate fluids, and since peripheral edema, pulmonary edema, and congestive heart failure result from fluid overload, maintaining desired fluid balance is essential. Fluid losses are increased in patients with respiratory distress, fever, high urinary output, increased ostomy output, diarrhea, and vomiting, as well as other conditions. These excessive fluid losses must be estimated and replaced daily along with maintenance fluids which contain electrolytes comparable to the body fluid being lost. For assistance in identifying, providing, and maintaining fluid balance, see the standard calculations for fluid and electrolyte requirements in Chapter 8: Fluid and Electrolyte Therapy.

TPN solutions generally provide adequate maintenance fluids for most patients. Supplemental intravenous (IV) fluid may be required to administer antibiotics or blood products to patients with substantial fluid losses, or to patients unable to eat or drink a partial diet. Additional fluids may be piggy-backed into the TPN line, if they are compatible, or administered via a separate site.

ENERGY ASSESSMENT
Adults

In general, energy requirements may be approximated in adults with normal liver and renal function according to the guidelines listed in Table 10–1.

A more specific method for determining a patient's energy needs may be calculated using the Harris-Benedict equation.[1]

$$\text{Resting Energy Expenditure} = \text{REE}$$

$$\text{REE}_{\text{Male}} = 66 + (13.7 \times \text{Weight in kg}) + (5 \times \text{Height in cm}) - (6.8 \times \text{Age in yr})$$

$$\text{REE}_{\text{Female}} = 655 + (9.6 \times \text{Weight in kg}) + (1.7 \times \text{Height in cm}) - (4.7 \times \text{Age in yr})$$

For patients who have lost more than 10% of their usual weight over a six month time period, use the usual weight. For grossly obese patients (50% > reference weight),

REE will be less than that estimated by the Harris-Benedict equation. Once the REE is calculated, it can be modified based on an activity or stress factor which results in the following equation:

$$\text{Energy Requirement} = \text{REE} \times (\text{Activity Factor}) \times (\text{Stress Factor})$$

The activity factor for patients *in bed* is 1.2 and 1.3 while *out of bed*. Stress factors are described in Table 10–2.[2]

Indirect Calorimetry

Indirect calorimetry is a more "precise" clinical measurement of energy expenditure (REE).[3] A mass spectrometer is required for on-line O_2 and CO_2 analysis. This method documents actual non-protein calorie needs using the Weir equation:

$$\text{Caloric Expenditure} = [(3.78 \times \text{VO}_2 \text{ L/min}) + (1.16 \times \text{VCO}_2 \text{ L/min})] \times 1440 \text{ min/day}$$

Where: VO_2 = Oxygen Consumption

VCO_2 = Carbon Dioxide Consumption

Remember: VO_2 is invalid in patients on ventilators with chest tubes (pneumothorax), in patients on continuous positive airway pressure (CPAP) with chest tubes, and/or when the FIO_2 is >50%. If the nutritional regimen has changed within 24 hours or the patient is not in steady-state equilibrium (e.g., labile blood pressure), these values will not be accurate.

Known oxygen consumption allows estimation of the respiratory quotient ($\text{RQ} = \text{VCO}_2 / \text{VO}_2$) which may be the only objective measure of overfeeding. Excess CO_2 production may have important consequences for patients with severe obstructive pulmonary disease and impaired ventilatory capacity.

The numbers in Table 10–3 should be interpreted in terms of individual patients and may not be valid for infants or very small children where a large amount of unphysiologic "dead space" is present.

TABLE 10–1: General Calorie Requirements[a]

Normal maintenance and elective surgery	25 kcal/kg/day
Trauma, acute pancreatitis, inflammatory bowel disease	30 kcal/kg/day
Sepsis, minor burns	35 kcal/kg/day
Major burns, severe trauma	40 kcal/kg/day

[a] Patients rarely require >3000 kcal/day.

TABLE 10–2: Stress Factor

Mild starvation	0.85–1.00
Postoperative	1.00–1.05
Cancer	1.10–1.45
Peritonitis	1.05–1.25
Long bone fracture	1.15–1.30
Severe infection and/or multiple trauma	1.30–1.55
Burns (10%–30% body surface)	1.50
Burns (30%–50% body surface)	1.75
Burns (>50% body surface)	2.00

Pediatrics

Energy requirements for infants and children vary with age and growth rate. Caloric demands during growth stages are at least 5 kcal/gm of weight gained. Normal growth proceeds at a rate of approximately 25 to 30 gm/day for the first six months; 13 to 18 gm/day for the next six months, and 5 to 7 gm/day thereafter.

TPN therapy in infants which is aimed at inducing rapid "catch-up" growth can be hazardous and often results in hepatic steatosis, edema, and excessive fat deposition. Therefore, moderate gains are advised, particularly since children seem to be more at risk for developing hepatic complications associated with TPN therapy.

The recommended dietary allowance (RDA) is the main source of information concerning the enteral caloric requirements of normal, active, growing children. The RDA serves as a guideline for many children requiring TPN (see Table 10–4).

Parenteral calories of 90 to 110 kcal/kg for a premature infant are usually sufficient for good growth. An intravenous regimen providing 60 to 70 non-protein kcal/kg with 2.5 gm/kg protein will result in a positive nitrogen balance. Additionally, caloric requirements of infants and children will be decreased by inactivity, mechanical ventilation (in

TABLE 10–3: Respiratory Quotient (RQ) Findings

RQ	Metabolic "Set"	Response
0.7	Fat catabolism	Increase calories
0.8	Protein catabolism for energy	Increase calories
0.9	Normal RQ-mixed fuel utilization	No change
1.0	Carbohydrate catabolism	OK versus impending overfeeding
>1.0	Fat synthesis/overfeeding	Decrease calories

TABLE 10–4: RDA Caloric Requirements for Children to Adolescents[a]

	Age	RDA: Enteral Energy (kcal/kg/day)	RDA: Enteral Protein (gm/kg/day)	TPN Protein (gm/kg/day)
Infants	Premature	110–150	3.0–4.0	2.0–2.5
	0–6 months	115	2.2	2.5–3.0
	6–12 months	105	2.0	2.5–3.0
Children	1–3 yr	100	1.8	1.5–2.5
	4–6 yr	90–85	1.5	1.5–2.5
	7–10 yr	85–80	1.2	1.5–2.5
Males	11–14 yr	60	1.0	1.0–1.5
	15–18 yr	42	0.85	
	19+ yr[b]	40	0.80	
Females	11–14 yr	47	1.0	1.0–1.5
	15–18 yr	38	0.84	
	19+ yr[b]	35	0.80	

[a] Reprinted with permission. Benitz WE, Tratos DS. Pediatric Handbook, 2nd ed., Chicago, IL: Mosby Yearbook Publishers, Inc.: 1988;339–47.

[b] Use adult energy assessments.

the child with pulmonary/respiratory problems), a comatose state, and a warm environment (e.g., infants in an isolette). Likewise, *basal* calories will be increased by:

>> **Fever.** 12% for each degree above 37 °C.

>> **Cardiac Failure.** 15% to 25%.

>> **Major Surgery.** 20% to 30%.

>> **Burns.** Up to 100%.

>> **Severe Sepsis.** 40% to 50%.

>> **Long-Term Growth Failure**. 50% to 100%.

>> **Protein Calorie Malnutrition.** 25% to 50%.

PARENTERAL SOLUTION CONSTITUENTS

Parenteral nutrition solutions are composed of a variety of constituents ranging from protein, fat, and carbohydrates as energy sources to electrolytes, vitamins, and trace elements.

Protein

Patient's protein requirements depend upon their clinical state. To prevent catabolism of muscle mass, adequate calories must be provided as protein. This can be accomplished by providing protein as crystalline amino acids which provide 4 kcal/gm. Protein requirements are *increased* in patients with severe burns, sepsis, multiple trauma with long bone fracture, and high output fistula losses.

However, some individuals have a limited capacity to handle even greatly *reduced* protein loads due to renal or hepatic compromise. Typical protein demands are listed in Table 10–5.

Renal patients must receive special consideration to achieve optimal nutritional support without aggravating uremic symptoms.[4] Nondialysis patients start low (0.5 gm/kg/day) and increase according to protein tolerance using BUN as an endpoint. For patients on dialysis, requirements for protein increase due to amino acid losses in dialysate. The use of essential amino acids (EAA) as the sole protein source has been suggested for use in renal failure patients. The beneficial effects of EAA may be due to the body's ability to reutilize urea nitrogen as a source of non-EAA synthesis; however, further study is needed.

A more patient-specific assessment of protein status can be determined using various biochemical markers.[5] Abnormalities in certain parameters may indicate protein deficiency (see Table 10–6).

Newborn and premature infants have immature renal and hepatic enzyme systems and may be unable to tolerate full protein requirements. Therefore, the initial intake of 1 gm/kg/day protein with increases of 0.5 gm/kg/day may improve tolerance.[6] Similarly, amino acids currently absent from most commercial mixtures may be essential for the premature infant. These include: cysteine, taurine, tyrosine, and carnitine. Preparations which contain cysteine are available for addition to TPN solutions.

Historically, hyperammonemia and hyperchloremia occur in pediatric patients receiving TPN; however, these complications are now less common with the improved formulations of protein solutions. Interestingly, most metabolic complications (including azotemia and acidosis), are related to amino acids in the solutions and occur when infants receive >4 gm/kg/day of protein. These complications are rarely encountered with the recommended intake of 2 to 3 gm/kg/day.

TABLE 10–5: Adult Protein Requirements

Normal	0.8 gm/kg/day
Moderately stressed	1.1–1.6 gm/kg/day
Severely stressed	1.6–3.0 gm/kg/day
Acute renal failure	
Non-dialyzed	0.5–0.6 gm/kg/day
Hemodialyzed	1.0–1.2 gm/kg/day
Peritoneal dialyzed	1.2–1.5 gm/kg/day
Acute liver failure	0.25–0.5 gm/kg/day or less
Subacute chronic liver dysfunction	Will vary; may approximate 0.5 gm/kg/day up to 1 gm/kg/day

TABLE 10–6: Biochemical Markers for Assessment of Protein Status

Parameter	Half-life (days)	Normal
Albumin	20	3.5–4.5 gm/dL
Transferrin	8	200–400 mg/dL
Pre-albumin	2	15–30 mg/dL
Retinol binding protein	0.5	2.5–7.5 mg/dL
Total lymphocyte count	—	800–4000/mm^3 (15%–45% WBC)

When providing protein, consider the patient's nitrogen balance. The goal of maintaining the proper calorie to nitrogen ratio allows nitrogen calories to be used for anabolism rather than as an energy source. This is known as "protein sparing." In addition, nitrogen utilization varies with altered states of metabolism (e.g., in renal and/or hepatic disease, sepsis, or trauma.) To maximize nitrogen utilization for anabolism, total caloric requirements must be met. Use of a carbohydrate supplied as dextrose or a combination of fat emulsion and dextrose can accomplish this. The kcal:nitrogen ratios listed in Table 10–7 can be used for various adult metabolic states; however, the optimal kcal:nitrogen ratio for children of various ages, stages of growth, and disease states needs further study. However, the optimal non-protein kcal:nitrogen ratio for infants is approximately 150 to 200:1.[7,8]

To provide the appropriate calorie to nitrogen ratio for a patient's clinical condition, crystalline free amino acids in various concentrations are available. Further, additional amino acids may be piggy-backed into the main TPN solution if necessary. Patients with hepatic failure must maintain lean body mass and prevent or reverse symptoms of hepatic encephalopathy which may be a manifestation of protein intolerance. The abnormal plasma amino acid patterns characteristic of liver disease show increased aromatic and decreased branched chain amino acids (BCAA). BCAA such as leucine, isoleucine, and valine are metabolized in the kidney and muscle rather than the liver. The use of protein solutions with increased BCAA amounts may decrease symptoms. Special solutions of BCAA are available and are generally reserved for use in patients with hepatic encephalopathy, severe acute trauma, or in a catabolic state.

TABLE 10–7: kcal to Nitrogen Ratio by Patient Condition

Adult Patient Condition	Ratio Non-Protein cal:gm Nitrogen
Adult medical patient (stable)	125–150:1
Minor catabolic state	125–180:1
Severe catabolic state	80–100:1
No renal function	250–400:1

Protein needs can be quantified by determining nitrogen balance (i.e., the amount of nitrogen intake minus nitrogen output).[9] Generally, a nitrogen balance of +2 to +5 is required to restore depleted protein mass. Nitrogen balance studies are inaccurate in cases of renal failure, with the noted exception of nephrotic syndrome.

$$\text{Nitrogen Balance} = N_{in} - (N_{out} + 2)$$

The constant 2 is added to cover average fecal and other losses (e.g., wound exudate, fistula drainage).

$$N_{in} = \frac{\text{gm of Protein Taken In}}{6.25}$$

N_{out} = gm of Nitrogen in a 24-hr Urine Collection

Where: 1 gm Nitrogen = 6.25 gm Protein

A 24-hour determination of protein intake is necessary if the patient is on oral or tube feedings. Any changes in protein intake should be followed by a 24 to 48 hour period before further nitrogen balance studies are performed.

Carbohydrate

The primary energy source in TPN is carbohydrates delivered in the form of hypertonic dextrose. Each gram of dextrose monohydrate provides 3.4 kcal. To prevent intolerance, the dextrose is administered as a slow constant infusion with gradual increases. Excess carbohydrate calories are stored as glycogen and fat and can cause fatty infiltration of the liver. The incidence of this complication can be reduced by replacing some of the carbohydrate calories with intravenous fat.

A minimum of 20% to 30% of calories should be provided as dextrose to assure adequate fuel for brain metabolism. The maximum glucose oxidation rate is 5 mg/kg/min in adults which translates into about 24.5 kcal/kg/day, the amount of carbohydrate recommended as an energy source. This may be increased to 7 mg/kg/min or 34.3 kcal/kg/day in postoperative patients. However, overutilization of glucose as the caloric source, increases CO_2 production and may exacerbate a patient's respiratory distress.

Carbohydrate tolerance is related to intake per kg, not the concentration of solution being administered. Children tolerate 25 to 30 gm/kg/day,[7] with the noted exceptions of very low birth weight and premature infants. To minimize glucose intolerance, lower dextrose concentrations are advised with more gradual increases. This can be accomplished by starting glucose at 5 mg/kg/min and gradually increasing to 15 mg/kg/min (20 to 25 gm/kg/day) over several days.

In renal patients with fluid limitations, 70% dextrose can be used to meet protein restrictions and provide adequate calories. If the patient is severely glucose intolerant, consider using 50% dextrose and providing the remaining calories as intravenous fat.

Fat

Parenteral fat emulsion can be used to deliver calories (9 kcal/gm), but it is primarily indicated to treat or prevent essential fatty acid deficiency (EFAD). EFAD has been reported in patients on fat-free, long-term TPN and in premature infants within a few days of life. To prevent EFAD, a minimum of 4% of the total energy intake should be supplied as essential fatty acids or 8% of total energy by fat emulsion. To treat EFAD,

15% to 20% of the total calories are provided as fat emulsion. For most adult patients, the equivalent of 250 mL of 20% fat emulsion twice weekly is sufficient to prevent EFAD. Amounts vary with children, depending upon individual caloric requirements.

Specific indications for the use of fat emulsion as a calorie source include: severe fluid restriction, peripheral parenteral nutrition, pulmonary failure with CO_2 retention, and patients with fatty liver infiltrates secondary to excess carbohydrate calories in relation to lipid and protein calories.

When used as a calorie source, parenteral fat should not exceed 60% of the total calories administered. The maximum recommended daily dose is 3 gm fat/kg body weight in adults and 4 gm fat/kg in children or infants.

Fat emulsion 10% provides 1.1 kcal/mL, while fat emulsion 20% provides 2.0 kcal/mL. Parenteral fat emulsion is compatible with TPN and may be administered as an intermittent piggyback with TPN or mixed with the TPN solution and given continuously. Ideally, TPN is administered through a central venous catheter to avoid thrombophlebitis and pain associated with infusion of a hypertonic solution through a peripheral vein. If peripheral nutritional support is necessary, the maximum concentration of dextrose tolerated is 10% which provides insufficient non-protein calories. Therefore, fat emulsion given continuously with a TPN solution not only decreases the venous complication of other hypertonic components, but provides a concentrated calorie source. However, rapid fat administration which may exceed the body's rate of hydrolysis, can result in hypertriglyceridemia and hyperlipidemia. In addition, the maximum recommended hang time of each lipid bottle is 24 hours due to the risk of bacterial or fungal contamination. Complications are generally avoided if these guidelines are observed:

>> **Adults.** Fat emulsion 20%; 250 mL should be administered at a rate not exceeding 50 mL/hr.

>> **Infants and Children.** Fat emulsions should *not* run at a rate exceeding 4 to 5 mg/kg/min.

>> **Uremic Patients.** These patients show a decreased capacity to clear triglycerides. Monitor serum levels while on liquids.

In the premature and newborn infant with immature enzyme systems, it is recommended that 10% intravenous lipid, which contains a smaller particle size, be initiated. The appropriate rate is 1 gm/kg/day with increases of 0.5 gm/kg/day as tolerated. In young infants, lipids are administered over an 18 to 24 hour period with serum triglycerides (TG) checked after the first 24 hours and after any increase in dose. Adjust the amount of lipid infused as follows:

>> **TG <100 mg/dL.** Infusion may be increased.

>> **TG = 100 to 150 mg/dL.** No change.

>> **TG >200 mg/dL.** Decrease infusion.

In older infants and children, the TG should be checked four to six hours after an 18 to 20 hour infusion. The therapeutic goal is to keep the TG <200 mg/dL.

Neonates with significant hyperbilirubinemia should not receive intravenous lipid emulsions. The lipids displace bilirubin from albumin binding sites resulting in further increases in bilirubin. However, lipids can be started when the bilirubin is <10 mg/dL (direct bilirubin <2 mg/dL). For a bilirubin >10 mg/dL, check the free fatty acid to albumin ratio. If the molar ratio is 4, bilirubin displacement is unlikely.

Electrolytes

Usual daily electrolyte requirements are listed in Table 10–8. (See Chapter 8: Fluid and Electrolyte Therapy for a more detailed discussion.)

Electrolyte requirements will vary with the disease states or medical conditions listed below, and may require more frequent monitoring. Note: Parentheses indicate the electrolytes which vary with the condition.

>> Severe diarrhea (Na^+, K^+, Mg^{++}).

>> Vomiting (Na^+, Cl^-, H^+).

>> Nasogastric losses (Na^+, Cl^-, H^+).

>> Fistula losses (specific deficits depend upon the part of GI tract from which fistula drains).

>> Congestive heart failure (Na^+).

>> Renal failure (K^+, Mg^{++}, PO_4).

>> Depleted/abnormal electrolyte imbalances before TPN (phosphate depletion).

>> Respiratory failure (low serum phosphate can precipitate respiratory depression).

Electrolytes can cause compatibility problems in parenteral nutrition. Commonly encountered situations include:

>> Bicarbonate is incompatible with TPN solutions; therefore, acetate on a mEq for mEq basis can be substituted for bicarbonate.

>> To avoid precipitation of calcium with phosphorus in the parenteral nutrition solution, the sum of calcium (mEq/L) and phosphorus (mmol/L) should be <45. With lower amounts of protein in solution, the maximum sum of calcium and phosphorus allowable before precipitation results will be decreased.

>> Calcium and magnesium also have the potential to precipitate in solutions at concentrations higher than 10 mEq/L of calcium and 16 mEq/L magnesium (as a sulfate salt). The exact limits are unknown; however, at usual daily doses and concentrations, precipitation is not a problem.

Vitamins

Commercially available multivitamin supplements [e.g., MVC-12 (adults) and MVI-Peds] meet the minimum required daily allowance (RDA) and American Medical Association (AMA) requirements (see Table 10–9). Therefore, the daily addition of a standard multivitamin dose to a TPN solution will generally prevent deficiencies. Recommended doses are:

>> **MVI Peds.** 5 mL for children <11 yr; 3 mL for infants <3 kg.

>> **MVC-12.** 10 mL for children >11 yr and for adults, plus phytona-
dione 1 mg/day in TPN or SQ 10 mg/week. Additional phytonadione up to 10 mg/day can be added if clinical conditions warrant.

Several medical conditions require additional vitamin supplementation. For example,
higher doses are needed for dialysis patients (ascorbic acid folate, B vitamins), surgical patients requiring wound healing (zinc, ascorbic acid), alcoholic patients (vitamin
B_6, thiamine), those with drug-nutrient interactions (isoniazid with vitamin B_6,
phenytoin with folate), and patients with other metabolic abnormalities (anemia,
malignancy, or deficiency states).

Trace Elements

The essential trace elements (chromium, copper, manganese, and zinc) are required
by patients on parenteral nutrition therapy. Table 10–10 on page 10–13 and Table
10–11 on page 10–14 list the suggested daily IV intake of these trace elements.

To provide trace elements, a standard trace element solution that contains zinc 3 mg,
copper 1.2 mg, chromium 12 μg, and manganese 0.3 mg in 3 mL of solution is recommended.

The dosage of trace element solution is 0.1 mL/kg/day up to 3 mL/day. Again, requirements need adjustment in the following circumstances: hemodialysis, severe diarrhea
(serum zinc and selenium need to be checked before supplementation), and long-term
TPN.

The recommended selenium dose to reverse a deficiency is 100 μg/day which may be
added to a TPN.[11] Iron administration is unnecessary if the patient receives blood
transfusions; otherwise, iron is also indicated for patients receiving prolonged TPN
therapy.

Patients receiving parenteral nutrition for long periods of time (>2 weeks) may be at
risk for developing deficiency states of trace elements needed for optimal metabolism
(see Table 10–11).[12] These deficiencies usually develop due to inadequate intake;
however, there are certain diseases which may predispose patients to depletion.

TABLE 10–8: Electrolyte Requirements Per 24 Hr

Component	Pediatric	Neonate	Adult
Sodium	3–4 mEq/kg	3–5 mEq/kg	50–120 mEq
Potassium	2–3 mEq/kg	2–3 mEq/kg	40–60 mEq
Magnesium	0.25–0.6 mEq/kg	0.25–0.6 mEq/kg	10–20 mEq
Phosphorus	1.0–1.5 mmol/kg	1–2 mmol/kg	20–45 mmol
Calcium	0–1 mEq/kg	1 mEq/kg	10–15 mEq
Acetate[a]	Varies	Varies	80–120 mEq
Chloride[a]	Varies	Varies	150–180 mEq

[a] Varies with acid base status. Ideally, chloride content should not exceed sodium content to avoid metabolic acidosis. Acetate and phosphate salts can be used to balance chloride against sodium ions.

TABLE 10–9: RDA and AMA Vitamin Requirements

Vitamins	Adult RDA 11 yr male	Adult AMA 11 yr old	Pediatric RDA <1 yr	Pediatric RDA >1 yr	Pediatric AMA 1 yr	Commercially MVC-12 10 mL	MVI PED 5 mL
Vitamin A (IU)	3300	3300	1400	1400–2300	2300	3300	2300
Vitamin D (µg)	10	5	10	10	10	5	10
Vitamin E (mg)	10	10	4	5–7	7.0	10	7
Thiamine (mg) (Vitamin B_1)	1.4	3.0	0.3–0.5	0.7–1.2	1.2	3	1.2
Riboflavin (mg) (Vitamin B_2)	1.7	3.6	0.5	0.8–1.4	1.4	3.6	1.4
Pyridoxine (mg) (Vitamin B_6)	2.2	4.0	0.3–0.6	0.9–1.6	1.0	4	1.0
Niacin (mg)	18	40	8	9–16	17	40	17.0
Pantothenate (mg)	4–7	15	2–3	3–5	5	15	5.0
Biotin (µg)	100–200	60.0	35–50	65–120	20	60	20
Folic acid (µg)	400	400	30–45	100–300	140	400	140
Cyanocobalamin (µg) (Vitamin B_{12})	3.0	5.0	0.5–1.5	2.0–3.0	1.0	5	1
Vitamin K (mg) (Phytonadione)	0.07–0.14	0.07–0.14	0.01–0.02	0.015–0.06	0.2	—	0.2
Ascorbic acid (mg) (Vitamin C)	60	100	35	45	80	100	80

Serum levels of zinc and copper are usually monitored initially and every two weeks. A progressive fall in serum levels suggests intake is inadequate and indicates that additional supplements may need to be added to the TPN solution. Serum levels of other trace elements are unavailable, and it is suggested that additional supplements of these minerals not be added to nutrition solutions unless a clinical deficiency is suspected.

Insulin

Insulin supplementation is sometimes necessary for patients receiving parenteral nutrition. Historically, all TPN therapy provided the majority of calories as carbohydrate which often required insulin supplementation to maintain glucose control. With the increased use of lipid emulsion and the curtailment of overfeeding, the need for insulin supplementation has dropped appreciably. Interestingly, the onset or escalation of glucose intolerance in a previously tolerant or well controlled patient suggests an impending septic episode or other deterioration in the patient's status. Hypoglycemia can also be seen in this situation.

There are several approaches to administering insulin. It may be given on a PRN basis via the subcutaneous (SC) or IV routes on a "sliding scales" schedule. Blood glucoses should be checked every six hours for the first 24 hours (by the laboratory or a portable glucose meter) and managed with an adjustable insulin scale. Table 10–12 on page 10–15 presents an example of insulin doses for a patient who has never before received insulin.

For patients who may exhibit poor subcutaneous absorption (e.g., hypotensive patients) or for stressed patients with varying needs, a separate continuous infusion of regular insulin may be justified. When administered via continuous infusion the standard concentration is 1 U regular insulin/mL of IV fluid. The infusion, usually consisting of 250 U of regular insulin in 250 mL of 5% dextrose in water, is initiated at 0.1 mL/kg/hr and titrated to the desired serum glucose concentration.

Regular insulin is compatible with the TPN solution and may be added directly to the solution if the sliding scale or separate infusion needs are fairly consistent. It is rec-

TABLE 10–10: Trace Elements

Element	Pediatrics (µg/kg)[a]	Stable Adult	Adult in Acute Catabolic State	Stable Adult With Intestinal Losses[b]
Zinc	300,[c] 100[d]	2.5–4.0 mg	Additional 2.0 mg	15–30 mg/L of diarrheal or ileostomy output
Copper	20	0.5–1.5 mg	—	—
Chromium	0.14–0.2	10–15 µg	—	200 mg
Manganese	2–10	0.15–0.8 mg	—	—

[a] Limited data are available for infants <1500 gm. Their requirements may be more than the recommendation because of their low body reserves and increased requirements for growth.

[b] Monitoring of blood levels in these patients is essential to provide proper dosage.

[c] Premature infants (weight <1500 gm) up to 3 kg of body weight. Thereafter, the recommendations for full-term infants apply.

[d] Full-term infants and children up to 5 years old. Thereafter, the recommendations for adults apply (up to a maximum dosage of 4 mg/day).

TABLE 10-11: Trace Elements: Requirements and Deficiencies

Trace Elements/Daily Dose	Factors Predisposing to Deficiency	Clinical Manifestations of Depletion
Zinc *Adults:* 2.5–4.0 mg; additional 2 mg in acute catabolic state, intestinal losses, and small bowel fluid loss $\approx$12.2 mg/L;[a] stool or ileostomy output $\approx$17.1 mg/L *Peds:* 0.3–4 mg/kg/day	Alcohol, alcoholic cirrhosis, pancreatitis, inflammatory bowel disease, celiac disease, short bowel syndrome, ileal-jejunum bypass, pancreatic insufficiency, cystic fibrosis, nephrotic syndrome, hemolytic anemia, anorexia nervosa, chronic anemia, large amounts of GI losses	Growth retardation, diarrhea, hypogonadism, alopecia, skin lesions, immune deficiencies, behavioral disturbances, night blindness, low sperm count, impaired taste acuity, impaired wound healing
Copper *Adults:* 0.5–1.5 mg	Short bowel syndrome, ileal-jejunal bypass, celiac disease, tropical sprue, nephrotic syndrome	Anemia, neutropenia, skeletal demineralization (children), depigmentation of skin and hair, defective elastin formation (aneurysms), CNS abnormalities, hypotonia, hypothermia
Chromium *Adults:* 10–15 µg/day; with major intestinal losses 20 µg/day	Long-term TPN (i.e., months to years)	Glucose intolerance, peripheral neuropathy, metabolic encephalopathy, increased susceptibility to cardiovascular disease
Molybdenum Dose unknown	Long-term TPN	Headache, night blindness, irritability, lethargy, coma, abnormal purine metabolism, abnormal metabolism of sulfur amino acids
Manganese 0.15–0.8 mg/day	Long-term TPN	Defective growth, bony anomalies, reproductive dysfunction, CNS abnormalities
Selenium *Adults:* 20–40 µg/day *Peds:* 3–5 µg/kg/day up to 60 µg/day	Long-term TPN	Myalgia and muscle tenderness, increased red cell fragility, pancreatic degeneration

[a] Amount of zinc loss per liter of fluid.

10–14

TABLE 10–12: Insulin Sliding Scale

| Serum Glucose (mg/dL) | Insulin (Regular U-100) | Administered | |
		SQ	IV
180–240	0.5 U/kg/day	Divide dose by 6 and administer Q 4 hr	Use $1/2$ of SQ dose
240–320	1.0 U/kg/day		
>320	1.5 U/kg/day		

a Renal patients exhibit decreased insulin clearance and should be dosed conservatively.

ommended that insulin doses added to the TPN solution be on the conservative side, since more insulin can always be added to the TPN or administered to the patient directly. Otherwise, decreasing the insulin dose in a previously prepared solution will likely cause a costly waste of solutions. The minimum amount to be added to a TPN container is 10 U (regular U-100) due to adsorption to glass/plastic and tubing.

PROFILE: PARENTERAL NUTRITION FORMULAS

Historically, many institutions have relied upon standardized recipes or formulas to avoid the expense of TPN waste. Standard concentrations are: dextrose 100 gm/L, 175 gm/L, 250 gm/L, 350 gm/L, and protein 25 gm/L, 50 gm/L. Combinations of these will provide the kcal and kcal ratios listed in Table 10–13. Standard electrolyte packages are also commercially available (see Table 10–14.)

Additional electrolytes may be added to standard solutions listed in Table 10–14 or non-standard formulations to meet specific patient needs or requirements. It is important to make sure the cation and anion amounts balance. Concentrations of several commercially available electrolyte solutions are listed in Table 10–15 on page 10–17.

To meet patient demands, new systems have been researched and experience demonstrates that a computerized admixture of all components is technically feasible and clinically more desirable.[13] Complex individualized nutrient solutions are possible because of computerized admixture equipment which enables pharmacy staff to select varied amounts of specific components using large volume concentrates of protein, carbohydrate, fat, electrolytes, etc. To be cost effective, these expensive solutions must be carefully evaluated for each patient on a daily basis.

COMPLICATIONS

For all patients receiving TPN, it is important to prevent, detect, and correct complications through monitoring. Complications that occur may be related to physical access or metabolic disturbances. Table 10–16 on page 10–18 outlines possible management approaches for the various venous access complications and Table 10–17 on page 10–19 describes the metabolic complications. Remember: The subclavian route is preferred because of its proximity to the superior vena cava (SVC) and the ease of maintaining sterility.

One of the most common complications of total parenteral nutrition is infection. The source of infection may be related to contamination of the catheter, administration apparatus, or infusate. An infected catheter, wound, or tunnel site may play a major role in the potential for sepsis.

TABLE 10–13: Standard Protein/Dextrose Formulas

Combinations	Non-protein kcal/gm nitrogen	Protein (kcal/L)	CHO[a] (kcal/L)	Total (kcal/L)
25 gm protein and 100 gm dextrose	85	100	340	440
25 gm protein and 175 gm dextrose	149	100	595	695
25 gm protein and 250 gm dextrose	212	100	850	950
25 gm protein and 350 gm dextrose	298	100	1190	1290
50 gm protein and 100 gm dextrose	43	200	340	540
50 gm protein and 175 gm dextrose	74	200	595	795
50 gm protein and 250 gm dextrose[b]	106	200	850	1050
50 gm protein and 350 gm dextrose	149	200	1190	1390

[a] CHO = Carbohydrates
[b] Most frequently ordered (kcal:N ratio suited for moderately stressed patients).

TABLE 10–14: Electrolyte Concentration of Standard Solutions

Electrolyte	Protein Concentrate 25 gm and NaPhos 5 mL	Protein Concentrate 50 gm and NaPhos 5 mL
Potassium	20 mEq	20 mEq
Sodium	45 mEq	45 mEq
Magnesium	5 mEq	5 mEq
Calcium	5 mEq	5 mEq
Chloride	40 mEq	50 mEq
Acetate	47 mEq	69 mEq
Phosphate	15 mmol	15 mmol

TABLE 10–15: Electrolyte Composition/mL of Solution

Sodium chloride	4.0 mEq/mL sodium and 4.0 mEq/mL chloride
Sodium acetate	2.0 mEq/mL sodium and 2.0 mEq/mL acetate
Sodium phosphate	4.0 mEq/mL sodium and 3.0 mmol/mL phosphate
Potassium chloride	2.0 mEq/mL potassium and 2.0 mEq/mL chloride
Potassium acetate	2.0 mEq/mL potassium and 2.0 mEq/mL acetate
Potassium phosphate	4.4 mEq/mL potassium and 3.0 mmol/mL phosphate
Calcium gluconate	0.48 mEq/mL calcium and 0.48 mEq/mL gluconate (1 gm = 4.8 mEq CaGluconate)
Magnesium sulfate	4.0 mEq/mL magnesium and 4.0 mEq/mL sulfate (1 gm = 8 mEq $MgSO_4$)

Although the precise mechanism responsible for sepsis and its interrelatedness to multiple other facets may not always be clear or adequately studied, the following factors play a significant role in the prevention of infection:

>> Quality control processes to ensure sterility in the admixture area.

>> Strict aseptic technique during catheter insertion.

>> Procedures to prevent in-use contamination.

>> Stringent routine aseptic care of the catheter insertion site.

>> Proper care of other parts of the TPN system.

To reduce the risk of infection, consider the following issues:

>> Change administration sets every 72 hours and/or with catheter site changes.

>> Make every effort to avoid using TPN lines for multiple purposes (e.g., blood drawing, administration of medications).

>> *Patients with unexplained fever or signs of systemic sepsis or any signs of local inflammation near the catheter site should always have the catheter removed and cultured by semiquantitative technique.* Hickman, Raaf, and Broviac catheters are the exceptions to this rule. These three catheters may be left in place in septic patients to allow for a trial of appropriate antimicrobial therapy to eradicate catheter-related infections. In general, remove the catheter if the subcutaneous tunnel is obviously infected or if the patient responds unsatisfactorily to antimicrobial therapy and the catheter is thought to be the probable source of septicemia. Systemic fungal infections may prompt early removal of the catheter.

TABLE 10–16: Complications of TPN Therapy

Complication	Signs and Symptoms	Treatment
Pneumothorax	None or shortness of breath (SOB), chest pain	Expectant if small; tube thoracostomy if large
Thrombosis	Neck/shoulder pain; superior vena cava syndrome; progressive thrombosis blocked catheter; 30%–50% of cases subclinical	Usually, remove catheter; approaches might include giving heparin, then streptokinase. If still blocked, flush with urokinase
Catheter occlusion	Blocked catheter	Remove catheter; other approaches might include those stated above
Infection (might be 10% to 15% in septic patients)	Fever, bacteremia	Treat infection (may remove catheter)
Arterial injury	Usually minimal; occasionally hemothorax	
Hydrothorax (TPN effusion)	SOB, abnormal chest x-ray	
Air embolism	Cardiac arrest or sudden neurologic change during insertion or dressing change	Cardiopulmonary resuscitation (CPR), aspirate air from right ventricle. Patient in Trendelenburg position, left side down
Catheter embolus	Minimal	Remove catheter
Skin erosion	Obvious	Remove catheter; if site must be maintained may clear up with careful wound care
Catheter tear or break	Leakage	Use repair kit

TABLE 10–17: Guidelines for Metabolic TPN Problems

Problems	Management
Hyperglycemia Serum glucose >200 mg/dL Urine glucose 4+	1) *Determine Cause*: infusion rate, diabetes, sepsis, stress, steroids, K+ depletion. 2) *Treatments*: slow infusion rate temporarily, give insulin, treat sepsis or stress situation, replace K+ stores, consider replacing carbohydrate calories with fat.
Hyperosmolar Dehydration Serum glucose >600 mg/dL Urine glucose 4+ Serum osmolality >350 Serum sodium >140 mmol/L Somnolence Lethargy Coma	1) Discontinue TPN solution. 2) Give hypotonic saline solution. 3) Give IV insulin by drip 0.1 U/kg/hr. 4) Monitor glucose until under control.
Hypoglycemia Serum glucose <50 mg/dL Hypothermia Lethargy or somnolence Seizure Vasoconstriction	1) Discontinue insulin in infusion. 2) Increase infusion rate of TPN solution. 3) Give 50 cc $D_{50}W$ bolus. 4) Monitor glucose Q 4 hr until problem solved.
Azotemia Elevated BUN Elevated creatinine Lassitude Asterixis	1) Increase kcal/nitrogen ratio.

(Continued)

TABLE 10–17: Guidelines for Metabolic TPN Problems *(Continued)*

Problems	Management
Hyperammonemia Seen in children <10 yr and patients with liver disease Elevated ammonia level Somnolence Lethargy Asterixis Coma	1) Increase kcal/nitrogen ratio. 2) Use only branched chain amino acids (if available) with high kcal/N ratio (e.g., D_{35} Hepatamine 4%).
Hyperchloremic Metabolic Acidosis Decreased pH and/or pCO_2 Decreased serum (HCO_3^-) Base excess <-3 Relatively increased chloride No anion gap	1) Substitute acetate for chloride in the TPN solution. 2) Give bicarbonate via peripheral IV.
Hypokalemia Serum K^+ <3.5 mmol/L Ileus Muscle weakness Cardiac arrhythmias (PVC)	1) Give extra K^+ via peripheral IV. 2) Increase K^+ in TPN solution.
Hyperkalemia Serum K^+ >6 mmol/L Heart block Idioventricular rhythm	1) Discontinue or decrease K^+ in TPN solution. 2) If severe, give insulin and/or Kayexalate PO or by enema. 3) If combined with renal failure, consider dialysis.

(Continued)

TABLE 10–17: Guidelines for Metabolic TPN Problems *(Continued)*

Problems	Management
Hyponatremia Serum Na <125 mmol/L Lethargy Confusion Seizure	1) Define etiology: Dehydration with ADH release or fluid overload with CHF and excessive ADH. 2) Give normal saline with or without a diuretic. 3) Restrict fluid and increase Na$^+$ in TPN solution.
Hypophosphatemia Serum phosphate <1.5 mmol/L Paresthesias Mental confusion Lethargy Coma Weakness Increased affinity of hemoglobin for oxygen	1) Increase phosphate in the TPN solution. 2) If severe, give Na or K phosphate via separate IV. 3) Monitor phosphate closely.
Hypomagnesemia Serum Mg <2 mg/dL Vertigo Weakness Distention Positive Chvostek sign Tetany Seizure	1) Increase Mg^{++} in TPN solution. 2) If severe, give MgSO$_4$ IM or via separate IV infusion.

(Continued)

TABLE 10-17: Guidelines for Metabolic TPN Problems *(Continued)*

Problems	Management
Hypercalcemia High to normal serum Ca in presence of normal to low albumin Obstructive nephropathy (with hyperphosphatemia)	1) Omit or reduce Ca in TPN. 2) Give NS + a diuretic if symptomatic.
Excessive Weight Gain Weight gain >2 kg/wk Edema Positive I&O (Intake versus Output)	1) Give a diuretic PRN to maintain neutral water balance. 2) Monitor electrolytes.
Zinc Deficiency Poor wound healing Dermatitis Diarrhea	1) Follow serum zinc levels. 2) Administer supplemental zinc in TPN.
Elevated LFTs and Cholestatic Jaundice Increased alkaline phosphatase Increased AST Hepatomegaly	1) *Clarify Liver Disease.* Rule out fatty liver (evaluated carbohydrate) calorie intake—too much? Evaluate EFA intake (too little)? Rule out drug-induced liver function changes. Underlying liver disease. Evaluate prothrombin time (PT), bilirubin. 2) Treat accordingly.
Anemia Decreased Hct Decreased Hgb Abnormal indices	1) Evaluate intake of B_{12}, folic acid, iron, pyridoxine, copper. 2) Supplement as needed.
Essential Fatty Acid (EFA) Deficiency Scaly dermatitis Alopecia Hepatomegaly	1) Evaluate fat intake; must be at least 500 mL of 10% fat emulsion twice weekly. 2) Evaluate high carbohydrate continuous infusion leading to high insulin levels and decreased mobilization of endogenous fatty acids. 3) Supplement with fat emulsion or topical safflower oil, 8% to 10% of total daily calories.

Fluid requirements are altered in various clinical conditions. TPN regimens should be designed to provide adequate caloric and protein intake within the administered fluid volume. Other IV sites should be utilized to fine tune fluid balance. Intracellular electrolyte deficiencies may develop with initiation of TPN. With refeeding, there is a shift from the catabolic to the anabolic state resulting in increased intracellular demand for potassium, magnesium, and phosphate (see Chapter 8: Fluid and Electrolyte Therapy for manifestations of abnormal serum electrolytes).

Hepatotoxicity eventually occurs with TPN therapy. There is a higher incidence in infants, especially premature infants, and long-term therapy in all age groups. Onset is gradual, starting with cholestatic jaundice and hepatomegaly, accompanied by elevated liver function tests (LFTs). Possible etiologies relate to immaturity of hepatic excretory function in infants, prolonged enteral fasting, or excess protein and/or nutrients. Avoid excess calories, cycle the TPN, or begin early minimal enteral feedings along with intravenous nutrition to manage this problem.

CYCLIC TPN

Cyclic TPN occurs when TPN therapy is administered on an intermittent basis. Indications for use of cyclic therapy include:

>> The lack of an IV line for administration of multiple blood products or antibiotics incompatible with TPN.

>> Provision of freedom for the patient to perform physical activity, work, or attend school. It also is indicated for long-term TPN or home parenteral nutrition (HPN) therapy.

>> The need to decrease risk of liver complications which may occur with continuous TPN.

When administering cyclic TPN, the non-infusion period may range from 6 to 12 hours, but not all patients can tolerate the metabolic fluctuations of going on and off cyclic TPN. In particular, cyclic TPN should be avoided in patients with compromised renal or cardiovascular function, unstable fluid status, and poor glucose control.

To initiate the cycle, the infusion time should be gradually decreased over three to five days. A sample schedule for attaining intermittent TPN is outlined in Tables 10–18 and 10–19.

TABLE 10–18: Cyclic TPN Schedule

	Pre-Cyclic TPN	Day 1[a]	Day 2[a]	Day 3[a]
Total TPN volume	X[b] mL	X mL	X mL	X mL
Rate/Hour	X ÷ 24	X ÷ 20	X ÷ 18	X ÷ 16
Off Time	0	4 hr	6 hr	8 hr

[a] Glucose should be initially monitored TID, including 30 minutes after the glucose infusion stopped. TPN should be tapered at one-half the hourly rate for one hour at the beginning and end of the infusion. A more gradual taper may be necessary for those patients receiving TPN with >25% dextrose.
[b] X represents the desired volume.

Table 10–19: Conversion From Continuous to Cyclic TPN[18]

Volume (L)	Day 1 (24 hr)	Day 2 (18 hr)			Day 3 (12 hr)			Day 4 (10 hr)		
		1st hr	16 hr	Last hr	1st hr	10 hr	Last hr	1st hr	8 hr	Last hr
2.5	105 mL/hr	75 mL/hr	145 mL/hr	75 mL/hr	115 mL/hr	225 mL/hr	115 mL/hr			
2.0	85 mL/hr	60 mL/hr	120 mL/hr	60 mL/hr	90 mL/hr	180 mL/hr	90 mL/hr			
1.5	65 mL/hr	45 mL/hr	90 mL/hr	45 mL/hr	70 mL/hr	135 mL/hr	70 mL/hr	85 mL/hr	165 mL/hr	85 mL/hr
1.0	40 mL/hr	30 mL/hr	60 mL/hr	30 mL/hr	45 mL/hr	90 mL/hr	45 mL/hr	55 mL/hr	110 mL/hr	55 mL/hr

PERIPHERAL PARENTERAL NUTRITION (PPN)

Although central venous access is recommended for TPN, there are cases where PPN is indicated. For example:

>> In mildly catabolic, mildly malnourished patients requiring parenteral supplementation of only five to ten days duration.

>> In patients at high risk for fungal or bacterial catheter sepsis or those whose central lines have been pulled due to positive cultures.

>> To supplement tube feedings where poor tolerance necessitates slow progression to full volume/strength.

PPN offers advantages over TPN since most complications associated with central venous catheterization are avoided. The major complication of PPN is thrombophlebitis which results from infusion of solutions with osmolarities in excess of 600 to 800 mOsm/L. Concentrations of PPN solution that remain within the range of 600 to 800 mOsm/L are:

>> 2.5% amino acids (238 mOsm/L) and 5% dextrose (250 mOsm/L).

>> 2.5% amino acids (238 mOsm/L) and 10% dextrose (505 mOsm/L).

>> 5% amino acids (475 mOsm/L) and 5% dextrose (250 mOsm/L).

A maximum of 10% to 12.5% dextrose can be infused into a peripheral vein. Continuous infusion of lipids (piggyback) is recommended to reduce the osmolarity and protect the vein by coating the venous epithelium. To prevent infections, infusion sites should be changed every 72 hours.

PPN is contraindicated in: fluid restricted patients, patients who cannot tolerate high volume lipid infusions, hypermetabolic patients whose daily caloric needs exceed 2500 to 3000 calories, and patients with thrombophlebitis or limited venous access.

TERMINATING TPN

Transition from full TPN to enteral alimentation is a gradual process. It occurs with a slow return (one week) of normal GI function and a decrease in severe anorexia associated with an active illness. Initially, the TPN rate is gradually decreased as tube or oral feedings advance.

Daily calorie counts are recorded and the TPN rate is adjusted according to intake (i.e., a 20 mL/hr decrease in standard TPN = 500 kcal/day). TPN is discontinued when oral intake approximates two-thirds of the patient's estimated needs. If the patient's nutritional needs are not being met within three to five days after initiation of enteral feedings, supplemental PPN may be added. However, if GI function is adequate, oral intake should be supplemented with tube feedings. For patients on long term TPN, tube feedings may be poorly tolerated initially. To improve tolerance, the feedings should begin at one-quarter strength and gradually advance in strength as tolerated. (See Chapter 9: Enteral Nutrition for formula selection and administration.)

CLINICAL MONITORING CHECKLIST

Clinical monitoring of TPN consists of monitoring the patient's clinical and laboratory data. Table 10–20 details various clinical parameters and monitoring frequencies.

TABLE 10–20: TPN Clinical Monitoring Parameters

Parameters	Suggested Frequency
Patient Examination	Daily
Vital Signs	At least every shift, more often as indicated
Blood Glucose (bedside)	Every 6 hr with initiation of TPN as indicated
Fluid Balance	Daily
Nutrient Balance	Daily
Body Weight	Daily
Liver Function Tests (LFTs)	Baseline/weekly/monthly
Hematology	
Full blood count	Two times weekly/monthly
Prothrombin time	Two times weekly
Folate and B_{12}	As clinically indicated
Iron, transferrin	As clinically indicated
Albumin	Weekly
Blood Chemistries	
Chemistry panel	Baseline, 3 times weekly
Electrolytes	Baseline, daily for 5 days, then 3 times weekly
Glucose	Baseline, every 6 hr x 24 hr then daily or as indicated
Phosphate	Daily x 5 days then with chemistry panel
Magnesium	Baseline, 3 times for first week, then weekly
Zinc	Every 2 months or as indicated
Triglycerides	*Premature and newborn infant:* 6 hr into initial infusion and after increase in fat emulsion *Infants and small children:* 4 –6 hr post 18 to 20 hr infusion and after any significant increases in dosage (i.e., from 2 to 3 gm/kg/day) *Adolescents and adults:* 8–12 hr after initial infusion
Selenium	After 2 months of TPN and every 2 months thereafter
Urine Tests	
Nitrogen balance	At 2 wk and repeat weekly if negative
Electrolytes	As clinically indicated

Additional clinical chemistries that may be useful for more detailed nutritional monitoring include individual vitamins, minerals, trace element levels and rapid turnover proteins (e.g., pre-albumin, retinol binding protein, triene/tetraene ratio).

TPN THERAPY: SUMMARY SEQUENCE OF EVENTS

Remember: Parenteral nutrition solutions are nutritional products which cannot be ordered on a STAT basis. Therefore, it is important to establish an organized approach to the use of TPN.

1) Establish the need for TPN.

2) Review the patient's status regarding activity and stress levels. Assess the nutritional state; calculate energy and protein needs.

3) Obtain appropriate baseline lab tests.

4) Choose appropriate protein, dextrose, lipids, vitamins, trace elements, and insulin as required.

5) Initiate TPN with slow taper up to appropriate rate. For example, 25 mL/hr every four to six hours or as tolerated.

6) Monitor patient and laboratory tests daily.

7) Avoid breaks in therapy, but if necessary run 10% or 5% dextrose, unless able to properly taper TPN or use cyclic therapy.

Meeting the patient's fluid and nutritional needs is the first requirement. While the cost of any TPN therapy is expensive, it is much more cost effective to prescribe a standard TPN formulation versus a non-standard formulation or some other specialty solution.

Given the cost of materials involved, avoid wastage whenever possible. Before changes in therapy are initiated, evaluate the use of existing solutions whenever possible to decrease wastage.

REFERENCES

1. Roza AM, Shizgal HM. The Harris Benedict equation reevaluated: Resting energy requirements and the body cell mass. Am J Clin Nutr. 1984;40:168–82.

2. MacBarney MW. Rational decision making in nutritional care. Surg Clin N Am. 1981;61(3):571–81.

3. Jequier E. Measurement of energy expenditure in clinical nutritional assessment. JPEN. 1987;11:86s–89s.

4. Mirtallo JM et al. Nutritional support of patients with renal disease. Clin Pharm. 1984;3:253–63.

5. Ingenbleek Y et al. Albumin, transferrin and the thyroxin-binding prealbumin/retinol-binding protein complex in assessment of malnutrition. Clin Chem Acta. 1975;63:61–67.

6. Cochran EB et al. Therapy review: Parenteral nutrition in pediatric patients. Clin Pharm. 1988;7:351.

7. Easton. Parenteral nutrition in the newborn, a practical guide. Ped Clin N Am. 1982;29:1171.

8. Manual of Pediatric Parenteral Nutrition. John Kerner, ed. Wiley Medical Publication; 1983.

9. Long C. Metabolic response to injury and illness: estimation of energy and protein needs from indirect calorimetry and nitrogen balance. JPEN. 1979;3:452.

10. Youssef H. Hypophosphatemic respiratory failure complicating TPN: An iatrogenic potentially lethal hazard. Anesthesiology. 1982;57:246–53.

11. Baptista RJ et al. Utilizing selenious acid to reverse selenium deficiency in total parenteral nutrition patients. Am J Clin Nutr. 1984;39(5);816–20.

12. Triplett WC. Clinical aspects of zinc, copper, manganese, chromium and selenium metabolism. Nutr Int. 1985;1(2):60.

13. Drisco DF. Clinical issues regarding the use of total nutrient admixtures. Drug Intell Clin Pharm. 1990;24:296–303.

14. Silk DBA. Nutritional Support in Hospital Practice. Blackwell Scientific Publications. St. Louis;1983:139.

15. Silberman H et al. Parenteral and Enteral Nutrition for the Hospitalized Patient., 2nd ed. Appleton-Lange. East Norwalk, CT, 1989.

16. Enteral and Parenteral Nutrition. Grant A , Todd E, eds. Blackwell Scientific Publications. St. Louis, MO;1982:89.

17. Total Parenteral Nutrition. 2nd ed. Fisher JE, ed. Little, Brown, and Company. Boston, MA;1991.

18 Adult Parenteral Nutrition Handbook. University of Wisconsin Hospital and Clinics. 1992 February; Madison, WI.

ACKNOWLEDGMENTS

The author acknowledges the contributions of Bill R. Check, James L. Stehley, Peter A. Underwood, Timothy D. Wolf, and the TPN Subcommittee and Dietary Committee at the University of Wisconsin Hospital and Clinics.

Common Pharmaceutical Calculations

Susan L. Bathke

Familiarity and accuracy with mathematical manipulations are critical to ensuring the safe and effective use of medications. This chapter includes calculations frequently used in pharmacy practice, however, it is not intended to be all inclusive. Each commonly encountered problem is accompanied by examples of mathematical calculations. The use of the metric system is emphasized.

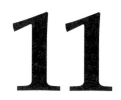

HEIGHT CONVERSION

The metric system of measurement is encountered with increasing frequency in the United States. Since most patients report their height in inches, rather than in centimeters, the following conversion is very useful. Height can also be estimated for hospitalized patients by the length of a patient bed or, for ambulatory patients, by the door frame or counter height.

$$1 \text{ inch} = 2.54 \text{ centimeters}$$
$$1 \text{ centimeter} = 0.3937 \text{ inches}$$

To convert height in inches to height in centimeters:

$$\text{Height in cm} = \text{Height in inches} \times \frac{2.54 \text{ cm}}{1 \text{ inch}}$$

Example: A patient is 5'10". What is his height in cm?

$$\text{Height in cm} = 70 \text{ inches} \times \frac{2.54 \text{ cm}}{1 \text{ inch}}$$
$$= 177.8 \text{ cm}$$

Example: A child is 24 inches. What is his height in cm?

$$\text{Height in cm} = 24 \text{ inches} \times \frac{2.54 \text{ cm}}{1 \text{ inch}}$$
$$= 61 \text{ cm}$$

See Feet to Centimeter Conversion Chart on page 11–2.

HEIGHT CONVERSION CHART
FROM INCHES TO CENTIMETERS

1' 0" = 30.5 cm	2' 0" = 61 cm	3' 0" = 91.4 cm
1" = 33 cm	1" = 63.5 cm	1" = 94 cm
2" = 35.6 cm	2" = 66 cm	2" = 96.5 cm
3" = 38.1 cm	3" = 68.6 cm	3" = 99.1 cm
4" = 40.6 cm	4" = 71.1 cm	4" = 101.6 cm
5" = 43.2 cm	5" = 73.7 cm	5" = 104.1 cm
6" = 45.7 cm	6" = 76.2 cm	6" = 106.7 cm
7" = 48.3 cm	7" = 78.7 cm	7" = 109.2 cm
8" = 50.8 cm	8" = 81.3 cm	8" = 111.7 cm
9" = 53.3 cm	9" = 83.8 cm	9" = 114.3 cm
10"= 55.9 cm	10"= 86.4 cm	10"= 116.8 cm
11"= 58.4 cm	11"= 88.9 cm	11"= 119.4 cm

4' 0" = 121.9 cm	5' 0" = 152.4 cm	6' 0" = 182.9 cm
1" = 124.5 cm	1" = 154.9 cm	1" = 185.4 cm
2" = 127 cm	2" = 157.4 cm	2" = 188 cm
3" = 129.5 cm	3" = 160 cm	3" = 190.5 cm
4" = 132.1 cm	4" = 162.6 cm	4" = 193 cm
5" = 134.6 cm	5" = 165.1 cm	5" = 195.6 cm
6" = 137.2 cm	6" = 167.6 cm	6" = 198.1 cm
7" = 139.7 cm	7" = 170.2 cm	7" = 200.7 cm
8" = 142.2 cm	8" = 172.7 cm	8" = 203.2 cm
9" = 144.8 cm	9" = 175.3 cm	9" = 205.7 cm
10"= 147.3 cm	10"= 177.8 cm	10"= 208.3 cm
11"= 149.9 cm	11"= 180.3 cm	11"= 210.8 cm

WEIGHT CONVERSION

Most patients report their weight in pounds, rather than kilograms. To convert from pounds to kilograms the following relationships are used.

$$1 \text{ pound (lb)} = 0.454 \text{ kilograms (kg)}$$
$$1 \text{ kilogram (kg)} = 2.204 \text{ pounds (lb)}$$

To convert weight in pounds to weight in kilograms:

$$\text{Weight in kg} = \text{Weight in lb} \times \frac{1 \text{kg}}{2.2 \text{ lb}}$$

Example: A patient weighs 170 lb. What is her weight in kg?

$$\text{Weight in kg} = 170 \text{ lb} \times \frac{1 \text{ kg}}{2.2 \text{ lb}}$$
$$= 77.3 \text{ kg}$$

Example: A child weighs 30 lb. What is his weight in kg?

$$\text{Weight in kg} = 30 \text{ lb} \times \frac{1 \text{ kg}}{2.2 \text{ lb}}$$
$$= 13.6 \text{ kg}$$

See Pound to Kilogram Conversion Chart on page 11–4.

TEMPERATURE CONVERSION

Depending upon your familiarity with temperature scales and the type of thermometer being used, the conversion from Fahrenheit to Centigrade and vice versa can be helpful in interpreting a particular value.

$$32° \text{ Farenheit (°F)} = 0° \text{ Centigrade (°C)}$$
$$212° \text{ Farenheit (°F)} = 100° \text{ Centigrade (°C)}$$

To convert temperature in degrees Fahrenheit to temperature in degrees Centigrade:

$$°C = \frac{5}{9} \left(°F - 32 \right)$$

To convert temperature in degrees Centigrade to temperature in degrees Fahrenheit:

$$°F = \frac{9}{5} °C + 32$$

Example: A patient's temperature is 98.6° F. What is her temperature in °C?

$$°C = \frac{5}{9} (98.6 - 32)$$
$$= 37.0 \; \textit{Note: This is considered normal}$$
$$\textit{oral body temperature}$$

WEIGHT CONVERSION CHART
FROM POUNDS TO KILOGRAMS

lb		kg	lb		kg	lb		kg	lb		kg
1	=	0.4	29	=	13.2	57	=	25.9	85	=	38.6
2	=	0.9	30	=	13.6	58	=	26.4	86	=	39.1
3	=	1.4	31	=	14.1	59	=	26.8	87	=	39.5
4	=	1.8	32	=	14.5	60	=	27.3	88	=	40
5	=	2.3	33	=	15	61	=	27.7	89	=	40.4
6	=	2.7	34	=	15.4	62	=	28.2	90	=	40.9
7	=	3.2	35	=	15.9	63	=	28.6	91	=	41.4
8	=	3.6	36	=	16.4	64	=	29.1	92	=	41.8
9	=	4.1	37	=	16.8	65	=	29.5	93	=	42.3
10	=	4.5	38	=	17.3	66	=	30	94	=	42.7
11	=	5	39	=	17.7	67	=	30.4	95	=	43.1
12	=	5.4	40	=	18.2	68	=	30.9	96	=	43.6
13	=	5.9	41	=	18.6	69	=	31.4	97	=	44.1
14	=	6.4	42	=	19.1	70	=	31.8	98	=	44.5
15	=	6.8	43	=	19.5	71	=	32.3	99	=	45
16	=	7.3	44	=	20	72	=	32.7	100	=	45.4
17	=	7.7	45	=	20.4	73	=	33.6	101	=	45.9
18	=	8.2	46	=	20.9	74	=	33.9	102	=	46.5
19	=	8.6	47	=	21.4	75	=	34.1	103	=	46.8
20	=	9.1	48	=	21.8	76	=	34.5	104	=	47.2
21	=	9.5	49	=	22.3	77	=	35	105	=	47.7
22	=	10	50	=	22.7	78	=	35.4	106	=	48.1
23	=	10.4	51	=	23.2	79	=	35.9	107	=	48.6
24	=	10.9	52	=	23.6	80	=	36.4	108	=	49
25	=	11.4	53	=	24.1	81	=	36.8	109	=	49.5
26	=	11.8	54	=	24.5	82	=	37.3	110	=	50
27	=	12.3	55	=	25	83	=	37.7	111	=	50.4
28	=	12.7	56	=	25.4	84	=	38.2	112	=	50.9

(Continued)

WEIGHT CONVERSION CHART
FROM POUNDS TO KILOGRAMS (Continued)

lb		kg	lb		kg	lb		kg	lb		kg
113	=	51.3	142	=	64.6	171	=	77.7	200	=	90.9
114	=	51.8	143	=	65	172	=	78.2	201	=	91.4
115	=	52.2	144	=	65.5	173	=	78.6	202	=	92
116	=	52.7	145	=	65.9	174	=	79.1	203	=	92.4
117	=	53.1	146	=	66.4	175	=	79.5	204	=	92.7
118	=	53.6	147	=	66.8	176	=	80	205	=	93.2
119	=	54	148	=	67.3	177	=	80.5	206	=	93.6
120	=	54.5	149	=	67.7	178	=	80.9	207	=	94.1
121	=	55	150	=	68.2	179	=	81.4	208	=	94.5
122	=	55.4	151	=	68.6	180	=	81.8	209	=	95
123	=	55.9	152	=	69.1	181	=	82.3	210	=	95.5
124	=	56.5	153	=	69.5	182	=	82.7	211	=	96
125	=	56.8	154	=	70	183	=	83.2	212	=	96.4
126	=	57.3	155	=	70.5	184	=	83.6	213	=	96.9
127	=	57.7	156	=	70.9	185	=	84.1	214	=	97.3
128	=	58.2	157	=	71.4	186	=	84.5	215	=	97.8
129	=	58.6	158	=	71.8	187	=	85	216	=	98.2
130	=	59.1	159	=	72.3	188	=	85.5	217	=	98.7
131	=	59.5	160	=	72.7	189	=	85.9	218	=	99.1
132	=	60	161	=	73.2	190	=	86.4	219	=	99.6
133	=	60.5	162	=	73.6	191	=	86.8	220	=	100.1
134	=	60.9	163	=	74.1	192	=	87.3	221	=	100.5
135	=	61.4	164	=	74.6	193	=	87.7	222	=	101
136	=	61.8	165	=	75	194	=	88.2	223	=	101.4
137	=	62.3	166	=	75.5	195	=	88.6	224	=	101.9
138	=	62.7	167	=	75.9	196	=	89	225	=	102.3
139	=	63.2	168	=	76.4	197	=	89.5			
140	=	63.6	169	=	76.8	198	=	90			
141	=	64.1	170	=	77.3	199	=	90.5			

Example: A patient's temperature is 37.5° C. What is his temperature in °F?

$$°F = \frac{9}{5}(37.5) + 32$$
$$= 99.5$$

It is sometimes difficult to recall whether you should multiply by 9/5 or 5/9 and add 32 to or subtract 32 from the Fahrenheit temperature or the centigrade temperature. Most Americans recognize that temperatures in Fahrenheit are in numbers greater than temperatures in Centigrade. Therefore, it is easy to remember that °C temperature needs to be multiplied and "32" needs to be added. If you only want to remember one formula for temperature conversion, the following formula is useful:

$$°F = 1.8° C + 32$$

The reverse calculation is then an algebraic manipulation, as shown below:

$$°F = 1.8° C + 32$$
$$°F - 32 = 1.8 °C$$
$$\frac{°F - 32}{1.8} = °C$$

See Temperature Conversion Chart on page 11–7.

IDEAL OR LEAN BODY WEIGHT CALCULATION (IBW OR LBW)[1]

When patients are not obese, ideal body weight (IBW) is equal to the lean body weight (LBW). Obesity is actual body weight ≥20% of the ideal body weight. The LBW is often used to calculate drug dosages (e.g., aminoglycosides) and in the calculation of creatinine clearance (Cl_{Cr}).

Males

IBW = 50 kg + 2.3 (height in inches over 5 ft)

Alternate Formula
IBW = 110 lb + 5 lb (height in inches over 5 ft), then
use lb to kg conversion (See page 11–4)

Example: A male patient is 5'10". What is his IBW?

$$IBW = 50 \text{ kg} + 2.3(10 \text{ inches})$$
$$= 73 \text{ kg}$$
or
$$IBW = 110 \text{ lb} + 5(10 \text{ inches})$$
$$= 160 \text{ lb} \times \frac{1 \text{ kg}}{2.2 \text{ lb}}$$
$$= 72.7 \text{ kg}$$

TEMPERATURE CONVERSION CHART
FROM FAHRENHEIT TO CENTIGRADE

°F	°C	°F	°C	°F	°C	°F	°C
95.0° = 35.0°		98.8° = 37.1°		102.6° = 39.2°		106.4° = 41.3°	
95.2° = 35.1°		99.0° = 37.2°		102.8° = 39.3°		106.6° = 41.4°	
95.4° = 35.2°		99.2° = 37.3°		103.0° = 39.4°		106.8° = 41.5°	
95.6° = 35.3°		99.4° = 37.4°		103.2° = 39.5°		107.0° = 41.6°	
95.8° = 35.4°		99.6° = 37.5°		103.4° = 39.6°		107.2° = 41.8°	
96.0° = 35.5°		99.8° = 37.6°		103.6° = 39.8°		107.4° = 41.9°	
96.2° = 35.6°		100.0° = 37.7°		103.8° = 39.9°		107.6° = 42.0°	
96.4° = 35.7°		100.2° = 37.9°		104.0° = 40.0°		107.8° = 42.1°	
96.6° = 35.9°		100.4° = 38.0°		104.2° = 40.1°		108.0° = 42.2°	
96.8° = 36.0°		100.6° = 38.1°		104.4° = 40.2°		108.2° = 42.3°	
97.0° = 36.1°		100.8° = 38.2°		104.6° = 40.3°		108.4° = 42.4°	
97.2° = 36.2°		101.0° = 38.3°		104.8° = 40.4°		108.6° = 42.5°	
97.4° = 36.3°		101.2° = 38.4°		105.0° = 40.5°		108.8° = 42.6°	
97.6° = 36.4°		101.4° = 38.5°		105.2° = 40.6°		109.0° = 42.7°	
97.8° = 36.5°		101.6° = 38.6°		105.4° = 40.8°		109.2° = 42.9°	
98.0° = 36.6°		101.8° = 38.7°		105.6° = 40.9°		109.4° = 43.0°	
98.2° = 36.8°		102.0° = 38.8°		105.8° = 41.0°		109.6° = 43.1°	
98.4° = 36.9°		102.2° = 39.0°		106.0° = 41.1°		109.8° = 43.2°	
98.6° = 37.0°		102.4° = 39.1°		106.2° = 41.2°		110.0° = 43.3°	

Females

IBW = 45 kg + 2.3 (height in inches over 5 ft)

Alternate Formula

IBW = 100 lb + 5 lb (height in inches over 5 ft), then
use lb to kg conversion (See page 11–4)

Example: A female patient is 5'4". What is her IBW?

$$IBW = 45 \text{ kg} + 2.3(4 \text{ inches})$$
$$= 54.2 \text{ kg}$$

or

$$IBW = 100 \text{ lb} + 5 (4 \text{ inches})$$
$$= 120 \text{ lb} \times \frac{1 \text{ kg}}{2.2 \text{ lb}}$$
$$= 54.5 \text{ kg}$$

CHILDREN AND ADULTS < 5 FEET TALL

The ideal body weight for children and adults less than 5 feet tall is described on page 11–12. For adults less than 5 feet tall, actual body weight may be used if <45 kg for females or <50 kg for males.

LEAN BODY WEIGHT CORRECTED FOR OBESITY (LBW)

When patients weigh ≥20% more than their IBW, the percent of additional body weight that is not fat must be accounted for. This corrected LBW is used to dose medications like aminoglycosides and in the calculations of creatinine clearance.

$$LBW = Ideal\ Body\ Weight + 0.2\ (Actual\ Body\ Weight - IBW)$$

Example: A patient's IBW is 73 kg. Actual body weight (ABW) is 90.9 kg. What is the LBW?

$$LBW = 73\ kg + 0.2\ (90.9\ kg - 73\ kg)$$
$$= 73\ kg + 3.6\ kg$$
$$= 76.6\ kg$$

BODY SURFACE AREA (BSA)

Body surface area, rather than body weight, is used often for chemotherapy and pediatric dose calculations. Body surface area can be determined by a nomogram or calculation; however, the results are not identical by each method.

By Nomogram

Separate nomograms are used for children and adults. Using the nomogram to determine body surface area from height and weight, a straight line connecting the patient's height and weight intersects at the individual's BSA. For BSA determination by nomogram see: BSA Nomograms for Children and Adults on pages 11–19 and 11–20.[2]

Example: An adult patient is 165 cm tall and weighs 75 kg. Using a straight edge, connect height and weight on the *adult's* BSA nomogram. BSA = 1.82 m^2.

Example: A pediatric patient is 61 cm tall and weighs 9 kg. Using a straight edge, connect height and weight on the *children's* BSA nomogram. BSA = 0.36 m^2.

By Calculation[3]

BSA can also be determined by calculation. The same calculation is used for adults and children.

$$BSA\ in\ m^2 = \sqrt{\frac{height\ in\ cm \times weight\ in\ kg}{3600}}$$

Example: An adult patient is 165 cm tall and weighs 75 kg. What is his BSA?

$$BSA\ in\ m^2 = \sqrt{\frac{165\ cm \times 75\ kg}{3600}}$$
$$= 1.85\ m^2$$

Example: A pediatric patient is 61 cm tall and 9 kg in weight. What is her BSA?

$$\text{BSA in m}^2 = \sqrt{\frac{61 \text{ cm} \times 9 \text{ kg}}{3600}}$$

$$= 0.39 \text{ m}^2$$

CALCULATED CREATININE CLEARANCE (Cl_{Cr}) (AN ESTIMATE OF RENAL FUNCTION)

The normal values for creatinine clearance are: 70 to 110 mL/min. A patient's renal function can be estimated by calculating his creatinine clearance utilizing the Cockroft-Gault equation:[4]

$$\text{Cl}_{\text{Cr}} \text{ in mL/min (males)} = \frac{(140 - \text{Patient's Age in yr}) \text{ (IBW)}}{(72) \text{ (Serum Creatinine)}}$$

For female patients, multiply the above formula by 0.85. The answer in either case should be rounded off to nearest mL/min. For children and adults <5 feet tall see page 11–12.

For adults <5 feet tall, the pediatric ideal body weight formula can be used, or the actual body weight can be used if <45 kg for females or <50 kg for males. When the patient's actual body weight (ABW) is less than LBW, ABW is preferred. Similarly, use the patient's corrected LBW if the ABW is at least 20% more than IBW.

If a patient's serum creatinine is less than 0.8 mg/dL, the Cl_{Cr} may appear higher than it actually is (e.g., in patients with decreased muscle mass, such as bedridden or spinal cord injury patients). A calculated creatinine clearance is either normal or below normal; if it is >110 mL/min, the patient's Cl_{Cr} is *normal*.

Note: Elderly patients will have a lower calculated Cl_{Cr}. However, this still indicates that their renal function is below normal and should be assessed as such.

Example: A 30-year-old male has an IBW of 70 kg (ABW 70 kg) and a serum creatinine of 1.0 mg/dL. Calculate his Cl_{Cr}.

$$\text{Cl}_{\text{Cr}} \text{ in mL/min} = \frac{(140 - 30) \text{ (70 kg)}}{(72) \text{ (1.0 mg/dL)}}$$

$$= 107 \text{ mL/min}$$

Example: A 55-year-old female has an IBW of 50 kg (ABW 80 kg) and a serum creatinine of 1.3 mg/dL. Calculate her Cl_{Cr}.

First, a corrected LBW should be calculated.

$$\text{LBW} = 50 \text{ kg} + 0.20 \, (80 \text{ kg} - 50 \text{ kg})$$

$$= 56 \text{ kg}$$

$$\text{Cl}_{\text{Cr}} \text{ in mL/min} = \frac{(140 - 55) \text{ (56 kg)}}{(72) \text{ (1.3 mg/dL)}} \times 0.85$$

$$= 43 \text{ mL/min}$$

Example: A 21-year-old male has an IBW of 75 kg (ABW 60 kg) and a serum creatinine of 0.5 mg/dL. Calculate his Cl_{Cr}.

This patient's ABW should be used because it is less than the IBW. When the serum creatinine is <0.8 mg/dL, the calculation will show an increased Cl_{Cr}. This increased value can be used to determine if the patient's renal function appears normal, or a value of 1.0 mg/dL can be substituted for serum creatinine.

$$Cl_{Cr} \text{ in mL/min} = \frac{(140 - 21)(60 \text{ kg})}{(72)(0.5 \text{ mg/dL})}$$

$$= 198.3 \text{ mL/min}$$

or

$$Cl_{Cr} \text{ in mL/min} = \frac{(140 - 21)(60 \text{ kg})}{(72)(1.0 \text{ mg/dL})}$$

$$= 99 \text{ mL/min}$$

In either case, this patient's renal function appears within the normal range. His renal function estimate could be verified with a 24-hour urine collection for creatinine. Again, it should be noted that renal function is either normal or below normal, not better than normal.

CREATININE CLEARANCE
BASED UPON URINE COLLECTION

A creatinine clearance based upon urine collection is considered a more accurate reflection of renal function than the calculated creatinine clearance. The urine can be collected over various time intervals, ranging from as little as 2 hours up to 24 hours, and the concentration of creatinine in the urine can be quantifiably measured. The urine collection must be a complete collection (all urine collected), or the Cl_{Cr} could appear less than it actually is. If a patient's bladder is intermittently catheterized, consider the catheterization interval when determining how long to collect the urine.

$$Cl_{Cr} \text{ in mL/min} = \frac{UV}{PT}$$

Where:

   U = Urine Concentration of Creatinine in mg/dL

   V = Urine Volume in mL

   P = Plasma Concentration of Creatinine in mg/dL

   T = Collection Period in min

Example: B.D., a 60-year-old, 70 kg male, has a serum creatinine of 1.1 mg/dL, a urine creatinine concentration of 70 mg/dL, and a 24-hour urine collection volume of 1400 mL. (24 hours = 1440 minutes.) What is his Cl_{Cr}?

$$Cl_{Cr} \text{ in mL/min} = \frac{70 \text{ mg/dL} \times 1400 \text{ mL}}{1.1 \text{ mg/dL} \times 1440 \text{ min}}$$

$$= 62 \text{ mL/min}$$

Example: A patient has a serum creatinine of 0.9 mg/dL, a urine creatinine concentration of 60 mg/dL, and a 4-hour urine collection volume of 400 mL. (4 hours = 240 minutes.) What is her Cl_{Cr}?

$$Cl_{Cr} \text{ in mL/min} = \frac{60 \text{ mg/dL} \times 400 \text{ mL}}{0.9 \text{ mg/dL} \times 240 \text{ min}}$$

$$= 111 \text{ mL/min}$$

CREATININE PRODUCTION VERIFICATION[5]

These calculations use a laboratory determination of a 24-hour urine collection to verify the reported Cl_{Cr}. If the urine collection is incomplete, the Cl_{Cr} can appear less than it actually is.

Amount of Creatinine Excreted = (Urine Volume per 24 hr in mL) (Urine Creatinine Concentration in mg/100 mL)

$$\text{Apparent Rate of Creatinine} = \text{Creatinine Production/day}$$

$$= \frac{\text{Amount of Creatinine Excreted}}{\text{Patient's Weight}}$$

$$= \frac{\text{mg/24 hr}}{\text{kg}}$$

$$= \text{mg/kg/day}$$

This apparent rate of creatinine production can be compared to the expected amount of creatinine production to determine if the urine collection was complete.

Expected Daily Creatinine Production for Males[5]

TABLE 11–1: Daily Creatinine Production

Age (yr)	Male mg/kg/day
20–29	24
30–39	22
40–49	20
50–59	19
60–69	17
70–79	14
80–89	12
90–99	9

Example: Using patient B.D. from page 11–10, the urine collection volume was 1400 mL in 24 hours. The urine creatinine concentration was 70 mg/100 mL. Was the urine collection complete?

$$\text{Amount of Creatinine Excreted} = \frac{(1400 \text{ mL}) (70 \text{ mg})}{(24 \text{ hr}) (100 \text{ mL})}$$

$$= 980 \text{ mg/24 hr}$$

$$\text{Apparent Rate of Creatinine Production} = \frac{980 \text{ mg/24 hr}}{70 \text{ kg}}$$

$$= 14 \text{ mg/kg/day}$$

From Table 11–1, expected daily creatinine production for a 60-year-old male is 17 mg/kg/day. It would be suspected that the urine collection was incomplete and the collection should then be repeated.

MATHEMATICAL CALCULATIONS FOR PEDIATRIC PATIENTS

Mathematical calculations of ideal body weight and creatinine clearance must be adjusted for children <12 years of age or patients <5 feet tall. Once a child is adult sized, these calculations may not be accurate.

Ideal Body Weight[6]

$$\text{IBW in kg} = \frac{(\text{height in cm})^2 (1.65)}{1000}$$

Example: A child is 85 cm tall. What is the child's IBW?

$$\text{IBW} = \frac{(85 \text{ cm})^2 (1.65)}{1000}$$

$$= 11.9 \text{ kg}$$

Creatinine Clearance[6]

$$\text{Cl}_{Cr} \text{ in mL/min} = \frac{(0.48) (\text{Height in cm})}{\text{Serum Creatinine}}$$

Example: A child is 105 cm tall and has a serum creatinine of 0.7 mg/dL. What is her creatinine clearance?

$$\text{Cl}_{Cr} \text{ in mL/min} = \frac{(0.48) (105 \text{ cm})}{(0.7 \text{ mg/dL})}$$

$$= 72 \text{ mL/min}$$

INTRAVENOUS DRIP RATES

Many intravenous solutions are administered by pump delivery devices; however, intravenous drip rates may need to be calculated when these devices are unavailable. Intravenous tubing by different manufacturers delivers different amounts of fluid and, therefore, knowledge of which product is being used before calculating intravenous drip rates is required.

McGaw and Abbott Adult Maxi-Drip IV Tubing

$$\frac{15 \text{ Drops}}{1 \text{ mL}} \times \frac{\text{Rate in mL}}{\text{hr}} \times \frac{1 \text{ hr}}{60 \text{ min}} = \text{Drops/min}$$

Or, to simplify and quickly calculate drops/min, divide the rate of infusion in mL/hr by 4.

Example: The rate of an IV is 100 mL/hr. At what rate in drops/min should the IV be run?

$$\text{Rate in Drops/min} = \frac{15 \text{ Drops}}{1 \text{ mL}} \times \frac{100 \text{ mL}}{\text{hr}} \times \frac{1 \text{ hr}}{60 \text{ min}}$$
$$= 25 \text{ Drops/min}$$

Travenol and All Blood Tubing

$$\text{Rate in Drops/min} = \frac{10 \text{ Drops}}{1 \text{ mL}} \times \frac{\text{Rate in mL}}{\text{hr}} \times \frac{1 \text{ hr}}{60 \text{ min}}$$

Or, to simplify and quickly calculate it, divide the rate of infusion by 6.

Minidrip Tubing

$$\text{Rate in Drops/min} = \frac{60 \text{ Drops}}{1 \text{ mL}} \times \frac{\text{Rate in mL}}{\text{hr}} \times \frac{1 \text{ hr}}{60 \text{ min}}$$

Hint: Drops/min = mL/hr

INTRAVENOUS DRIP
CONCENTRATION AND RATE DETERMINATION

The intravenous drip concentration and rate determination are usually calculated based upon the pharmacodynamic characteristics of individual drugs. Many institutions utilize standard drip concentrations for various drugs as indicated below. This facilitates the modification of doses without requiring preparation of a new solution.

Example: A patient must have IV heparin administered at 1000 U/hr. If a standard heparin drip contains 25,000 U of heparin sodium in 500 mL of 5% Dextrose, at what rate should the IV be run?

$$\text{Rate in mL/hr} = \frac{500 \text{ mL}}{25000 \text{ U}} \times \frac{1000 \text{ U}}{1 \text{ hr}}$$

$$= 20 \text{ mL/hr}$$

Example: A 70 kg patient is to be given IV dobutamine at 4 μg/kg/min. If a standard dobutamine drip contains 1.25 gm in 375 mL of 5% Dextrose, at what rate should the IV be run?

$$\text{Rate in mL/hr} = 4 \text{ μg/kg/min} \times 70 \text{ kg} = 280 \text{ μg/min}$$

$$= 280 \text{ μg/min} \times 60 \text{ min/1 hr}$$

$$= 16800 \text{ μg/hr} \times 1 \text{ mg/1000 μg}$$

$$= 16.8 \text{ mg/hr}$$

$$\text{Rate in mL/hr} = 16.8 \text{ mg/1 hr} \times 375 \text{ mL/1250 mg}$$

$$= 5 \text{ mL/hr}$$

Example: A 70 kg patient is to be given IV nitroprusside and/or nitroglycerin at 0.5 μg/kg/min. If a standard drip contains 50 mg in 250 mL of 5% Dextrose, at what rate should the IV be run?

$$\text{Rate in mL/hr} = 0.5 \text{ μg/kg/min} \times 70 \text{ kg} = 35 \text{ μg/min}$$

$$= 35 \text{ μg/min} \times 60 \text{ min/1 hr}$$

$$= 2100 \text{ μg/hr} \times 1 \text{ mg/1000 μg}$$

$$= 2.1 \text{ mg/hr}$$

$$\text{Rate in mL/hr} = 2.1 \text{ mg/1 hr} \times 250 \text{ mL/50 mg}$$

$$= 10.5 \text{ mL/hr}$$

CORRECTION OF SERUM CALCIUM FOR LOW SERUM ALBUMIN[7]

When a patient's serum albumin is low, the serum calcium may actually be higher than reported. This formula attempts to correct the problem and identify patients with the potential risk of hypercalcemia.

$$\text{Corrected Serum Calcium} = \text{Serum Calcium} + (4.0 - \text{Patient's Serum albumin}) \, 0.8$$

The reference value for serum calcium is: 8.8 to 10.4 mg/dL.
The reference value for serum albumin is: 3.5 to 5.0 mg/dL.

Example: A patient's serum calcium is reported at 9.8 mg/dL. The serum albumin is reported at 3.0 gm/dL. What is the corrected serum calcium?

$$\text{Corrected Serum Calcium} = 9.8 \text{ mg/dL} + (4.0 - 3.0 \text{ gm/dL}) (0.8)$$

$$= 10.6 \text{ mg/dL}$$

CORRECTION OF
MAGNESIUM FOR ELEVATED BILIRUBIN

The serum magnesium value may also be falsely lowered when the patient's bilirubin is elevated. For every 3 mg/dL the total bilirubin is above 10 (mg/dL), the magnesium concentration will be falsely lowered by 0.1 mg/dL.

The reference value for total serum bilirubin is: 0.4 to 1.4 mg/dL
The reference value for serum magnesium is: 1.7 to 2.3 mg/dL

Example:

$$\text{Corrected Magnesium (Mg)} = \left[\frac{\text{Bil} - 10}{3} \right] (0.1) + \text{Reported Mg}$$

$$\text{Reported Mg} = 1.5 \text{ mg/dL}$$
$$\text{Total Bilirubin} = 22 \text{ mg/dL}$$

$$\text{Therefore Corrected Mg} = \left(\frac{22 - 10}{3} \right) (0.1) + 1.5$$
$$= 1.9 \text{ mg/dL}$$

USING STRENGTH RATIO TO CALCULATE
INGREDIENT CONCENTRATION OF A SOLUTION[8]

Strength ratio solutions refer to gm of solute per mL of solution. This means that a 1:100 solution contains 1 gm of solute per 100 mL of solution.

Example: An epinephrine injection 1:1000 (Adrenalin) contains how many mg of epinephrine per mL?

$$1:1000 = \frac{1 \text{ gm Epinephrine}}{1000 \text{ mL}} = \frac{1000 \text{ mg}}{1000 \text{ mL}} = \frac{1 \text{ mg}}{1 \text{ mL}}$$

Example: An epinephrine injection 1:200 (Sus-Phrine) contains how many mg of epinephrine per mL?

$$1:200 = \frac{1 \text{ gm Epinephrine}}{200 \text{ mL}} = \frac{1000 \text{ mg}}{200 \text{ mg}} = \frac{5 \text{ mg}}{1 \text{ mL}}$$

STRENGTH RATIO AND PERCENT STRENGTH[8]

Strength ratio solutions refer to gm of solute per mL of solution. Percent weight to volume solutions refer to number of gm of solute per 100 mL of solution. A 1% w/v solution contains 1 gm of solute in 100 mL of solution. The strength ratio of the same solutions would be ^{1}gm/100 mL or 1:100.

Example: A potassium permanganate ($KMnO_4$) solution is in a strength of 1:5000. What would the percent strength be?

$$1 : 5000 \ = \ \frac{1 \text{ gm } KMnO_4}{5000 \text{ mL}} \ = \ \frac{0.02 \text{ gm}}{100 \text{ mL}} \ = \ 0.02\% \ \frac{W}{V}$$

Example: Acetic acid solution is ordered in a W/V strength of 0.25%. What would the strength ratio be?

$$0.25\% \ = \ \frac{0.25 \text{ gm Acetic Acid}}{100 \text{ mL}} \ = \ \frac{1 \text{ gm}}{400 \text{ mL}} \ = \ 1 : 400 \text{ Strength Ratio}$$

GRAIN TO MILLIGRAM CONVERSION

Some drugs (e.g., phenobarbital, thyroid, aspirin) may be ordered or labeled in grains.

$$1 \text{ grain} \ = \ 64.8 \text{ mg}$$

To convert dosage in grains to dosage in mg:

$$\text{Dosage in mg} \ = \ \text{Number of gr} \times \frac{64.8 \text{ mg}}{1 \text{ gr}}$$

> *Note:* Grain is abbreviated as gr. Take care not to confuse this with gm, the abbreviation for gram.

Example: A patient takes 5 gr of aspirin. What is this dosage in mg?

$$\text{Dosage in mg} \ = \ 5 \text{ gr} \times \frac{64.8 \text{ mg}}{1 \text{ gr}}$$

$$= \ 324 \text{ mg}$$

Example: A patient takes $^1/4$ gr phenobarbital. What is this dosage in mg?

$$\text{Dosage in mg} \ = \ \frac{1}{4} \text{ gr} \times \frac{64.8 \text{ mg}}{1 \text{ gr}}$$

$$= \ 16.2 \text{ mg}$$

> *Note:* This is often labeled as 15 mg. Many people use a conversion of 1 gr = 60 mg. This should be kept in mind when interpreting gr to mg conversions.

DRUG DOSAGE VOLUME CALCULATIONS

These are usually calculated on an individual basis. A dosage ordered may not be standard and needs to be prepared.

Example: A syringe contains 50 mg/mL of meperidine (Demerol). A physician orders a dose of 20 mg for a pediatric patient. How much should be administered?

$$\text{Volume in mL} \ = \ 20 \text{ mg} \times \frac{1 \text{ mL}}{50 \text{ mg}}$$

$$= \ 0.4 \text{ mL}$$

The final volume of the syringe should be 0.4 mL. The 0.6 mL of Demerol should be disposed of properly. Check at your practice site for appropriate procedures.

Example: A vial of vancomycin (Vancocin) contains 500 mg in 10 mL. A physician orders a 1 gm dose for an adult patient. How much should be administered?

$$\text{Volume in mL} = 1000 \text{ mg} \times \frac{10 \text{ mL}}{500 \text{ mg}}$$
$$= 20 \text{ mL}$$

SPECIAL DILUTIONS

A special dilution is prepared when a dosage of a drug is required in a larger dilution than is commercially available. These are most often used for pediatric dosages, ophthalmic injections, and skin testing (e.g., penicillin serial dilutions).

Example: An intravitreal ophthalmic injection of gentamicin 400 µg/0.1 mL is ordered. Gentamicin is commercially available in a strength of 40 mg/1 mL. How is this dose prepared?

One method is to start with a 1 mL aliquot of gentamicin; this would be 40 mg of drug.

$$\frac{400 \text{ µg}}{0.1 \text{ mL}} = \frac{40 \text{ mg}}{x}$$
$$x = 10 \text{ mL}$$

To end up with the desired concentration, the 40 mg must be diluted to a total volume of 10 mL. Thus, 9 mL of diluent must be added to the 1 mL of gentamicin to achieve the desired concentration.

ABSOLUTE NEUTROPHIL COUNT (ANC)

This calculation is often used for patients who receive chemotherapy or who are immuno-suppressed. Neutrophils are the most common type of white blood cell (WBC) and are important for fighting infections. When their value is low, the patient is at increased risk of an infectious complication.

If absolute neutrophil count is <500, neutropenic precautions should be taken.

$$\text{ANC} = [\% \text{ segs} + \% \text{ bands} + (\% \text{ metamyleocytes if present})] \times \text{WBC}$$

Segs, bands, metamyleocytes or types of neutrophils are reported as percentages of the WBC count.

Reference value for neutrophils is 1600 to 7000/µL.
Reference value for WBC is 3500 to 10,000/µL.

Example: An adult medicine patient's WBC is 5.7 K/uL (5700/uL). Segs = 48%, bands = 12%, and metamyleocytes = 0. What is the patient's ANC?

$$\text{ANC} = (0.48 + 0.12)(5700)$$
$$= 3420$$

Example: A hematology patient has a WBC of 0.3 K/uL (300/uL). Segs = 0%, bands = 0%, and metamyleocytes = 0. What is the patient's ANC?

$$ANC = (0 + 0)(300)$$
$$= 0$$

Neutropenic precautions should be followed for this patient.

REFERENCES

1. Devine BJ. Clinical pharmacy case studies–gentamicin therapy. Drug Intell and Clin Pharm. 1974; 8:650–655.

2. Diem K, Lentner C, eds. Scientific tables. Documenta Geigy, 7th ed. Basle, Switzerland: J.R. Geigy, S. A; 1970.

3. Lam TK, Leung O. More on simplified calculation of body surface area. N Eng J Med. 1988; 318:1130.

4. Cockroft DW, Gault MH. Prediction of creatinine clearance from serum creatinine. Nephron. 1976; 16:31–41.

5. Young LY, Koda-Kimble MA, eds. Applied Therapeutics: The Clinical Use of Drugs. 5th ed. Vancouver: Applied Therapeutics, Inc.; 1992.

6. Payne RB et al. Interpretation of serum total calcium: effects of adjustment for albumin concentrations on frequency of abnormal values and on detection of change in the individual. J Clin Pathol. 1979; 32:56–60.

7. Traub SL, Johnson CE. Comparison of methods of estimating creatinine clearance in children. Am J Hosp Pharm. 1980; 37:195–201.

8. Stoklosa MJ, Ansel HC. Pharmaceutical Calculations. 7th ed. Philadelphia: Lea and Febiger; 1980.

ACKNOWLEDGMENT

The author acknowledges and thanks the decentral pharmacists at the University of Wisconsin Hospital and Clinics for their helpful comments.

Body Surface Area of Children

Nomogram for determination of body surface area from height and weight

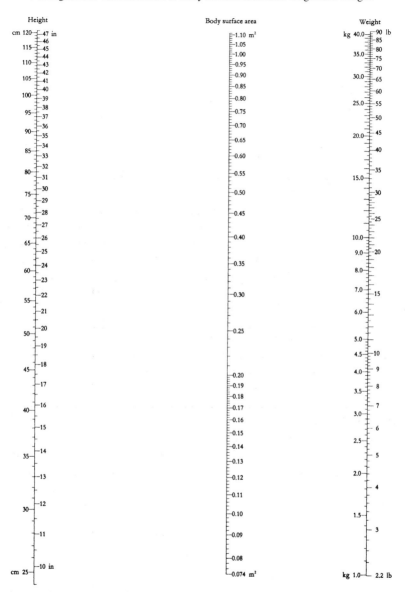

From the formula of Du Bois and Du Bois, *Arch. intern. Med.*, 17, 863 (1916): $S = W^{0.425} \times H^{0.725} \times 71.84$, or $\log S = W \times 0.425 + \log H \times 0.725 + 1.8564$ (S = body surface in cm², W = weight in kg, H = height in cm)

Body Surface Area of Adults

Nomogram for determination of body surface area from height and weight

Height	Body surface area	Weight

cm 200 — 79 in
— 78
195 — 77
— 76
190 — 75
— 74
185 — 73
— 72
180 — 71
— 70
175 — 69
— 68
170 — 67
— 66
165 — 65
— 64
160 — 63
— 62
155 — 61
— 60
150 — 59
— 58
145 — 57
— 56
140 — 55
— 54
135 — 53
— 52
130 — 51
— 50
125 — 49
— 48
120 — 47
— 46
115 — 45
— 44
110 — 43
— 42
105 — 41
— 40
cm 100 — 39 in

— 2.80 m²
— 2.70
— 2.60
— 2.50
— 2.40
— 2.30
— 2.20
— 2.10
— 2.00
— 1.95
— 1.90
— 1.85
— 1.80
— 1.75
— 1.70
— 1.65
— 1.60
— 1.55
— 1.50
— 1.45
— 1.40
— 1.35
— 1.30
— 1.25
— 1.20
— 1.15
— 1.10
— 1.05
— 1.00
— 0.95
— 0.90
— 0.86 m²

kg 150 — 330 lb
145 — 320
140 — 310
135 — 300
130 — 290
125 — 280
120 — 270
115 — 260
110 — 250
105 — 240
100 — 230
95 — 220
90 — 210
85 — 200
80 — 190
75 — 180
70 — 170
65 — 160
60 — 150
55 — 140
50 — 130
45 — 120
40 — 110
35 — 105
— 100
— 95
— 90
— 85
— 80
— 75
— 70
kg 30 — 66 lb

From the formula of Du Bois and Du Bois, *Arch. intern. Med.*, 17, 863 (1916):
$S = W^{0.425} \times H^{0.725} \times 71.84$, or $\log S = W \times 0.425 + \log H \times 0.725 + 1.8564$ (S = body surface in cm², W = weight in kg, H = height in cm)

Pharmacokinetics

Steven C. Ebert
Marilyn G. Bufton

USE OF SERUM DRUG LEVELS (SDLS) IN THERAPEUTIC DRUG MONITORING

12

Rationale for SDLs

SDLs are obtained for the following reasons:

>> To ensure that the patient's serum concentrations of drug are consistent with serum concentrations that usually are associated with the desired pharmacological effect.

>> To ensure that the patient's serum concentrations are not likely to cause drug toxicity.

>> To serve as a guide for adjustment of doses or to confirm the adequacy of a prior dose adjustment.

>> To serve as an objective measure of patient compliance.

The cost to assay the concentration of a drug in serum is typically about $20 to $50; therefore, SDLs should not be obtained without due consideration for the cost. SDLs should be determined at a time that will yield the desired information (e.g., steady state, peak, trough).

"Therapeutic Range" for an SDL

A *therapeutic range* represents serum concentrations that define the upper and lower limits of the desired drug concentration. Serum drug concentrations below or above the usual therapeutic range are usually associated with decreased drug efficacy or increased drug toxicity, respectively. The "therapeutic range" for a drug is affected by the condition being treated and the time of sample in relationship to when the drug was administered, as well as by the pharmacokinetic parameters specific for the drug being monitored.

Many drugs possess a *wide therapeutic range* (i.e., the *toxic serum concentrations* are *much* higher than the *therapeutic* serum concentrations). When the dose of a drug with a wide therapeutic range (e.g., penicillin) appears to be insufficient, a larger dose can be administered without undue concern for toxicity because there is a wide margin of safety; thus, the dose can be adjusted based upon the *clinical response* rather than serum concentration.

The serum concentrations of some drugs with narrow therapeutic ranges are not monitored because a *consistent relationship* between a particular serum *concentration* and the incidence of *toxicity* is lacking. In some situations, patients are more tolerant of the drug than others, or the adverse effects may be *reversible*. Under these conditions, the dose can be decreased based upon reversal of an adverse effect rather than on the serum drug concentration.

The SDL is an *indirect* reflection of the desired effect. An SDL within a therapeutic range simply increases the likelihood of success; it does not guarantee success. Therefore, patients occasionally can be well-controlled with "subtherapeutic" SDLs or can experience toxicity with "therapeutic" SDLs.

The Desired SDL

A drug can be indicated for the treatment of different medical conditions, and different clinical conditions may require different serum concentrations of the drug. For example, higher serum concentrations of digoxin often are needed for the treatment of atrial fibrillation than for the treatment of congestive heart failure. Likewise, higher serum concentrations of aspirin are required for anti-inflammatory effects than for analgesia. When adjusting the dose of a drug by use of SDLs, it is important to know the clinical condition that is being treated.

Sampling Times

The accepted therapeutic range for SDLs is based upon *steady-state* conditions (i.e., the rate of drug elimination equals the rate of drug administration). Clinically, a drug is assumed to be at steady state in plasma after four to five half-lives. For example, a drug with a half-life of 6 hours would not be in a steady-state condition for at least 24 to 30 hours.

Occasionally, a clinician will not have the luxury of time to wait for a steady-state condition before a SDL is needed to assess whether therapeutic serum levels are achievable (e.g., in a life-threatening infection). In this case, the presteady-state SDL should be used to assist in the calculation of volume of distribution and elimination rate in order to estimate the steady-state SDL. Presteady-state SDLs should not be obtained *unless* these values can be used to calculate the SDLs at a steady-state.

Caution: If the patient has been on a drug for an extended period of time and a recent dose has been omitted four to five half-lives must pass before SDLs return to steady state.

SDLs for Drugs Given Via Continuous Infusion

When drugs such as theophylline or lidocaine are administered by continuous intravenous infusion, the serum concentration of that drug will be at steady state four to five half-lives after initiation of the infusion, and a subsequent SDL is deemed to be at steady state. It is often wise to review nursing notes and even the volume of fluid left in the IV bag to ensure that drug administration has not been interrupted and that the rate of drug delivery has been recorded accurately in the chart.

Predose (Trough) SDLs for Drugs Administered Intermittently (Oral Dosing or Intermittent Infusion)

The lowest serum concentration, or "trough" SDL, is of importance in *two situations*:

1) When the serum concentration of a drug should not be less than a specific serum concentration because of possible recurrence of symptoms (e.g., quinidine-SDLs below a therapeutic value might result in arrhythmias).

2) When the patient's serum concentration should be less than a specific level because accumulation of drug could lead to toxicity (e.g., aminoglycoside-induced nephrotoxicity).

The trough SDL should be obtained just before the next dose. If it is obtained earlier (e.g., one hour before the dose) the *true* trough concentration should be calculated, based upon the patient's elimination rate of the drug. Therefore, knowledge of not only *when* the drug is *administered,* but also *exactly when the SDL is obtained* is important.

Postdose (Peak) SDLs for Drugs Given Intermittently (Oral Dosing or Intermittent Infusion)

The postdose or "peak" SDL is measured to assure that serum concentrations are therapeutic and not in the toxic range. The precise time of sampling for the postdose SDL depends upon the "distribution phase" of the drug. Soon after the intravenous administration of a drug there is an initial rapid decrease in the serum concentration. During this "distribution phase," the drug in the serum is equilibrating into extravascular sites. You are interested in the concentration of the drug at the *target site*, and the serum concentration will better reflect the target site concentration *after* distribution than *during or before* distribution. For some drugs, such as the *aminoglycosides or theophylline,* the distribution time is very short; postdose SDLs may be obtained within 15 to 30 minutes after the conclusion of an IV infusion of the drug. For other drugs, such as *digoxin or vancomycin,* the distribution phase is longer; therefore, postdose SDLs should not be obtained until after two hours have elapsed for vancomycin, or until 6 to 12 hours have elapsed after IV administration for digoxin. If SDLs are obtained before distribution is complete, the values may be falsely elevated and dosage adjustments may be inappropriate.

When drugs are administered IM or PO, an *absorption phase* occurs; therefore, the peak serum concentration can be delayed. For drugs with *no appreciable distribution phase*, peak SDLs following IM or PO dosing can be measured 30 minutes to 2 hours after the dose. Again, as with predose SDLs the *time* that the drug is *administered* and the time the serum sample is assayed must be noted accurately. *If* the serum sample for the postdose SDL is delayed, the true postdose SDL can be calculated if the elimination rate is known.

Predose and Postdose Measurements of SDLs

For most drugs, either the predose or postdose SDL is monitored. Aminoglycoside therapy, however, is often monitored with both predose *and* postdose SDLs. These two values can be used to calculate both *volume of distribution* and *elimination rate*. The *volume of distribution* is used to calculate the *size* of the dose (e.g., 80 mg, 120 mg, 200 mg). The *elimination rate* is used to calculate the *frequency* of dosing (e.g., Q 6 hr, Q 8 hr, Q 12 hr).

Summary

When ordering and interpreting a SDL the following information must be known:

>> The clinical condition being treated.

>> Whether the information obtained would affect therapeutic interventions.

>> Whether adequate time has elapsed to ensure a steady-state condition.

>> The exact time the drug was administered and the exact time of completion of the drug administration process.

>> The exact time of sampling and the relationship of the dose to the sampling time.

>> Factors that can influence the SDL when the results are inconsistent with expectations.

>> The methods to adjust doses (e.g., change in size of dose, change in dose frequency, or both).

DRUG MONOGRAPHS

*The following drug monographs are excerpted from **Basic Clinical Pharmacokinetics** by Dr. Michael E. Winter. For a more extensive discussion of these drugs, see Dr. Winter's book.*

FIGURE 12–1: Matthew-Rumak Nomogram for Interpretation of Severity of Acetaminophen Poisoning. Reprinted with permission. Pediatrics, 1975;871:55.

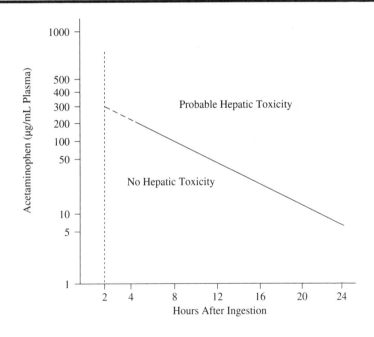

Acetaminophen

Acetaminophen is primarily used as an analgesic and an antipyretic and pharmacokinetic monitoring is unnecessary. Serum levels of acetaminophen are, however, critical in the mangement of acute overdoses of acetaminophen because of the potential for fatal centrilobular hepatic necrosis.

Clinical Pearls

>> Hepatic injury is possible if the serum concentration at 4 hours is >150 µg/mL.

>> The nomogram is used for **ACUTE** ingestion and not chronic intoxication.

>> Draw levels 4 hours after the ingestion as this will usually indicate a peak concentration.

>> The nomogram measures plasma free acetaminophen levels. Identify how the laboratory reports the results.

>> The nomogram should be used with caution in patients receiving chronic therapy with enzyme inducing products such as phenytoin.

Aminoglycoside Antibiotics

The aminoglycosides are bactericidal antibiotics used in the treatment of serious gram-negative infections. Since absorption from the gastrointestinal tract is poor, the aminoglycosides must be administered parenterally. In most instances, the aminoglycosides are administered by intermittent intravenous infusions. The choice of an aminoglycoside dose is influenced by the specific agent (e.g., gentamicin versus amikacin), infection (e.g., site and organism), renal function, and weight of the patient. The three most commonly monitored aminoglycoside antibiotics are gentamicin, tobramycin, and amikacin. The usual daily dose for gentamicin and tobramycin is 3 to 5 mg/kg/day in three divided doses, administered over 30 to 60 minutes. The total daily dose of gentamicin or tobramycin is increasingly being administered in a single daily dose or in two daily divided doses. The dose of amikacin usually is 15 mg/kg/day in two daily divided doses.

The clearance, volume of distribution, and half-life of all the aminoglycosides are similar.[1] Therefore, the same pharmacokinetic model can be used for all of the aminoglycosides and the principles that govern the dosing for any given aminoglycoside generally are applicable to all aminoglycosides. The aminoglycosides have different ranges of "therapeutic" serum concentrations and have different potential for interaction with penicillin compounds.

Therapeutic and Toxic Plasma Concentrations. Peak plasma concentrations for gentamicin and tobramycin are in the range of 4 to 8 mg/L.[2-4] Peak plasma concentrations of less than 2 to 4 mg/L are less likely to be effective [3] against some organisms and successful treatment of serious cases of gram-negative sepsis may require peak concentrations of 8 mg/L.[2] These peak and trough serum concentrations for gentamicin and tobramycin are merely guidelines and the validity of these guidelines is being re-evaluated in light of the new once-a-day and twice-a-day dosing regimens. Desirable peak concentrations for amikacin are usually 20 to 30 mg/L and trough concentrations are usually less than 10 mg/L.[1]

Almost all available data correlating aminoglycoside concentrations with oto- and nephrotoxicity refer to trough plasma concentrations, although some data suggest a correlation between peak concentrations and toxicity.[5,6] Although gentamicin trough concentrations of greater than 2 mg/L have been associated with renal toxicity, the high trough concentrations may be the result, and not the cause, of renal dysfunction. In fact, the use of elevated trough concentrations as an indication of early renal dam-

AMINOGLYCOSIDES: KEY PARAMETERS

Therapeutic Plasma Concentrations

Gentamicin, Tobramycin	*peak:*	4–8 mg/L
	trough:	<2 mg/L
Amikacin	*peak:*	20–30 mg/L
	trough:	<10 mg/L

Vd should be adjusted for obesity and/or alterations in extracellular fluid status	0.25 L/kg

Cl

Normal renal function	Equal to Cl_{Cr}
Functionally anephric patients	0.0043 L/hr/kg
Anephric patients	0.0021 L/hr/kg
Hemodialysis	1.8 L/hr

Half-Life

Normal renal function	2–3 hr
Functionally anephric patients	30–60 hr

Reprinted with Permission. Winter ME. Basic Clinical Pharmacokinetics.
Vancouver: Applied Therapeutics; 1988.

age has been suggested by some investigators.[7,8] Fortunately, most patients who develop renal dysfunction during aminoglycoside therapy appear to regain normal renal function after the drug has been discontinued.[9]

Ototoxicity has been associated with trough plasma concentrations of gentamicin exceeding 4 mg/L for more than 10 days. When the trough concentration is multiplied by the number of days of therapy, the risk of ototoxicity is increased when the product exceeds 40 mg-days/L. Aminoglycoside-ototoxicity also seems to be most prevalent in patients who have existing impaired renal function or have received large doses during the course of their treatment.[5-7,10,11]

Clinical Insights.

>> The expansion of aminoglycoside dosing intervals from 8-hour intervals to 12– or to 24 hour interals has become more commonplace, even in patients with normal renal function. The same total daily dose of drug is still dependent on the predicted drug clearance (i.e., renal function) and the dosing interval merely is extended with this new approach. As a result, peak serum concentrations would be much higher than would normally be considered "therapeutic." For example, in patients with normal renal function receiving a full daily dose of gentamicin or tobramycin as a single daily dose, peak serum concentrations of 20 μg/mL are considered equivalent to older "standard" concentrations of 5–7 μg/mL using every 8 hour dosing. It is apparent that future dosing guidelines for aminoglycosides will focus on achieving a desired AUC as a primary goal, rather than a given peak serum concentration.[114]

>> Vd is increased in CHF, liver disease/ascites, peritonitis, sepsis, and postoperative patients. Vd tends to contract as the patient's clinical status improves from these conditions.

>> If adequate penetration into bronchial secretions (e.g., cystic fibrosis) is necessary, aerosolization may be considered; however, the efficacy by aerosol is controversial.

>> Ototoxicity usually involves high frequency hearing impairment that can progress to the lower frequency ranges.

>> Nephrotoxicity rarely occurs within the first 4 days of therapy, and presents as a nonoliguric acute tubular necrosis. Patients with liver disease may be at increased risk.

>> Serum concentrations should be monitored early in therapy if there is a reasonable expectation that the aminoglycoside will be continued for more than a few days.

Carbamazepine

Carbamazepine is an antiepileptic drug that is structurally similar to the tricyclic antidepressant agents. It has been the drug of choice for the treatment of trigeminal neuralgia, and for the treatment of generalized as well as complex partial seizures. Carbamazepine is available as a 200 mg oral and a 100 mg chewable tablet.

Carbamazepine is eliminated primarily by the metabolic route, with one of the metabolites (10,11-epoxide) having some anticonvulsant activity.[12] Carbamazepine is bound to plasma protein to a significant extent. The free fraction is approximately 0.2, indicating that alterations in serum albumin may affect the therapeutic range or the relationship between the measured carbamazepine concentration and its pharmacologic effect.

Therapeutic and Toxic Plasma Concentrations. The range of therapeutic serum concentrations for carbamazepine is 4 to 12 mg/L. Many patients, however, will develop symptoms of toxicity when plasma concentrations exceed 9 mg/L. The most common adverse effects associated with carbamazepine involve the central nervous system (CNS): nystagmus, ataxia, blurred vision, and drowsiness.[12] There are a number of dermatologic and hematologic side effects that are not dose-related, the most serious of which are the rare, but potentially fatal aplastic anemia and Stevens-Johnson syndrome.[12]

Clinical Insights

>> A baseline CBC with differential, platelet count, serum sodium, and liver function tests should be obtained before the initiation of therapy. The neurological examination should include a baseline evaluation of gait and nystagmus for future comparisons.

>> Rare, but potentially fatal blood dyscrasias (asplastic anemia, agranulocytosis, thrombocytopenia and leukopenia) have been reported. Watch for signs of bone marrow toxicity (e.g., fever, sore throat, easy bruising). Frequent laboratory monitoring of blood counts and platelets after the patient is stabilized on carbamazepine are unnecessary and unlikely to detect toxicity.

>> The chew tablet or suspension achieve peak concentrations quickly and should be administered on a divided (QID) schedule of smaller doses. Larger, less frequent doses tend to cause uncomfortable side effects.

>> The suspension should be diluted with water (1:1) for rectal administration. Although the rectal route of administration is viable, absorption is too slow for acute control of seizures.[115]

>> The metabolite, carbamazepine-10, 11-epoxide concentration can contribute to toxicity.

>> Erythromycin combined with carbamazepine may cause additive hepatotoxicity.

>> SIADH occurs occasionally with carbamazepine and the patient may therefore present with a decreased serum sodium.

Digoxin

Digoxin is an inotropic agent which is primarily used in the treatment of congestive heart failure and atrial fibrillation. It is incompletely absorbed and a substantial fraction of an absorbed dose is cleared by the kidneys. An oral digoxin loading dose of approximately 1.0 to 1.5 mg/70 kg is administered prior to the initiation of a usual maintenance dose of 0.25 mg/day. Because of a relatively long elimination half-life, it is generally prescribed orally as tablets and is given once daily. Dosage adjustments are critical in any patient who is being converted from parenteral to oral therapy or vice versa; a patient who has concurrent renal impairment, congestive heart failure, or thyroid abnormalities; or a patient who is also taking quinidine.

DIGOXIN: KEY PARAMETERS

Therapeutic Plasma Concentrations		1–2 µg/L
F	*Tab:*	0.7
	Elixir:	0.8
	Gelatin cap:	1.0
S		1.0
Vd[a] (after distribution complete)		7.3 L/kg
Cl[a,b]		57 mL/min + 1.02 Cl_{Cr}
β Half-Life		2 days

[a] Altered by renal disease, thyroid disease, and quinidine.
[b] Altered by congestive heart failure.

Reprinted with Permission. Winter ME. Basic Clinical Pharmacokinetics. Vancouver: Applied Therapeutics; 1988.

Therapeutic Plasma Concentrations. While there is considerable variation between patients, plasma digoxin concentrations of approximately 1 to 2 µg/L (ng/mL) are considered to be within the therapeutic range.[13,14] The use of pharmacokinetics to adjust the dosing regimen can reduce the incidence of digoxin toxicity.[14-17]

Clinical Insights.

›› Onset of action is 15–30 minutes following IV administration for supraventricular tachyarrhythmias (SVT). Time to peak effect is 1.5–5 hours. Rate control of SVT often requires high digoxin concentrations in the range of 1.5–2.5 ng/mL.

›› Sampling for digoxin serum concentrations must take into account the prolonged distribution phase of digoxin. Wait at lease six hours after an IV dose and 8 hours after an oral dose to obtain the blood sample. High concentrations obtained during the distribution phase are not correlated with clinical effect.

›› Digoxin loading doses are generally divided into 3 or 4 doses (e.g., one-half, one-quarter, one-quarter given Q6H) in order to assess the clinical effect of each dose prior to administration of the next. Patients with significant renal insufficiency often have a decreased Vd, decreased capacity to eliminate the drug, and require a smaller loading as well as less frequent or smaller mainenance doses.

›› Enterohepatic recycling of digoxin is significant. Bile salt sequestrants such as cholestyramine and colestipol can be used therapeutically to increase clearance and treat non-life threatening toxicity in patients who have supratherapeutic accumulation.

›› Bowel flora may significantly metabolize digoxin in approximately 10% of patients. This leads to poor bioavailability, a need for high dosing, and risk of serious toxicity in selected patients during concomitant antibiotic administration.

›› Check apical pulse before administering a dose to ensure that it is >50 beats/minute.

›› Digoxin concentrations are elevated for several days following administration of digoxin antibodies (Digibind). Digoxin concentrations in this setting don't correlate with toxicity.

›› Many drugs (e.g., varapamil, quinidine) interact with digoxin. Consult an updated text or database for current information.

Ethosuximide

Ethosuximide has been used primarily for the treatment of absence seizures. It is available as 250 mg capsules and as a solution containing 250 mg of ethosuximide per 5 mL. Ethosuximide is eliminated by metabolism to an inactive hydroxyethyl metabolite which is excreted in the urine as the glucuronide. About 20% of the unchanged drug is excreted in the urine. The usual dosage range is 15 to 30 mg/kg/day. Children 3 to 6 years of age usually receive a single daily dose of approximately 250 mg. Older children and adults generally receive their daily regimen in two divided doses, although some older patients appear to do well on once daily dosing.

Therapeutic and Toxic Plasma Concentrations. The range of therapeutic plasma concentrations for ethosuximide (measured just before the next dose) is 40 to 100 mg/L. Most patients with plasma concentrations in this range respond with a significant or complete reduction in seizure activity; patients with plasma concentrations below 40 mg/L are less likely to be well controlled.[18-21] The incidence of adverse effects associated with ethosuximide therapy is relatively low and does not correlate well with plasma concentrations. Many patients with plasma concentrations in excess of 100 mg/L experience no side effects.[22] Plasma levels are, therefore, primarily used to evaluate a patient's potential for clinical response and compliance.

Lidocaine

Lidocaine, a local anesthetic agent with antiarrhythmic properties, is commonly used for the acute treatment of severe ventricular arrhythmias. Lidocaine has poor oral bioavailability, is almost exclusively metabolized by the liver, and has a relatively short duration of action. For these reasons, one or more intravenous boluses of 1 to 2 mg/kg are administered initially to achieve an immediate response. These initial doses are followed by an infusion of 1 to 4 mg/min to maintain the therapeutic effect. Lidocaine has a narrow therapeutic index and toxic effects are generally dose- or concentration-related. Furthermore, concurrent conditions such as congestive heart failure and liver dysfunction may alter the kinetics of lidocaine and, therefore, the expected therapeutic responses of the usual doses. The application of pharmacokinetic principles to the individualization of lidocaine dosing can be invaluable. Nevertheless, lidocaine's short half-life and use in acute treatment require a short assay turnaround time for optimal therapeutic drug monitoring.

Therapeutic and Toxic Plasma Levels. Lidocaine plasma concentrations of 1 to 5 mg/L are usually associated with therapeutic control of ventricular arrhythmias.[23-25] Minor CNS side effects (e.g., dizziness, mental confusion, and blurred vision) can be

LIDOCAINE: KEY PARAMETERS

Therapeutic Plasma Concentrations		1–5 mg/L	
F		1.0 (IV)	
S		1.0	

	Normal	CHF	Cirrhosis
Vi	0.5 L/kg	0.3 L/kg	0.61 L/kg
Vd	1.3 L/kg	0.88 L/kg	2.3 L/kg
Half-Life			
α	8 min	8 min	8 min
β	100 min	100 min	300 min
Cl	10 mL/min/kg	6 mL/min/kg	6 mL/min/kg

Reprinted with Permission. Winter ME. Basic Clinical Pharmacokinetics.
Vancouver: Applied Therapeutics; 1988.

observed in patients with plasma concentrations as low as 3 to 5 mg/L. Although seizures have occurred when plasma concentrations of lidocaine were as low as 6 mg/L, they are usually associated with concentrations exceeding 9 mg/L.[23-26,27] Lidocaine does not usually cause hemodynamic changes, but hypotension associated with myocardial depression has been observed in a patient whose plasma lidocaine concentration was 5.3 mg/L.[28] In addition, there are reports of sinus arrest following rapid intravenous injection.[29]

Clinical Insights.

>> Lidocaine should not be administered to patients with hypovolemia or complete heart block.

>> MEGX (monoethylglycinexylidide) and GX (glycinexylidide) are active metabolites of lidocaine. GX can accumulate in renal failure and contribute to CNS toxicity.

>> Lidocaine is highly protein bound (70%) to alpha-1-acid glycoprotein (AAG) which is an acute phase reactant (protein which rises with stress or injury). AAG may increase in patients with an acute myocardial infarction, renal failure, cardiac surgery, malignancy or seizures. These patients may have a decreased free fraction of lidocaine temporarily due to enhanced protein binding. The dynamic rise and fall of AAG makes interpretation of time to steady state unpredictable in intensive care unit patients.

>> Drugs (e.g., oral contraceptives, heparin), diseases (e.g., hepatic cirrhosis, nephrotic syndrome), and age (e.g., neonates), have been associated with decreased protein binding. A greater free fraction of lidocaine may also occur with higher concentrations of the drug.

>> If bolus doses are administered faster than 50 mg/min, transient but life threatening toxicity may occur due to exposure of the heart and brain (central compartment) to toxic concentrations of lidocaine. Seizures and arrhythmias may occur and are not always heralded by a prodrome of toxic signs (e.g., confusion, dizziness).

>> Patients with decreased liver blood flow due to congestive heart failure, cardiogenic shock or concomitant administration of cimetidine or propranolol may have significantly decreased lidocaine clearance. These patients may present with serious toxicity at doses which are traditionally viewed to be "low" infusion rates of 1–2 mg/minute, especially if infusions continue for longer than 24 hours. Lidocaine infusion rates should be decreased (e.g., 0.25–0.5 mg/minute) for these patients and should be based on the decreased clearance.

>> Monitoring of lidocaine concentrations is warranted in patients with compromised liver blood flow or if confusion or disorientation ensues. Iatrogenic toxicity is easily missed and often is incorrectly attributed to other causes without investigation.

Lithium

Lithium salts have been used for a variety of psychiatric illnesses; however, they are most commonly used to treat patients with mania or patients with bipolar depression. Lithium is most commonly prescribed as the carbonate salt which contains 8.12 mEq of lithium per 300 mg tablet or capsule. It is also available as 300 mg (8.12 mEq) or 450 mg (12.18 mEq) extended-release capsules and as an oral solution which contains 8 mEq/5 mL. The usual adult dose for lithium carbonate ranges from 900 to 1200 mg/day. Lithium is not bound to plasma proteins and is distributed extensively in the intracellular compartment. Lithium elimination is influenced significantly by renal function as well as sodium loading or depletion.

Therapeutic and Toxic Plasma Concentrations. The usual range of therapeutic plasma concentrations for lithium in patients receiving chronic therapy is 0.8 to 1.2 mEq/L. Occasionally, in patients with acute mania, slightly higher plasma levels of 1 to 1.5 mEq/L are desirable; however, chronic therapy at these concentrations is not usually the goal.[30-32] In general, the lowest lithium concentration which controls the manic state is the desired endpoint.

The most common side effects associated with lithium therapy are nausea, vomiting, anorexia, epigastric bloating, and abdominal pain. These adverse effects seem to occur after large doses of rapidly-absorbed dosage forms are administered and may be due to high intragastrointestinal concentrations or high plasma concentrations. Many of these effects subside with continued therapy, but they occasionally persist. Gastrointestinal side effects may be minimized in some patients by use of the slow-release lithium dosage forms. Central nervous system side effects (e.g., lethargy, fatigue, muscle weakness, and tremor) are usually associated with plasma concentrations exceeding 1.5 mEq/L.[31,32]

Clinical Insights.

›› Lithium-induced fine hand tremor can be treated with beta blockers.

›› Trough serum concentrations are obtained twelve hours after the last dose.

›› Since lithium reabsorption follows sodium reabsorption in the proximal tubule, patients with precipitous changes in fluid balance or electrolytes due to drug therapy (e.g., diuretics) or changes in the environment or temperature are at increased risk of toxicity.

›› Serious lithium CNS toxicity may have an irreversible neurological component.

Methotrexate

Methotrexate is a folic acid antagonist which competitively inhibits dihydrofolate reductase, the enzyme responsible for converting folic acid to the reduced or active folate cofactors. Although methotrexate has been used as an anti-cancer agent for a number of years, there has been a resurgence in its use because moderate (500 to 1500 mg) and high (greater than 5 gm) dosage regimens have been introduced. Moderate- and high-dose regimens were developed because tumors responded poorly to low-dose regimens (20 to 100 mg). Currently, methotrexate is used to treat a number of neoplasms including leukemia, osteogenic sarcoma, Wilm's tumor, and non-Hodgkin's lymphoma. Methotrexate is always administered by the intravenous route when doses exceed 30 mg/m² because oral absorption is limited.[33] Current dosing regimens can range from as low as 20 to 50 mg to as high as 10 to 12 gm or more. These doses are administered over a period as short as 3 to 6 hours to as long as 40 hours.[34,35] Methotrexate in low oral doses (10 to 20 mg/week) is used in the management of patients with rheumatoid arthritis and in some cases of asthma.

Approximately, 50% of methotrexate is bound to plasma proteins.[33,34] Methotrexate has active metabolites, the most significant of which is the 7-hydroxy compound.

METHOTREXATE: KEY PARAMETERS[c]

Therapeutic Plasma Concentration	Variable
Toxic Concentration	
Plasma	$>1 \times 10^{-7}$ M for >48 hr; $>1 \times 10^{-6}$ molar at >48 hr requires increased rescue factor doses
CNS	Continuous CNS methotrexate concentrations $>10^{-8}$ M
F	
Dose <30 mg/m^2	100%
Dose >80 mg/m^2	Variable
Vi (initial)	0.2 L/kg
Vd AUC	0.7 L/kg
Cl	$[1.6][Cl_{Cr}]$
Half-Life[a]	3 hr
Half-Life[b]	10 hr

[a] Half-life of 3 hr generally employed with methotrexate plasma concentrations greater than 5×10^{-7} molar.

[b] Half-life 10 hr generally employed with methotrexate plasma concentrations of less than 5×10^{-7} molar.

c Data primarily based on high dose methotrexate regimens.

Reprinted with Permission. Winter ME. Basic Clinical Pharmacokinetics. Vancouver: Applied Therapeutics; 1988.

This metabolite has approximately 1/200th the clinical activity of methotrexate, and is one-third to one-fifth as soluble. As a result, the metabolite can precipitate in the renal tubules causing acute nephrotoxicity especially with high-dose regimens.[36] Patients receiving large doses of methotrexate, therefore, should be adequately hydrated and should receive sodium bicarbonate to maintain the urine pH above 7.[34,35]

Therapeutic and Toxic Plasma Concentrations. The therapeutic and toxic effects of methotrexate are closely linked to its plasma concentrations. Since the goal of therapy is to inhibit dihydrofolate reductase (DHFR) and ultimately, to deplete the reduced folate cofactors, the relative ability to inhibit DHFR and the time course required to deplete the cofactors is critical to the relationship between the drug's efficacy and toxicity.

Therapeutic Plasma Concentration. Most therapeutic regimens are designed to achieve concentrations above 1×10^{-7} M for less than 48 hours. Concentrations of methotrexate which have been associated with successful treatment of various neoplasms range from 10^{-6} up to 10^{-3} or 10^{-2} M. Although the relationship of the methotrexate concentration to tumor kill is somewhat empiric, methotrexate concentrations in the range of 16×10^{-6} M are more successful in the treatment of leukemic patients.[37] These high methotrexate levels are not usually associated with serious methotrexate toxicity as long as adequate hydration and renal function are maintained, and the methotrexate concentration falls below 1×10^{-7} M within 48 hours after the initiation of therapy or the discontinuation of rescue factor.

Toxic Plasma Concentration. Plasma concentrations exceeding 1×10^{-8} to 1×10^{-7} M for 48 hours or more are associated with methotrexate toxicity.[38] The most common toxic effects of methotrexate include myelosuppression, oral and gastrointestinal mucositis, and acute hepatic dysfunction.[33,34,38]

Leucovorin Rescue. Rescue factor (citrovorin factor or leucovorin) is administered every 4 to 6 hours in doses which range from 10 to 50 mg/m^2 in order to minimize methotrexate toxicity.[34,35,38] The usual course of rescue therapy is from 12 to 72 hours, or until the plasma concentration of methotrexate falls below the critical value of 1×10^{-7} M . In some rescue protocols, concentration values of less than 1×10^{-7} M (e.g., 5×10^{-8}) have been considered as the value appropriate for rescue to be considered complete.[35] Most protocols, however, have utilized the value of 1×10^{-7} M.

Methotrexate concentrations in excess of 1×10^{-6} M at 48 hours are associated with an increased incidence of methotrexate toxicity, even in the face of leucovorin rescue doses of 10 mg/m^2. When the methrotrexate concentration exceeds 1×10^{-6} M at 48 hours, increasing the leucovorin rescue dosage to 50 to 100 mg/m^2 or more reduces methotrexate toxicity.[38] Presumably this increased dose enables leucovorin factor to compete successfully with methotrexate for intracellular transport; it thereby rescues host tissues.

Although rescue regimens vary considerably, most employ a leucovorin dosing regimen of approximately 10 mg/m^2 administered every six hours for 72 hours. If the methotrexate concentration falls below the value of 1×10^{-7} M before the completion of the 72-hour rescue period, then the rescue factor can be discontinued. If the methotrexate concentrations are still greater than 1×10^{-7} M but less than 1×10^{-6} M at 48 hours, then rescue with leucovorin is continued at doses of approximately 10 mg/m^2 every six hours until the methotrexate concentration falls below the rescue value of 1×10^{-7} molar.

Clinical Insights.

>> High doses of methotrexate ($\approx$100 mg/m^2) usually require leucovorin therapy, though occasionally lower doses may require leucovorin therapy.

>> Oral or parenteral low doses of methotrexate ($\leq$50 mg/m^2) are associated with serum concentrations of approximately 1 μmol/L.

>> Urinary alkalinization with a pH $\geq$6.5 can be useful in minimizing MTX nephrotoxicity.

>> Aspirin and some nonsteroidal anti-inflammatory drugs can impair renal tubular secretion of methotrexate and increase in methotrexate toxicity.

Phenobarbital

Phenobarbital is a long-acting barbiturate which is used in the treatment of seizure disorders, insomnia, and anxiety. It is most commonly administered orally, but it may be administered intramuscularly or intravenously.

PHENOBARBITAL: KEY PARAMETERS

Therapeutic Plasma Concentrations	10–30 mg/L
F	>0.9
S (for Na salt)	0.9
Vd	0.6–0.7 L/kg
Cl[a]	4 mL/hr/kg (0.096 L/day/kg)
Half-Life	5 days
Fraction Free (α)	0.5

[a] Primarily metabolized by the liver. 20% cleared renally. Clearance in children >1 yr is approximately twice the adult value.

**Reprinted with Permission. Winter ME. Basic Clinical Pharmacokinetics.
Vancouver: Applied Therapeutics; 1988.**

The usual adult maintenance dose of 2 mg/kg/day produces a steady-state plasma concentration of approximately 20 mg/L. Phenobarbital has a half-life of 5 days; therefore, steady-state plasma concentrations are not achieved for two or three weeks following the initiation of a maintenance regimen. When therapeutic levels of 20 mg/L are required immediately, a loading dose of 15 mg/kg can be administered, usually in three divided doses of 5 mg/kg.

Therapeutic and Toxic Concentrations. In adults, phenobarbital concentrations of 10 to 30 mg/L are required for seizure control.[39] The upper end of the therapeutic range is limited by the appearance of side effects such as central nervous system depression and ataxia.[40] Occasionally, patients exhibit no symptoms of toxicity even when phenobarbital concentrations exceed 40 mg/L.[41] Phenobarbital concentrations in excess of 100 to 150 mg/L are considered potentially lethal, although patients with much higher concentrations have survived.[41-43]

Clinical Insights.

>> Due to phenobarbital's long half-life, a serum sample for assay of phenobarbital concentration can be obtained at any time during the dosing interval.

>> Serum concentrations should be obtained when initially titrating doses, when noncompliance or toxicity is suspected, when seizure frequency increases, when therapy with drugs known to interact with phenobarbital is begun, or when patients require hemodialysis or plasmapheresis.

>> Alkalinization of the urine can increase the rate of phenobarbital elimination.

>> Steady-state phenobarbital concentrations can be estimated by multiplying the daily dose in mg/kg by a factor of ten.

Phenytoin

Phenytoin is primarily used as an antiepileptic drug and is occasionally used in the treatment of certain types of cardiac arrhythmias.[44] It is usually administered orally in single or divided doses of 200 to 400 mg/day. When a rapid therapeutic effect is required, a loading dose of 15 mg/kg can be administered by the oral or intravenous route. Although phenytoin can be administered intramuscularly, this route should be avoided because of slow and erratic absorption.

Individualizing the dose of phenytoin is beset by two major problems. First, binding of phenytoin to plasma proteins is decreased in patients with renal failure or hypoalbuminemia. Second, the metabolic capacity for phenytoin is limited; therefore, modest changes in the maintenance dose result in disproportionate changes in steady-state plasma concentrations. The capacity-limited metabolism of phenytoin also eliminates the clinical usefulness of half-life as a pharmacokinetic parameter and makes estimates of the time required to achieve steady state difficult.

Therapeutic and Toxic Plasma Concentrations. Phenytoin plasma concentrations of 10 to 20 mg/L are generally accepted as therapeutic.[45-47] Plasma concentrations in the range of 5 to 10 mg/L can be therapeutic for some patients, but concentrations below 5 mg/L are not likely to be effective.[48]

A number of phenytoin side effects, such as gingival hyperplasia, folate deficiency, and peripheral neuropathy, do not appear to be related to plasma phenytoin concentrations. In contrast, central nervous system (CNS) side effects do correlate with plasma concentration. Far-lateral nystagmus is probably the most common CNS side effect and usually occurs in patients with plasma phenytoin concentrations greater than 20 mg/L. The concentration range associated with this side effect, however, is broad with some patients showing symptoms at concentrations of 15 mg/L and others having no nystagmus at concentrations greater than 30 mg/L. Other CNS symptoms such as ataxia and diminished mental capacity are frequently observed in patients with concentrations exceeding 30 and 40 mg/L, respectively.[46] In addition, precautions should be taken when phenytoin is administered by the intravenous route because the propylene glycol diluent has cardiac depressant properties.[45]

Alterations in Plasma Protein Binding. The usual phenytoin therapeutic range of 10 to 20 mg/L represents the total drug concentration which consists of unbound (or free) drug concentration plus phenytoin which is bound to plasma albumin. The usual alpha (α) or free fraction of phenytoin is approximately 0.1. Therefore, approximately 90% of phenytoin in the plasma is bound to serum albumin; about 10% is unbound and free to equilibrate with the tissues where the pharmacologic effects and metabolism occur.

There are two approaches one can use to interpret phenytoin levels when protein binding is significantly altered. The first is to adjust all the parameters (i.e., therapeutic range, volume of distribution, and "clearance") to those that would be observed in the presence of altered plasma binding. The second is to equate the measured or observed plasma concentration to that which would be observed under normal binding conditions ($Cp_{Normal\ Binding}$). In this second instance, parameters associated with normal plasma protein binding would also be used. While either of these approaches is acceptable, the second method probably is the least likely to result in calculation errors.

The three factors which are known to significantly alter the plasma protein binding of phenytoin are: hypoalbuminemia, renal failure, and displacement by other drugs.

Hypoalbuminemia. In patients with low serum albumin, the following equation can be used to determine the plasma concentration that would have been observed with a normal albumin concentration.

$$Cp_{Normal\ Binding} = \frac{Cp'}{(1-\alpha)\left[\dfrac{P'}{P_{NL}}\right] + \alpha}$$

Cp' is the observed plasma concentration reported by the laboratory; α is the normal free function of phenytoin ($\alpha = 0.1$);[49,50,51] P' is the patient's serum albumin in units of gm/dL; P_{NL} is the normal serum albumin (4.4 gm/dL); and $Cp_{Normal\ Binding}$ is the plasma drug concentration that would have been observed if the patient's serum albumin concentration had been normal. This equation is most useful when a patient has an unusual serum albumin concentration, but does not have significantly diminished renal function or is not taking other drugs known to displace phenytoin.

Renal Failure. In patients with end-stage renal disease, the free fraction of phenytoin increases from 0.1 to approximately 0.2 to 0.35.[49,52-55] Some of this change in plasma binding is due to the decrease in serum albumin concentration known to be associated with end-stage renal disease, and some of the binding changes are due to a change in the binding affinity of phenytoin to serum albumin. When the creatinine clearance is greater than 25 mL/min, the change in the binding affinity is minimal and no adjustment for renal function need be made. However, if the creatinine clearance is less than 10 mL/min and the patient is undergoing hemodialysis treatments, binding changes can be significant.[56]

In the latter circumstance, the previous equation can be altered to accommodate changes in both the serum albumin concentration and the affinity of phenytoin for serum albumin.

$$Cp_{Normal\ Binding} = \frac{Cp'}{(0.48)\,(1-\alpha)\left[\dfrac{P'}{P_{NL}}\right] + \alpha}$$

The above equation should only be used in patients with end-stage renal disease receiving hemodialysis treatments, because the factor which represents the decreased affinity (0.48) was derived from these types of patients. In patients not undergoing intermittent hemodialysis, binding affinity is unpredictably altered when the creatinine clearance is between 10 to 25 mL/min. The plasma concentration of drugs cannot be interpreted accurately for this latter group of patients.[56]

Drug Displacement. Drugs also can displace phenytoin from plasma-protein binding sites. It is usually difficult to estimate the extent of drug displacement from protein-binding sites because the concentration of the displacing agent is seldom known. One exception to this rule is the situation when valproic acid and phenytoin serum concentrations are both being monitored. When the serum valproic acid concentration is less than 35 mg/L, the displacement of phenytoin appears to be minimal and adjustment of the phenytoin concentration is probably not warranted. When the valproic acid concentration exceeds 50 mg/L, the extent of phenytoin displacement from plasma-protein binding sites increases; at valproic acid concentrations of approximately 70 mg/L, phenytoin serum concentrations decrease by 40%.[57,58]

Clinical Insights.

›› Oral phenytoin products should not be arbitrarily substituted for another due to variability in the oral absorption of different products.

›› An increase in the dose of phenytoin will likely result in disproportionate increases in serum concentration because the rate of metabolism of phenytoin is capacity-limited.

›› The concentration of unbound phenytoin can be measured in patients with known or suspected protein binding defects.

›› Oral bioavailability can be reduced by concomitant oral nutrition supplements, (e.g., osmolite).

›› Only Dilantin capsules and phenytoin sustained-release formulations should be dosed once daily.

›› Hypotension can occur with IV administration due to the propylene glycol diluent.

›› Metabolites can accumulate and interfere with assay in patients with renal failure.

Procainamide

Procainamide (PA) is used in the treatment of ventricular tachyarrhythmias, and is administered orally, intramuscularly, and intravenously. A loading dose of approximately 1000 mg (15 mg/kg) is generally followed by a maintenance dose of 250 to 500 mg every three to four hours. The short plasma half-life of procainamide dictates the use of three to four hour dosing intervals unless sustained-release drug products are used. Long-term administration has been associated with immunologic reactions.

Pharmacokinetic predictions are complicated because procainamide is cleared renally and it also is metabolized. In addition, the metabolite, N-acetylprocainamide (NAPA), which is an antiarrhythmic agent in its own right. Although the activity of

PROCAINAMIDE KEY PARAMETERS

Therapeutic Plasma Concentrations	4–8 mg/L
F	0.85
Vd^a	2 L/kg
Cl^b	
$\quad$ Cl$_{renal}$^{c}	[3][Cl$_{Cr}$]
$\quad$ Cl$_{acetylation}$ (average)	0.13 L/hr/kg
$\qquad$ Fast	0.19 L/hr/kg
$\qquad$ Slow	0.07 L/hr/kg
$\quad$ Cl$_{other}$	0.1 L/hr/kg
Half-Life	
$\quad$ α	5 min
$\quad$ β	3 hr
S (HCl salt)	0.87

^{a} Decreased by 25% in patients with low cardiac output.

^{b} Decreased by 25% to 50% in patients with low cardiac output.

^{c} Units of Cl$_{Cr}$ must be appropriate when Cl$_{renal}$ is added to Cl$_{acetylation}$ and Cl$_{other}$ (i.e., L/hr or L/kg/hr).

^{d} Half-life increased in patients with renal and/or cardiac dysfunction.

**Reprinted with Permission. Winter ME. Basic Clinical Pharmacokinetics.
Vancouver: Applied Therapeutics; 1988.**

the NAPA metabolite is limited, monitoring NAPA plasma concentrations may be appropriate in some patients[59] (e.g., those with diminished renal function), because NAPA is primarily eliminated by the kidneys.

Therapeutic and Toxic Plasma Concentrations. Procainamide plasma concentrations of 4 to 8 mg/L are usually considered therapeutic.[60,61] Minor toxicities such as gastrointestinal disturbances, weakness, mild hypotension, and changes in the electrocardiogram (10% to 30% prolongation of the PR, QT or QRS intervals) usually do not occur at plasma concentrations less than 8 mg/L. Toxicities may develop in as many as 30% of the patients when plasma concentrations exceed 12 to 13 mg/L.[61] Plasma concentrations in the range of 15 to 20 mg/L, however, may be appropriate in some patients.[62-64] Patients in whom unusually high target procainamide concentrations were needed suffered from severe arrhythmias that were difficult to control with conventional therapy. While the therapeutic range of procainamide is undergoing reevaluation, care should be taken to carefully evaluate the risk versus benefit of therapy in any patient with plasma concentrations above the usual therapeutic range.

Clinical Insights.

>> Antiarrhythmics which prolong the Q-T interval may predispose to arrhythromogenic effect or torsades de pointes when used in combination with terfenadine (Seldane).

>> Procainamide plasma concentrations peak 1 to 2 hours after regular release products and 3 hours after sustained release capsules. Sustained release procainamide formulations permit dosing at six hour intervals rather than at 3 to 4 hour intervals. This contrasts with the much longer sustained release formulations of other drugs.

>> Slow acetylators have drug concentrations of PA > NAPA; fast acetylators have NAPA > PA. Most laboratores report the concentrations of both entities since both PA and NAPA have antiarrhythmic effects.

>> Hypotension may occur if IV procainamide is given too quickly. Do not administer faster than 25 mg/minute.

>> Wax matrix carcasses or "skeletons" of the sustained release tablets may come through intact in the stool. This is not a concern because the drug is absorbed despite the recovery of the wax matrix.

>> Cautiously dose patients in renal failure and assess serum concentrations. NAPA accumulates to a much greater extent than the parent drug because of its longer half-life and greater reliance on renal elimination. Since both procainamide and NAPA accumulate in renal failure, but are cleared by hemodialysis to different extents, these patients may fluctuate between toxic and subtherapeutic levels. Consider using an antiarrhythmic which is metabolized to inactive metabolites in this setting if feasible.

Quinidine

Quinidine is used in the treatment of atrial fibrillation and other cardiac arrhythmias. It is administered orally as the sulfate, gluconate, or polygalacturonate salts and by intravenous infusions prepared from quinidine gluconate. Usual doses of quinidine are 200 to 300 mg given orally three to four times a day.[68,69]

An assessment of the specificity of the assay used by the clinical laboratory is essential to the interpretation of quinidine plasma concentrations.[70] Likewise, congestive heart failure, liver disease, nephrotic syndrome, or recent stress, can alter the protein binding and clearance of quinidine, and significantly influence the interpretation of plasma quinidine concentrations.

Therapeutic Plasma Concentrations. A number of quinidine assays of varying specificity are available. Each is associated with a different range of therapeutic plasma concentrations. Patients with quinidine plasma concentrations higher than the upper limit of the therapeutic range are at greater risk for toxicity. Most clinical laboratories currently use specific quinidine assay procedures.

Protein Precipitation Assay. This is one of the oldest of the quinidine assays. It measures the fluorescence of a protein-free plasma filtrate and is nonspecific, measuring many less active metabolites in addition to quinidine.[71,72] Assay concentrations of 4 to 8 mg/L correlate with therapeutic response.[73]

QUINIDINE: KEY PARAMETERS

Therapeutic Plasma Concentrations

Specific assays	1–4 mg/L	(1–4 µg/mL)
Benzene double extraction assay	2–5 mg/L	(2–5 µg/mL)
Protein precipitation assay	4–8 mg/L	(4–8 µg/mL)

	Vd (Specific Assays)[a]	Cl (Specific Assays)[a]	t$^{1/2}$ (Specific Assays)[a]
Normal	2.7–3.0 L/kg	4.7 mL/min/kg (0.28 L/hr/kg)	7 hr
Congestive heart failure	1.8 L/kg	3.0–3.9 mL/min/kg (0.17–0.23 L/hr/kg)	7 hr
Chronic liver disease	3.8 L/kg	Decreased	Increased
Nephrotic patients	Increased	Increased	7 hr

	S	F
Quinidine sulfate	0.82	0.73
Quinidine gluconate	0.62	0.70
Quinidine polygalacturonate	0.62	?

[a] Since the benzene extraction and protein precipitation assays report higher plasma concentrations of quinidine, the calculated values for Vd and Cl will both be reduced. The decrease in these calculated parameters can be seen from the relationship between plasma concentration and volume of distribution:

$$\downarrow Vd = \frac{Ab\ (or\ dose)}{\uparrow Cp}$$

(Continued)

QUINIDINE: KEY PARAMETERS (Continued)

and the relationship between plasma concentration and clearance:

$$\downarrow Cl = \frac{(S)\,(F)\,(Dose/\tau)}{\uparrow Cpss\ ave}$$

Furthermore, "quinidine" levels measured by the protein precipitation assay include both quinidine and its metabolites and this may result in pharmacokinetic calculations that are misleading. For example, with only about 20% of quinidine cleared by the renal route,[86] renal failure would not be expected to significantly prolong the half-life; yet, the accumulation of metabolites in renal failure has resulted in spuriously long estimates of quinidine half-life in patients with renal failure when the protein precipitate assay was used. This does not occur when the benzene double extraction assay is used.[76]

Reprinted with Permission. Winter ME. Basic Clinical Pharmacokinetics. Vancouver: Applied Therapeutics; 1988.

Benzene Double Extraction Assay. This assay eliminates many, but not all of the metabolites measured by the protein precipitation assay.[71,74,75] Quinidine plasma concentrations of 2 to 5 mg/L are considered to be in the usual therapeutic range with this assay.[76]

Specific Assays. These specific assays usually measure quinidine by high performance liquid chromatography,[77,78] thin layer chromatography coupled with a fluorometric procedure,[79] or enzyme immunoassay. When these specific assays are used, plasma quinidine concentrations of 1 to 4 mg/L are considered to be in the therapeutic range.[77]

Changes in *plasma protein binding* can alter the desired therapeutic concentrations of quinidine. Quinidine is a basic drug which is bound primarily to alpha1-acid glycoprotein.[81,82] Although some studies suggested that quinidine was 80% to 90% bound to plasma proteins (i.e., alpha or fraction free = 0.2 to 0.1 respectively),[81,83] the alpha or fraction free is approximately 0.1 for most patients.[80] Since only the free or unbound drug is active, a change in the plasma protein binding could change the desired plasma concentration.

The plasma protein binding of quinidine is reduced in patients with chronic liver disease, presumably because the alpha$_1$-acid glycoprotein concentration is decreased.[78,84] Therefore, the alpha or fraction free is increased and the desired quinidine plasma concentrations for patients with chronic liver disease will be lower than usual. Although the alpha or fraction free plasma concentration of quinidine would be expected to be increased in patients with nephrotic syndrome, studies have not been conducted in this type of patient. It is known, however, that nephrotic patients frequently have decreased alpha$_1$-acid glycoprotein concentrations in addition to hypoalbuminemia.[85] A decrease in plasma protein concentrations would result in lower therapeutic quinidine plasma concentrations.

The plasma protein binding of quinidine is increased following acute stress such as surgery.[81] Factors associated with alterations in alpha$_1$-acid glycoprotein concentrations appear to have in common tissue damage, would healing, or an inflammatory response (see Table 12–1). Such events would tend to increase the total drug concentration with relatively little change in the free drug levels. Since altered plasma binding may influence plasma quinidine concentrations, the relationship between the measured quinidine concentration (which represents both the bound and unbound drug) and clinical response should be assessed. For example, a patient with an unusually high quinidine concentration, should be evaluated for the presence of clinical factors known to alter quinidine binding. One should also carefully assess the clinical response of the patient to ensure that it is consistent with the elevated plasma concentration (e.g., increased PR, QRS, or QT intervals on ECG).

Clinical Insights.

>> Use of quinidine can be contraindicated in atrial fibrillation/flutter because it can enhance AV conduction and thereby, increase the ventricular rate. Administration of a loading dose of digoxin before quinidine administration should slow conduction through the AV node.

>> While quinidine may be safe when given by *slow* infusion, many clinicians are reluctant to administer quinidine by the parenteral routes because life threatening hypotension has occurred. Nevertheless, parenteral procainamide often is prescribed when lidocaine is unsuccessful in converting a ventricular arrhythmia.

>> Extended release tablet (ERT) may be broken in half to titrate dose.

>> May use diphenoxylate/atropine (Lomotil) or aluminum hydroxide gel to counteract diarrhea without affecting absorption. GI toxicity is related to direct GI irritation not to toxic levels. Patients usually develop GI tolerance if quinidine is slowly titrated to therapeutic levels over a week. Diarrhea may be severe enough to warrant discontinuation of therapy or may preclude patient acceptance of the regimen.

>> Quinidine can prolong the Q-T interval and many cases of torsades de pointes have been reported. High serum concentrations of terfenadine (Seldane) can potentiate Q-T prolongation.

Salicylates

Salicylates possess analgesic, anti-inflammatory, and antipyretic properties. Although salicylates are available in parenteral, rectal, and oral dosage forms, the oral dosage forms are used primarily in anti-inflammatory therapy. There are a number of ester and salt forms, as well as liquid, tablet, and capsule dosage forms of salicylates. Salicylates exhibit some capacity-limited plasma protein binding; therefore, serum albumin concentration is an important factor to consider when evaluating serum salicylate plasma levels.

Therapeutic and Toxic Plasma Concentrations. The therapeutic concentration of salicylic acid necessary for the anti-inflammatory activity ranges from 100 to 300 mg/L (10 to 30 mg/dL). Salicylates can produce a variety of side effects, including tinnitus, which generally occurs at concentrations greater than 200 mg/L. In the case of acute or chronic overdoses, serious acid-base imbalances can develop.[88,89]

TABLE 12–1: Factors Known to Alter Alpha$_1$-Acid Glycoprotein Concentrations[a]

Increased	Decreased
Tumors	Pregnancy
Rheumatoid arthritis	Oral contraceptives
Rheumatic fever	Cirrhosis
Pulmonary tuberculosis	Nephritis
Acute infections	
Obstructive liver disease	
Inflammatory bowel disease	
Burns	
Fractures	
Trauma	
Surgery	
Myocardial infarction	

[a] Adapted from references 82, 87.

SALICYLATES: KEY PARAMETERS

Therapeutic Range	100–300 mg/L or 10–30 mg/dL
F	100%
Vd[a]	0.2 L/kg
Cl[b]	0.012 L/hr/kg
Half-Life $(^1/_2)$[c]	10–24 hr
Fraction Free (α)	0.1–0.2

[a] The capacity-limited plasma protein binding results in a volume of distribution which increases with dose. On average, the Vd is approximately 0.2 L/kg at salicylate concentrations of 200 mg/L.

[b] The clearance of salicylates declines as the plasma concentrations increase from <5 to approximately 100 mg/L, but remains relatively stable between 100 and 300 mg/L.

[c] The half-life of salicylates reflects a complex relationship between the apparent volume of distribution and clearance. In the therapeutic range, most patients have a half-life of approximately 10–15 hours.

Reprinted with Permission. Winter ME. Basic Clinical Pharmacokinetics.
Vancouver: Applied Therapeutics; 1988.

Other more common side effects include gastrointestinal bleeding, alterations in renal function, and decreased platelet activity. Some of these effects may be dose-related, but there is no clear relationship that has been established between the salicylate plasma concentration and some of these adverse effects.

Clinical Insights.

›› Antiplatelet effects of aspirin last seven to 10 days, the lifetime of the platelet.

›› To achieve anti-inflammatory effects, doses greater than 3.6 grams per day may be necessary. At this dose, obtain plasma levels after 5 to 7 days.

›› Salicylate doses greater than 2 gm/day are uricosuric. Plasma uric levels <3.5 mg/dL may be observed in patients taking therapeutic anti-inflammatory doses of salicylates.

›› Urinary alkalinization may increase salicylic acid excretion.

›› Nomograms for monitoring and predicting salicylate concentration are based on acute *not* chronic intoxication.

Theophylline

Theophylline is a bronchial smooth muscle relaxant and is widely used in the treatment of bronchial asthma and other respiratory diseases. Theophylline is poorly soluble in water (about 1%), and is usually administered intravenously as the more soluble ethylenediamine salt of theophylline, aminophylline. Dilute solutions of theophylline (approximately 1 mg/L) also can be administered intravenously. There are numerous oral preparations of theophylline, aminophylline, and other theophylline salts. In addition, aminophylline and other theophylline salts are sometimes administered rectally as suppositories or rectal solutions. The rectal solutions are absorbed slowly and erratically, but tend to have better absorption characteristics than the suppositories.

Doses vary widely and should be based upon pharmacokinetic considerations and plasma theophylline concentrations. Aminophylline is the most widely used salt of theophylline. An aminophylline loading dose of 250 to 500 mg for an average 70 kg patient usually is administered by slow intravenous injection. The loading dose generally is followed by intravenous aminophylline infused at a rate of about 30 to 50 mg/hr. The usual oral maintenance dose of aminophylline tablets is 200 to 300 mg three to four times a day.

Therapeutic and Toxic Plasma Concentrations. The usual therapeutic plasma concentration for theophylline is to 10 to 20 mg/L;[90-92] however, improvement in respiratory function can be observed with plasma concentrations as low as 5 mg/L.[90]

Nausea and vomiting are the most common side effects of theophylline. Although these effects can occur at concentrations as low as 13 to 15 mg/L, they are observed more frequently at plasma concentrations exceeding 20 mg/L.[92,93] Cardiac symptoms such as tachycardia are usually minor within the therapeutic range;[94] premature atrial and ventricular contractions are less predictable, but are usually associated with theophylline levels greater than 40 mg/L.[95] Insomnia and nervousness are side effects which occur over a wide range of concentrations. More severe CNS manifestations such as seizures usually occur at plasma concentrations exceeding 50 mg/L,[95,96] but have occurred in patients with theophylline concentrations less than 30 mg/L.[96,97]

Side effects such as nausea and vomiting that usually occur at lower plasma concentrations cannot be used as reliable indicators of excessive theophylline concentrations. These less severe toxic effects are not always observed—even at high plasma concentrations. In a series of eight patients who suffered from theophylline-induced seizures, only one patient had premonitory signs such as nausea, vomiting, tachycardia, or nervousness which were recognized as a sign of toxicity.[96]

The bronchodilating effects of theophylline are proportional to the log of the theophylline concentration. This means that as the theophylline concentration increases, there will be a less than proportional increase in bronchodilation.[95] For this reason, many patients with theophylline concentrations greater than 20 mg/L will experience about the same therapeutic benefit as that associated with concentrations of less than 20 mg/L; these patients, however, will be at much higher risk for theophylline toxicity. Patients should always be maintained at the lowest possible theophylline plasma concentration that produces a satisfactory therapeutic endpoint.

Clinical Insights.

>> Newer antibiotics (ciprofloxacin, enoxacin, clarithromycin, azithromycin) may decrease metabolism of theophylline.

>> Neonates may metabolize an appreciable portion of theophylline to caffeine.

>> Saturable metabolism of theophylline may occur in some patients.

>> High fat foods may cause "dose dumping" of some extended release products (Theo-24, TheoDur Sprinkles).

>> Children metabolize theophylline rapidly, and may require 8 hourly dosing of sustained release products.

Valproic Acid

Valproic acid is currently used in the treatment of various seizure disorders. The mechanism of action for valproic acid is uncertain; it purportedly increases the brain concentrations of gamma aminobutyric acid (GABA), an inhibitory neurotransmitter in the central nervous system. The usual daily dose of valproic acid is 30 to 60 mg/kg/day, but initial doses are usually in the range of 10 to 20 mg/kg/day.[98-100] Valproic acid is interesting from a pharmacokinetic point of view for a number of reasons. First, valproic acid is known to influence the pharmacokinetics of a number of other drugs. Phenobarbital's metabolism is inhibited by valproic acid, and phenytoin is displaced from its albumin binding sites by high concentrations of valproic acid. In addition, valproic acid is highly bound to serum albumin, and at therapeutic plasma concentrations, saturates plasma protein binding sites.[98,101]

Therapeutic and Toxic Plasma Concentrations. The therapeutic range for valproic acid ranges from 50 to 100 mg/L;[98-100] however, valproic acid concentrations in excess of 100 mg/mL do not appear to be associated with obvious signs of toxicity. In most cases, the dose-limiting side effects are gastrointestinal (e.g., nausea, vomiting, diarrhea, and abdominal cramps). Sedation and drowsiness are relatively uncommon side effects that may, in part, be due to the interaction between valproic acid and other concomitant antiepileptic drugs. Other infrequent side effects include alopecia, a benign essential tremor, thrombocytopenia, and hepatotoxicity. Although not clearly established, elevated levels of valproic acid have been associated with hepatotoxicity.[98,102,103] While the hepatotoxicity associated with valproic acid is rare, it is a serious complication of therapy and should be considered in any patient with elevated liver enzymes.

Clinical Insights.

>> Protein-binding sites are saturable at high serum concentrations; the free fraction in serum may increase from 10% at 50 μg/mL to 30% at 80 μg/mL. Unbound drug concentration determinations may be helpful when the extent of protein binding is important.

>> The absorption of enteric-coated tablets is delayed which will subsequently delay the time to peak concentration.

>> If necessary, valproic acid solution can be administered rectally.

Vancomycin

Vancomycin is a bactericidal antibiotic with a gram-positive spectrum of activity that includes methicillin-resistant *Staphylococcus aureus*. It is also an alternative to penicillin in patients who have a history of serious penicillin allergy.[104-107]

Vancomycin is poorly absorbed orally and has been used to treat gastrointestinal overgrowths of gram-positive bacteria. When used to treat systemic infections, vancomycin must be given by the intravenous route. The usual dose is 500 mg administered over 30 to 60 minutes every six hours or 1 gm administered over 30 to 60 minutes every 12 hours.[107] Although 2.0 gm/day of vancomycin has been recommended historically, this dose can be excessive, particularly in the elderly and in patients with diminished renal function. In these individuals, doses should be adjusted. Vancomycin is not administered intramuscularly because it causes local irritation and a histamine reaction.

Therapeutic and Toxic Plasma Concentrations. The ideal vancomycin dosing regimen is one that results in peak vancomycin plasma concentrations that are less than 30 to 50 mg/L and trough concentrations that are in the range of 5 to 15 mg/L.[104,105,108-110] Peak concentrations above 50 mg/L have been associated with ototoxicity; however, vancomycin-induced ototoxicity has been primarily reported in

VANCOMYCIN: KEY PARAMETERS

Therapeutic Plasma Concentrations[a]

Peak:	<40–50 mg/L
Trough:	≈ 10 ± 5 mg/L
F	<5%
Vd	0.7 (0.5 to 1) L/kg
Cl	$[0.65][Cl_{Cr}]$
Half-Life	7 hr

[a] A peak concentration in the range of 30 mg/L is probably a reasonable target; however, to ensure efficacy trough concentrations should be maintained at or above 10 mg/L.

Reprinted with Permission. Winter ME. Basic Clinical Pharmacokinetics. Vancouver: Applied Therapeutics; 1988.

patients with vancomycin concentrations greater than 80 mg/L.[104,106,111] Other major side effects that are associated with vancomycin therapy include phlebitis and a histamine reaction (Red Man Syndrome) consisting of flushing, tachycardia, and hypotension. To minimize the histamine response, vancomycin should be infused slowly (1 gm over at least 60 minutes). Even at this rate of infusion, some patients will experience the flushing and tachycardia.[112,113] It occurs much less often in infected patients than in healthy volunteers. Although renal toxicity was originally associated with vancomycin, this was probably due to an impurity present in the original formulation; there have been no recent reports of vancomycin alone resulting in renal toxicity.[104,113]

The minimum inhibitory concentration for most strains of staphylococcus is below 5 mg/L; therefore, trough concentrations should be maintained in the range of 5 to 15 mg/L. Many clinicians recommend maintaining trough concentrations above 10 mg/L since there is evidence of increased efficacy in patients with endocarditis and there is no known increased risk of toxicity at these concentrations.[108,110]

Clinical Insights.

>> Some high-flux dialysis methods clear vancomycin more rapidly than previously reported, though post-dialysis rebound occurs.

>> One-compartment and two-compartment pharmacokinetic models appear equally useful for dose modification.

>> While trough serum concentrations >10 μg/mL may be correlated with nephrotoxicity, a much greater risk factor is the presence of concomitant therapy with an aminoglycoside.[116]

>> "Red Man Syndrome" may be managed by slowing the infusion rate and/or premedication with an antihistamine. It occurs much less often in infected patients than in healthy volunteers.

>> Data supporting an advantage of frequent versus infrequent dosing of vancomycin are unavailable. Serum concentration determinations are of questionable benefit in patients with normal renal function and no risk factors for therapeutic failure. [117]

REFERENCES

1. Pechere JC, Dugal R. Clinical pharmacokinetics of aminoglycoside antibiotics. Clin Pharmacokinet. 1979;4:170.

2. Noone P et al. Experience in monitoring gentamicin therapy during treatment of serious gram-negative sepsis. Br Med J. 1974;1:477.

3. Jackson GG, Riff LF. Pseudomonas bacteremia: pharmacologic and other basis for failure of treatment with gentamicin. J Infect Dis. 1971;124(Suppl):185.

4. Klastersky J et al. Antibacterial activity in serum and urine as a therapeutic guide in bacterial infections. J Infect Dis. 1974;129:187.

5. Cox CE. Gentamicin: a new aminoglycoside antibiotic: clinical and laboratory studies in urinary tract infections. J Infect Dis. 1969;119:486.

6. Jackson GG, Arcieri G. Ototoxicity of gentamicin in man: a survey and controlled analysis of clinical experience in the United States. J Infect Dis. 1971;124(Suppl):130.

7. Goodman EL et al. Prospective comparative study of variable dosage and variable frequency regimens for administrations of gentamicin. Antimicrob Agents Chemother. 1975;8:434.

8. Schentag JJ et al. Clinical and pharmacokinetic characteristics of aminoglycoside nephrotoxicity in 201 critically ill patients. Antimicrob Agents Chemother. 1982;5:721.

9. Wilfret JN et al. Renal insufficiency associated with gentamicin therapy. J Infect Dis. 1971;124(Suppl):148.

10. Mawer GE. Prescribing aides for gentamicin. Br J Clin Pharmacol. 1974;1:45.

11. Federspil P et al. Pharmacokinetics and ototoxicity of gentamicin, tobramycin, and amikacin. J Infect Dis. 1976;134(Suppl):200.

12. Bertilsson L. Clinical pharmacokinetics of carbamazepine. Clin Pharmacokinet. 1978;3:128.

13 Smith TW. Digitalis toxicity: epidemiology and clinical use of serum concentration measurements. Am J Med. 1975;58:470.

14 Smith TW, Harber E. Digoxin intoxication: the relationship of clinical presentation to serum digoxin concentration. J Clin Invest. 1970;49:2377.

15 Koch-Weser J et al. Influence of serum digoxin concentration measurements on frequency of digitoxicity. Clin Pharmacol Ther. 1974;16:284.

16. Sheiner LB et al. Instructional goals for physicians in the use of blood level data and the contribution of computers. Clin Pharmacol Ther. 1974;16:260.

17. Ogilvie RI, Ruedy J. An educational program in digitalis therapy. JAMA. 1972;222:50.

18. Browne, TR et al. Ethosuximide in the treatment of absence seizures. Neurology. 1975;25:515.

19. Sherwin AL et al. Improved control of epilepsy by monitoring plasma ethosuximide. Arch Neurol. 1973;27:178.

20. Penry JK et al. Ethosuximide: relation of plasma levels to clinical control. In: Woodbury DM, Penry JK, Schmidt RP, eds. Anti-epileptic Drugs. New York: Raven Press; 1972:431–441.

21. Sherwin AL, Robb JP. Ethosuximide: relation of plasma levels to clinical control. In: Woodbury DM, Penry JK, Schmidt RP, eds. Anti-epileptic Drugs. New York: Raven Press; 1972:443–448.

22. Sherwin AL et al. Plasma ethosuximide levels: a new aid in the management of epilepsy. Ann R Coll Surg Can. 1971;14:48.

23. Gianelly R et al. Effect of lidocaine on ventricular arrhythmias in patients with coronary heart disease. N Engl J Med. 1967;277:1215.

24. Jewett DE et al. Lidocaine in the management of arrhythmias after acute myocardial infarction. Lancet. 1968;1:266.

25. Seldon R, Sasahara AA. Central nervous system toxicity induced by lidocaine. JAMA. 1967;202:908.

26. Thompson PD. Lidocaine pharmacokinetics in advanced heart failure, liver disease, and renal failure in humans. Ann Intern Med. 1973;78:499.

27. Benowitz N. Clinical application of the pharamcokinetics of lidocaine. In: Melmon K, ed. Cardiovascular Drug Therapy. Philadelphia: FM Davis; 1974;77–101.

28. Stannard M, et al. Hemodynamic effects of lidocaine in acute myocardial infarction. Br Med J. 1968;2:468.

29. Cheng TO, Wadhwa K. Sinus standstill following intravenous lidocaine administration. JAMA. 1973;223:790.

30. Elizur A et al. Intra:extracellular lithium ratios and clinical course in affective states. Clin Pharm Ther. 1972;13:947.

31. Salem RB. A pharmacist's guide to monitoring lithium drug-drug interactions. Drug Intell Clin Pharm. 1982;16:745.

32. Amdisen A. Lithium. In: Evans WE, Schentag JJ, Jusko WJ, eds. Applied Pharmacokinetics: Principles of Therapeutic Drug Monitoring, 2nd ed. Vancouver: Applied Therapeutics; 1986:978–1002.

33. Wan SH et al. Effect route of administration and effusions on methotrexate pharmacokinetics. Cancer Res. 1974;34:3487.

34. Bleyer WA. The clinical pharmacology of methotrexate. Cancer. 1978;41:36.

35. Bleyer WA. Methotrexate, clinical pharmacology, current status and therapeutic guidelines. Cancer Treat Rev. 1977;4:87.

36. Shen DD, Azarnoff DL. Clinical pharmacokinetics of methotrexate. Clin Pharmacokinet. 1978;3:1.

37. Evans WE et al. Clinical pharmacodynamics of high-dose methotrexate in acute lymphocytic leukemia. N Engl J Med. 1986;314:471.

38. Stoller RG et al. Use of plasma pharmacokinetics to predict and prevent methotrexate toxicity. N Engl J Med. 1977;297:630.

39. Buchthal F et al. Relation of EEG and seizures to phenobarbital in serum. Arch Neurol. 1968;19:567.

40. Plass GL, Hine CH. Hydantoin and barbiturate blood levels observed in epileptics. Arch Int Pharmacodyn Ther. 1960;128:375.

41. Sushine I. Chemical evidence of tolerance to phenobarbital. J Lab Clin Med. 1957;50:127.

42. Baselt RC et al. Therapeutic and toxic concentrations of more than 100 toxicologically significant drugs in blood, plasma or serum: a tabulation. Clin Chem. 1975;21:44.

43. Kennedy AC et al. Successful treatment of three cases of very severe barbiturate poisoning. Lancet. 1969;1:995.

44. Bigger JT et al. Relationship between the plasma level of diphenylhydantoin sodium and its cardiac antiarrhythmic effects. Circulation. 1968;38:363.

45. Louis S et al. The cardiocirculatory changes caused by intravenous dilantin and its solvent. Am Heart J. 1967;74:523.

46. Kutt H et al. Diphenylhydantoin metabolism, blood levels and toxicity. Arch Neurol. 1964;11:642.

47. Lund L. Effects of phenytoin in patients with epilepsy in relation to its concentration in plasma. In: David DS, Prichard NBC, eds. Biological Effects of Drugs in Relation to Their Concentration in Plasma. Baltimore: University Park Press; 1972;227.

48. Lascelles PT et al. The distribution of plasma phenytoin levels in epileptic patients. J Neurol Neurosurg Psychiatry. 1970;33:501.

49. Odar-Cederlof I et al. Kinetics of diphenylhydantoin in uremic patients: consequence of decreased protein binding. Eur J Clin Pharmacol. 1974;7:31.

50. Koch-Weser J, Sellers EM. Binding of drugs to serum albumin. N Engl J Med. 1976;294:311.

51. Lund L et al. Plasma protein binding of diphenylhydantoin in patients with epilepsy. Clin Pharmacol Ther. 1972;13:196.

52. Adler DS et al. Hemodialysis of phenytoin in a uremic patient. Clin Pharmacol Ther. 1975;18:65.

53. Reidenberg MM et al. Protein binding of diphenylhydantoin and desmethylimipramine in plasma from patients with poor renal function. N Engl J Med. 1971;285:264.

54. Odar-Cederlof I. Plasma protein binding of phenytoin and warfarin in patients undergoing renal transplantation. Clin Pharmacokinet. 1977;2:147.

55. Reidenberg MM. The binding of drugs to plasma proteins and the interpretation of measurements of plasma concentrations of drugs in patients with poor renal function. Am J Med. 1977;62:466.

56. Liponi DL et al. Renal function and therapeutic concentrations of phenytoin. Neurology. 1984;34:395.

57. Mattson RH et al. Valproic acid in epilepsy; clinical and pharmacological effects. Neurology. 1978;3:20.

58. Monks A, Richens A. Effect of single dose of sodium valproate on serum phenytoin levels and protein binding in epileptic patients. Clin Pharm Ther. 1980;27:89.

59. Vlasses PH et al. Lethal accumulations of procainamide metabolite in renal insufficiency. Drug Intell Clin Pharm. 1984;18:493. Abstract.

60. Koch-Weser J. Pharmacokinetics of procainamide in man. Ann NY Acad Sci. 1971;169:370.

61. Koch-Weser J, Klein SW. Procainamide dosage schedules, plasma concentrations and clinical effects. JAMA. 1971;215:1454.

62. Engel TR et al. Modification of ventricular tachycardia by procainamide in patients with coronary artery disease. Am J Cardiol. 1980;46:1033.

63. Giardina EV et al. Efficacy, plasma concentrations and adverse effects of a new sustained release procainamide preparation. Am J Cardiol. 1980;46:855.

64. Greenspan AM et al. Large dose procainamide therapy for ventricular tachyarrhythmia. Am J Cardiol. 1980;46:453.

65. Kutt H. Pharmacodynamic and pharmacokinetic measurements of anti-epileptic drugs. Clin Pharmacol Ther. 1974;16:243.

66. Gallagher BB et al. The relationship of the anticonvulsant properties of primidone to phenobarbital. Epilepsia. 1970;11:293.

67. Booker HE. Primidone: toxicity. In: Woodbury DM, Penry JK, Schmidt RP, eds. Anti-epileptic Drugs. New York: Raven Press; 1972:377–383.

68. Thompson GW. Quinidine as a cause of sudden death. Circulation. 1956;14:757.

69. Wetherbee DG et al. Ventricular tachycardia following the administration of quinidine. Am Heart J. 1952;43:89.

70. Guentert TW et al. Divergence in pharmacokinetic parameters of quinidine obtained by specific and non-specific assay methods. Pharmacokinet Biopharm. 1979;7:303.

71. Hartel G, Harjanne A. Comparisons of two methods for quinidine determination and chromatographic analysis of the difference. Clin Chem Acta. 1969;23:124.

72. Conn HL, Luchi RJ. Some cellular and metabolic considerations relating to the action of quinidine as a prototype antiarrhythmic agent. Am J Med. 1969;37:685.

73. Sokolow M, Ball RE. Factors influencing conversion of chronic atrial fibrillation with special reference to serum quinidine concentration. Circulation. 1956;14:568.

74. Di Bonna GF. Measurement of plasma quinidine. N Engl J Med (Letter). 1974;290:1325.

75. Cramer G, Isakson B. Quantitative determination of quinidine in plasma. Scand J Clin Lab Invest. 1963;15:553.

76. Kessler KM et al. Quinidine elimination in patients with congestive heart failure or poor renal function. N Engl J Med. 1974;290:706.

77. Powers J, Sadee W. Determination of quinidine by high-performance liquid chromatography. Clin Chem. 1978;24:299.

78. Conrad KA et al. Pharmacokinetic studies of quinidine in patients with arrhythmias. Circulation. 1977;55:1.

79. Ueda CT et al. Absolute quinidine bioavailability. Clin Pharmacol Ther. 1976;20:260.

80. Chow MS et al. Pharmacokinetic data and drug monitoring: antibiotics and antiarrhythmics. J Clin Pharmacol. 1975;15:405.

81. Fremstad D et al. Increased plasma binding of quinidine after surgery. A preliminary report. Eur J Clin Pharmacol. 1976;10:441.

82. Piafsky KM. Disease-induced changes in the plasma binding of basic drugs. Clin Pharmacokinet. 1980;5:246.

83. Kessler KM. Blood collection techniques; heparin, and quinidine protein binding. Clin Pharmacol Ther. 1979;23:204.

84. Kessler KM et al. Quinidine pharmacokinetics in patients with cirrhosis, or receiving propranolol. Am Heart J. 1978;96:627.

85. Staprans I, Felts JM. The effect of alpha-1 acid glycoprotein on triglyceride metabolism in nephrotic syndrome. Biochem Biophys Res Commun. 1977;79:1272.

86. Ueda CT et al. Disposition kinetics of quinidine. Clin Pharmacol Ther. 1976;19:30.

87. Pike E et al. Binding and displacement of basic drugs, acidic and neutral drugs in normal and orsomucoid deficient plasma. Clin Pharmacokinet. 1981;6:367.

88. Mongan E et al. Tinnitus as an indication of therapeutic serum salicylate levels. JAMA. 1973;226:142.

89. Koch-Weser J. Serum concentrations as therapeutic guides. N Engl J Med. 1972;287:227.

90. Mitenko PA, Ogilvie RI. Rational intravenous doses of theophylline. N Engl J Med. 1973;289:600.

91. Bierman CW et al. Acute and chronic therapy in exercise induced bronchospasm. Pediatrics. 1977;60:845.

92. Jenne JW. Pharmacokinetics of theophylline: application to adjustment of the clinical dose of aminophylline. Clin Pharmacol Ther. 1972;13:349.

93. Jacobs MH et al. Clinical experience with theophylline: relationships between dosage, serum concentration and toxicity. JAMA. 1976;235:1983.

94. Ogilvie R et al. Cardiovascular response to increasing theophylline concentrations. Eur Clin Pharmacol. 1977;12:409.

95. Piafsky KM, Ogilvie RI. Dosage of theophylline in bronchial asthma. N Engl J Med. 1975;292:1218.

96. Zillich CW et al. Theophylline-induced seizures in adults. Ann Intern Med. 1975;82:784.

97. Yarnell PR, Chu NS. Focal seizures and aminophylline. Neurology. 1975;25:819.

98. Pinder RM et al. Sodium valproate: a review of its pharmacological properties in therapeutic efficacy in epilepsy. Drugs. 1977;13:81.

99. Graham L et al. Sodium valproate, serum level, and critical effect in epilepsy: a controlled study. Epilepsia. 1979;20:303.

100. Sherard ES et al. Treatment of childhood epilepsy with valproic acid: result of the first 100 patients in a 6-month trial. Neurology. 1980;30:31.

101. Gugler R et al. Disposition of valproic acid in man. Eur J Clin Pharm. 1977;12:125.

102. Suchy FJ et al. Acute hepatic failure associated with the use of sodium valproate. N Engl J Med. 1979;300:962.

103. Donat JT et al. Valproic acid and fatal hepatitis. Neurology. 1979;29:273.

104. Alexander MB. A review of vancomycin. Drug Intell Clin Pharm. 1974;8:520.

105. Kirby WMM et al. Treatment of staphylococcal septicemia with vancomycin. N Engl J Med. 1960;262:49.

106. Banner WN Jr, Ray CG. Vancomycin in perspective. Am J Dis Child. 1984;183:14.

107. Cunha BA, Ristuccia AM. Clinical usefulness of vancomycin. Clin Pharm. 1982;2:417.

108. Rotschafer JC et al. Pharmacokinetics of vancomycin: observations in 28 patients and dosage recommendations. Antimicrob Agents Chemother. 1982;22:391.

109. Blouin RA et al. Vancomycin pharmacokinetics in normal and morbidly obese subjects. Antimicrob Agents Chemother. 1982;21:575.

110. Mollering RC et al. Vancomycin therapy in patients with impaired renal function; a nonogram for dosage. Ann Intern Med. 1981;94:343.

111. Farber BF, Mollering RC Jr. Retrospective study of the toxicity of preparations of vancomycin from 1974 to 1981. Antimicrob Agents Chemother. 1983;23:138.

112. Newfield P, Roizen MF. Hazards of rapid administration of vancomycin. Ann Intern Med. 1979;91:581.

113. Cook FV, Farrar WE. Vancomycin revisited. Ann Intern Med. 1978;88:813.

114. Gilbert DN. Once-daily aminoglycoside therapy. Antimicrob Agents Chemother. 1991;35:399

115. Graves NM, Kriel RL. Rectal administration of antiepileptic drugs in children. Pediatr Neurol. 1987;3:321–326.

116. Rybak MJ et al. Nephrotoxicity of vancomycin, alone and with an aminoglycoside. J. Antimicrob Chemother 1990;25:679.

117. Rodvold KA et at. Routine monitoring of vancomycin serum concentrations: can waiting be justified? Clin Pharmacy 1987;6:655

Clinical Drug Monitoring

Marilyn G. Bufton
Larry E. Boh

13

Clinical drug monitoring is the systematic, prospective evaluation of a patient's drug regimen and clinical course. As a pharmacist, the major goal of monitoring is to optimize drug therapy by effectively assuring therapeutic efficacy, minimizing toxicity, and resolving problems that undermine a patient's access to, or compliance with, a particular drug therapy regimen. To accomplish this, the pharmacist's assessments and interventions performed while monitoring a patient's medication therapy are directed, throughout the entire course of therapy and not just at a single point in time, at fostering positive patient outcomes.

Often, at any one time, pharmacists routinely care for a high volume of patients on an ongoing basis (several days to weeks or years). Many patients require complex, intricate care due to: 1) the severity of their disease state and its associated complex drug therapy (e.g., liver transplantation with immunosuppressive drugs); 2) the chronicity of a particular disease state (e.g., IDDM for 20 yr); 3) the refractory nature of their disease (e.g., metastatic cancer, Crohn's disease unresponsive to conventional therapy, progressive rheumatoid arthritis); or 4) the predisposition to toxicity associated with the disease state or medication therapy (e.g., chronic renal disease, advanced age, cancer chemotherapy). To enable practitioners to successfully accomplish their goals, an organized, written method for rapid and concise monitoring becomes an essential tool.

By using a structured written note, practitioners can effectively and correctly organize, sequence, and interpret relevant information. This encourages timely and clinically appropriate interventions. These notes also facilitate better communication and continuity of care when more than one pharmacist provides care to a group (caseload) of patients. Further, this structured approach prevents duplication of efforts while ensuring that all patients requiring monitoring receive this service.

The location of these notes (patient chart, medication profile) is predicated on what is most functional for providing optimal *pharmaceutical care* in the particular health care facility or pharmacy. If the chart is routinely *unavailable* to pharmacists due to diagnostic procedures, physician note writing, or other health care professional charting, a pharmacy-based location like the medication profile quickly becomes the preferred choice.

Timely, *patient specific* clinical notes documented by the pharmacist, are as essential as notes traditionally written by the physician or nurse. This is especially true with the volume and complexity of patients and when the potential benefit, risk of toxicity, and economical considerations of today's drug therapy regimens are considered. Historically, the practice of a pharmacist keeping a list of "problems for the day to be resolved" and tossing the note at the end of the shift/day has failed to provide a systematic, patient specific, ongoing approach to monitoring. With the outmoded reminders and fragmented notes, true continuity of care could not be maintained. Ultimately, the optimal pharmaceutical care for patients was not achieved and a more structured approach was sought.

THE MONITORING PROCESS

The monitoring process involves four major steps:

1) Data gathering,

2) Data assessment,

3) Problem formulation, and

4) Intervention and follow-up assessment.

The monitoring process begins, irrespective of the type of pharmacy practice (e.g., inpatient unit, outpatient clinic, ambulatory pharmacy, or home health care program), when you see a patient for the first time. The first step involves interviewing the patient to obtain baseline information for generating a patient specific data base. This is then followed by concise documentation of the relevant clinical information.

Step 1: Data Gathering

Demographic Data. The first components of any patient data base are the patient's name; history or account number; address; home or work telephone; sex; date of birth (DOB), as opposed to the patient's age which requires constant updating to keep current; and insurance information, especially as it relates to prescription medication coverage. The patient's weight and height should also be determined at this time, as they will be needed for dosing and renal function calculations. The next step requires performing a patient's medication history interview. The information obtained during this interview typically focuses on identifying the patient's current and past medication use of both prescription and nonprescription medication, allergy or adverse drug reaction history, social drug use (alcohol, cigarette smoking, illicit drugs), and addressing any concerns regarding efficacy, toxicity, or compliance with the current regimen.

Medication History.

›› **Source/Compliance:** A typical medication history should first describe and document the source of information for the history. It should be noted whether the information was provided by the patient, a family member, or friend or whether it was obtained by contacting the patient's pharmacy. Documentation of the reliability of the information that was obtained can usually be determined by listening to the information being provided and attempting to understand whether the name of the medication is noted and if it is consistent with the dosage form, color, or shape of the manufactured product. Further, clarifying information that identifies what the medication is being used for and how this compares with previously documented information in the patient's records or chart, can also provide an appreciation of the patient's understanding of her drug therapy regimen. Finally, the identification of any potential disabilities that may ultimately lead to noncompliance or require special patient counseling (e.g., hearing or visual impairment) should be recorded. This information will be used later to assist in planning a counseling strategy to maintain continuity of care.

>> **Current Prescription Use.** The next stage of the medication history interview requires that the current prescription medication use (past 3 to 6 months) be identified. This includes the name of the product (brand and generic), the dose, dosage form, regimen, and when and why it was started. If the patient is hospitalized, it may also be important to document how many doses where taken that day and when the last dose was given. This information provides the opportunity to administer additional doses of medications such as prednisone, cardiac medications, or antibiotics that were scheduled to be administered that day, thus preventing important doses from being omitted. When documenting the use of current prescription medications, it is always important to ask questions about medications that you suspect a patient of a particular age, sex, or given disease state may be taking. For example, in a 20-year-old female, it is important to ask about the use of oral contraceptives; or in a patient with a renal transplant or rheumatoid arthritis whether he is taking an immunosuppressant such as prednisone. Ideally, the practitioner should identify whether the patient feels the medication is effective or if particular problems are being encountered with the medication. Further, information regarding proper use (e.g., inhalers, nasal sprays, insulin injections) or compliance related issues should be identified at this time. This allows for intervention by the pharmacist to correct medication compliance or drug administration issues. Finally, the documentation of prior medication use may be required to establish previous treatment failures or potential toxicities; however, this should be individualized based upon the patient, disease state, clinical status, and the potential need for this information in the future.

>> **Current Nonprescription Drugs.** Documentation of any nonprescription (OTC) medication use is the next component of a medication interview. Specifically, patients should be questioned about the use of antacids, analgesics, sleep medications, cough and cold medications, vitamins, topical creams, ophthalmic products, laxatives, or antidiarrheals. The reason for use, dose being administered, and frequency either per day or per week should also be recorded. Careful attention to the actual dose being used is extremely important for many medications that are available in different strengths (e.g., Tylenol 325 mg or 500 mg). As before, patients should be questioned to establish whether the particular product is working for them or if they are experiencing any particular toxicity. Similarly, patients with certain disease states, drug therapy, or of a particular age group should be questioned about specific nonprescription medications which you might expect them to use. For example, the use of antacids in a patient

taking a nonsteroidal anti-inflammatory medication like ibuprofen (Motrin) or the use of a laxative in patients being treated with antidepressants or narcotic pain medications.

>> **Allergic/Adverse Drug Reactions.** The third component documented during the interview is a history of allergic or adverse drug reactions. This requires an accurate and complete history of allergic or adverse reactions of the patient to medications and foods. Exposure to commonly used medications such as penicillin, sulfa drugs, aspirin, local anesthetics, iodine, narcotics, and radio-contrast dyes should be identified. Additionally, information on the type of reaction, when the reaction occurred, how it was managed, and if the patient has been rechallenged should be recorded. Finally, food allergies should also be identified since they alert the practitioner to potential problems with medications. For example, an allergy to eggs might be a contraindication to some vaccines or an allergy to fish might make calcitonin an unwise choice.

>> **Social Use/Substance Abuse.** Finally, the last component of the interview should identify any substance abuse. This includes the use of alcohol, tobacco products, or potential drugs of abuse. Alcohol use should be identified based upon the quantity consumed and how long it has been consumed (e.g., 5 beers per day for the past 20 years). Likewise, cigarette use may be expressed as two packs per day for the past 20 years (2 PPD x 20 yr). Finally, depending upon the patient and the disease state, it may be important to question the use of illegal substances such as marijuana, cocaine, or other illicit drugs. This is important because smoking marijuana will affect the clearance of some drugs (e.g., theophylline) and cocaine use in previously healthy adults may be the cause of presenting symptoms.

Renal/Hepatic Function. The last two components in establishing a patient data base require identification of the patient's renal and hepatic function. These two components are extremely critical both initially and in the future as they provide insight into whether a particular dosage may require modification. Identification of the patient's renal function status, using serum creatinine to calculate creatinine clearance or using an actual measured creatinine clearance, is critical to providing dosing adjustments for medications extensively eliminated by the kidney. At the same time, establishment of whether this renal function is stable or changing (e.g., reduced function in a dehydrated patient) should be identified.

For hepatic function, specific laboratory tests commonly referred to as liver enzymes (e.g., AST, ALT) provide a poor indication of function: these tests measure the release of enzymes into the serum and not liver function with respect to drug metabolism. Therefore, to provide a more meaningful assessment, these parameters must be used in concert with the patient's past medical history of liver disease and signs of liver dysfunction observed during the physical examination. Additionally, special laboratory tests like albumin and prothrombin time may also be used to reflect the metabolic/synthetic capacity of the liver.

Step 2: Data Assessment

After obtaining the patient data base, assess the data. Successful assessment of the data is often the most difficult aspect of drug therapy monitoring for the new practitioner. It requires a complete and thorough understanding of the disease state, drug therapy, and interrelationship of the clinical data such as laboratory tests, physical examination, and diagnostic procedures. Without an appreciation of this, you quickly become confused and feeling overwhelmed can rapidly lead to frustration. Therefore, to begin sorting out the data, it is useful to first review basic information about the disease state and drug therapy. Next, evaluate the patient's current medication use and "retrospectively" identify why he is receiving a particular medication. For example, if the patient is on a beta blocker is it because he has migraine headaches, angina, or hypertension? If you are unable to answer this question, speak with the patient or review the chart to identify what additional data (laboratory, physical examination, patient history) is required to confirm and establish a particular medical problem. Once you are able to assess the data, the next step in monitoring is to formulate a problem list.

Step 3: Problem List Formulation

The problem list should identify those active medical or psychosocial problems that require drug therapy or a pharmacist's intervention. It should reflect medication based issues and not focus on a diagnostic listing. (See Example Problem List above.)

Once equipped with a patient's problem list, pharmacists primarily seek to optimize the therapeutic regimen by monitoring medication therapy for *effectiveness* while attempting to minimize any potential drug-related *toxicity*. To accomplish this, relevant subjective and objective clinical patient data are gathered on an ongoing basis from a variety of sources (e.g., by observing and talking with the patient, from the laboratory data, from other health care professionals, or from data obtained during the medical team rounds).

The data should be categorized as either subjective or objective. Subjective data relate to comments or concerns expressed by the patient and are not directly measurable (e.g., "I have severe pain" or "I am nauseated"). Objective data refer to information that can be quantified (e.g., a laboratory test value, a blood pressure reading, or a pulse rate). Subjective evaluations of a patient (e.g., drowsiness) are usually considered objective data when assessed by a health care professional, because the assessment can be independently confirmed.

As new data become available, they must be organized and assessed for trends that reflect how well therapy is working (efficacy) and whether any signs or symptoms of toxicity have occurred. Since drug-related problems (e.g., interactions, inappropriate dosing for the degree of renal function, incorrect medication selected for a particular problem) present at variable times after treatment begins, thoroughly monitoring the course of the patient's therapy is hard work and often challenging! Therefore, a variety of monitoring approaches used to record critical data are described below. They will assist you in following a patient's progress as a result of drug therapy interventions or to identify other potential drug-related problems.

Step 4: Approaches to Intervention and Follow-up

SOAP Format. One traditional prose/text method used by physicians and pharmacists for following a patient with multiple diseases utilizes the SOAP format. SOAP stands for *S*ubjective *O*bjective *A*ssessment *P*lan.

Each active problem is numbered consecutively and relevant clinical information is noted under each problem daily when the note is written. Use of the SOAP outline logically organizes both the data and the clinician's thought process. The steps used in documenting the note are similar to the sequence used during rounds or at other times when the patient is interviewed and examined.

> **S: Subjective.** First, the patient's subjective status is assessed with questions (e.g., How do you feel? What are your symptoms?). Subjective symptoms are documented next to the letter *S* in the outline. These patient perceptions are aimed at assessing whether therapy is working and if potential adverse reactions are occurring. Again, the subjective observations are symptoms which the patient reports but which cannot be independently confirmed by the observer. Data under the S (Subjective) for the problem of aspiration pneumonia in a hospitalized patient might look like this:

> **Problem 1: Aspiration Pneumonia**
>
> S: Headache, feels chilled and short of breath, IV site burns during drug administration.

> **O: Objective.** After subjective symptoms are written in the note, the patient's objective symptoms, which assist in evaluating the efficacy or toxicity of therapy, are assessed and documented. Again, objective signs can be measured by the observer and include fever, vital signs, appearance of skin lesions, rebound tenderness on palpation of the abdomen, and laboratory values such as a potassium of 4.2 mmol/L.

During hospital work rounds, special attention usually focuses on diseased organ systems or organs thought to be the source of a patient's symptoms (i.e., complaints). For example, the heart, circulation, lungs, and ankles are assessed during the physical examination for patients with congestive heart failure (CHF). In the above example of aspiration pneumonia, objective parameters include: assessment of vital signs (i.e., heart rate, respiratory rate, temperature); results of auscultation of the chest/lungs; color of sputum; night sweats; infiltrates and effusions on chest x-ray; white blood cell count (WBC) and differential; and microbiological cultures and sensitivities (C&S). These parameters reflect the efficacy (or lack of efficacy) of the antibiotics used to treat the pneumonia. Equally important in the assessment and subsequent notes is the appearance of the vein where antibiotics and IV fluids are infusing. Since the patient complains of burning at the IV site, objective signs of toxicity must be assessed and documented by the pharmacist, physician, or nurse. The IV site should be evaluated for the redness, warmth, and edema that are indicative of thrombophlebitis caused by the IV fluid or antibiotic. The IV site should also be evaluated to determine whether extravasation (i.e., leakage of the IV fluid outside the vein) is causing local tissue irritation and damage. The S (Subjective) and O (Objective) data for the patient with aspiration pneumonia might look like this:

Problem 1: Aspiration Pneumonia

S: Headache, feels chilled and short of breath, IV site burns during drug administration.

O: T 38.6 x 2, productive cough, WBC 16,000 (segs 58%, bands 17%), infiltrate on chest x-ray but no effusion, IV site red and tender.

As you see, the information follows a logical sequence for easier integration and interpretation. Obviously, all the pertinent information (laboratory or diagnostic procedure) will not be available during patient care rounds and, therefore, may require additional searching after work rounds.

A: Assessment. Once the patient's course and status are known from the subjective symptoms and objective signs/clinical parameters, the pharmacist must make and document an assessment of the patient's medication therapy in terms of the therapeutic efficacy and toxicity. Questions to ask yourself include: Is the patient responding to therapy? Are there any signs of toxicity? Are there compliance or psychosocial issues interfering with the drug regimen? Are there any new *drug-related problems* which should be listed under this problem or added as a new problem in the problem list? Addition of this assessment to the note might look like this:

> **Problem 1: Aspiration Pneumonia**
>
> **S:** Headache, feels chilled and short of breath, IV site burns during drug administration.
>
> **O:** T 38.6 x 2, productive cough, WBC 16,000 (segs 58%, bands 17%), infiltrate on chest x-ray but no effusion, IV site red and tender.
>
> **A:** Day 2 of antibiotic therapy with 2 additional fever spikes and elevated WBC with left shift indicating poor response to antibiotic thus far (*efficacy assessment*); thrombophlebitis at IV site likely due to erythromycin (*toxicity assessment*).

P: Plan. Monitoring and documenting the "S-O-A" information are critical steps, but the plan for intervention and implementation is most important in optimizing a patient's care. The plan for further intervention or follow-up of all drug-related problems is written next to the "P" and might look like this:

> **Problem 1: Aspiration Pneumonia**
>
> **S:** Headache, feels chilled and short of breath, IV site burns during drug administration.
>
> **O:** T 38.6 x 2, productive cough, WBC 16,000 (segs 58%, bands 17%), infiltrate on chest x-ray but no effusion, IV site red and tender.
>
> **A:** Day 2 of antibiotic therapy with 2 additional fever spikes and elevated WBC with left shift indicating poor response to antibiotic thus far; thrombophlebitis at IV site likely due to erythromycin.
>
> **P:** Review C&S for antibiotic susceptibility/choice; change IV site and add lidocaine to erythromycin; repeat blood cultures if patient spikes a temperature >38°.

Subsequent Follow-Up. Subsequently, the information being documented each day reflects: 1) the patient's response to therapy, drug toxicities, and cooperation with treatment plans; 2) the assessment of the meaning of the clinical data and symptoms, and success of past interventions; and 3) the plan for interventions and follow-up warranted by the current status of the patient. The note on Day 3 of therapy reflects the changes over the past 24 hours.

Problem 1: Aspiration Pneumonia

S: Dull headache but otherwise more comfortable. No complaints about IV site.

O: Fever spike x 1, cough still produces 20 mL green sputum, WBC decreased slightly, new IV site on left looks good with IV infusing well.

A: Day 3 of erythromycin/ceftriaxone. 1 fever spike but decreased WBC. Blood C&S drawn with spike. Sputum C&S—*Klebsiella pneumoniae* sensitive to gentamicin, cefazolin, trimethoprim-sulfamethoxazole but resistant to ampicillin. DFA for Legionella negative.

P: DC (discontinue) erythromycin and recommend changing to cefazolin from ceftriaxone. Document good tolerance of cephalosporins despite history of allergy to penicillins. Continue to observe closely for delayed beta-lactam antibiotic allergy [serum sickness (e.g., arthralgias, rash)].

Although we simplified this example by only discussing **Problem 1: Aspiration Pneumonia**, *each problem* identified on the patient's problem list must be addressed in a similar fashion *each day* for hospitalized patients. For patients managed in an outpatient clinic or by a home health care program, notes are documented whenever the patient is seen or contacted by phone.

It is apparent from the length of the daily note that this type of documentation has some limitations. First, some of the symptoms and signs of patient status (subjective and objective parameters) may overlap between several different problems. This leads to redundancy in documenting or an arbitrary decision to record the information in one place rather than in several. Likewise the "S-O-A-P" note takes considerable time to write even if you are concise. While the course of the patient and daily progress should be evident when well planned and clear notes are composed each day, it is still time consuming and often a challenge for another clinician (e.g., pharmacist cross covering the service on weekends, holidays, or emergencies) to read and integrate all the information when the "S-O-A-P" format is used. This is particularly true when a patient has many problems being managed simultaneously. To minimize the shortcomings and circumvent the limitations of this approach we have devised another format for documenting the clinical course of a patient and the status of pharmacist interventions.

Clinical Monitoring Note (CMN). This method utilizes two forms which contain grids or tables to document patient specific information and a separate data base form to document information previously discussed in the data base section. Each patient has a laboratory/disease parameter grid for tracking the results of pertinent objective data [e.g., laboratory tests (Na^+, K^+, serum creatinine), physical exam (edema, rales, presence of a S_3 heart sound), and general patient care flowsheet findings (leg circumference, urine output, vital signs, temperature, heart rate, blood pressure)]. Each patient also has a daily note grid to organize the interventions by the medical problem. See Figures 13–1 through 13–3 for examples of the forms.

FIGURE 13–1: Clinical Monitoring Form—Patient Data Base Form.

ADDRESSOGRAPH	MR #8350781	UNIT	Medicine III
	Jones, Ralph Q	ATT.MD	Smith, Fred
	BD 10/26/42	PG1	
	GI/Med Male	Age 48	
		Wt (adm) 86 kg	
	5/26/90	Ht 5'9"	

SOURCE OF RX HISTORY: (PT)   FAMILY   OTHER:

RELIABLE?   YES   (NO)

DRUG THERAPY RISK FACTORS:

1. COMPLIANCE?   GOOD   (POOR)   UNCERTAIN   OK WITH ASSISTANCE

2. LIVES ALONE?   (YES)   NO   NEEDS HELP WITH MEDS?   (YES)   NO

3. FUNCTIONAL LIMITATIONS: (NO)
   YES:_____

4. ALLERGIES/ADR'S-ASA, PCN, SULFA, DYE, etc.(DRUG-ROUTE-TYPE-RXN-DATE)

   1) H/O PcN Allergy as a child—? Rash. No rechallenge.

   2) Itching with Iodine.

5. RENAL FUNCTION: $SrCr = 1.6$ $\downarrow Cl_{cr} = 58.4$

6. HEPATIC FUNCTION: $? \downarrow$ — significant ETOH Abuse History $PT = 15$

7. OTHER:_____

PROBLEM LIST:

   1) Aspiration pneumonia
   2) ETOH abuse $^{R}/o$ Withdrawal
   3) Chronic pancreatitis $\bar{c}$ Pain/? Narc seeking history
   4) Lacks insurance from medications/employed/$\downarrow$ compliance
   5) $^{R}/o$ Decreased Liver Metabolism ≥ 0 ETOH/Cirrhosis

PHARMACY: CLINIC/(RE-ADMIT)   CLINICAL QA   CASE MANAGEMENT
             TEACHING

             (Circle or highlight appropriate category)

(Continued)

ADDRESSOGRAPH   *Jones, Ralph Q.*

MEDS PTA—Dose, route, sched., duration, time last dose, total doses today	MEDICATION TAKEN HOME OR STORED

1) *Cephalexin 500 mg PO QID X*
    1 week. (10 Day Rx by LMD)
    No allergy to date. Last 830A   *D=1*
	Home

2) *Diazepam 5 mg PO PRN*
    "Nerves/Shakes" x 6 mos–Takes
    2–3/day + ETOH   *D = 2*
	Home

3) *Viokase Powder (Ran out of Cotazym-S*
    pancrelipase caps) shakes
    on food when he feels like it   *D = 0*
	Home

4) *Acetaminophen/Oxycodone PRN* *Last EA Ran out → ER* *D = 1*	*None*

<u>OTC</u>: Antacids, analgesics, vitamins, laxatives-diarrhea, cold-cough, topicals, sleeper, insulin, EENT products

Malox–Takes 1–2 laxatives—"swigs"/day and chews tabs chronically

Acetaminophen and/or ASA daily HA 1–2/Dose   2–3 Doses/Day

<u>DISCHARGE PLANNING</u>:

    Anticipated discharge date: *6/1/90*

    Insurance: *None*

    Follow-up or Referral: NO   (YES)

                                               AA/Social Work

    DC Meds: (Fill at Hospital)   DC Meds Located: TSA

                Get SW Payment Approval

         Other:

    Compliance devices: Self-administration sheet   Mediset   Special Labeling

      Ped Syringe/Cup   Nonsafety Caps

    Counseling by:_____

FIGURE 13–2: Clinical Monitoring Form/Laboratory/Disease Parameters.

Rationale	Test or Parameter	Date 1/24	Date 1/25	Date 1/26	Date 1/27	Date 1/28	Date 1/29	Date 1/30
ETOH Withdrawal	K+							
ETOH Withdrawal	Mg++							
Baseline	Creatinine							
Pneumonia ETOH W/D	Temp Tmax							
Pneumonia	WBC							
Pneumonia	BANDS							
Pneumonia	Chest x-ray							
R/O Cirrhosis	T. Bili.							
R/O Cirrhosis	AST (SGOT)							
Cirrhosis? Effect on metabolism?	PT							
Cirrhosis? Effect on metabolism?	Albumin							

13–12

FIGURE 13–3: The Clinical Monitoring Note (CMN) Assessment Planning Form.

Date/ RPH Sig.	Daily Opportunities	Problem 1 Aspiration Pneumonia	Problem 2 ETOH Abuse R/O ETOH Withdrawal	Problem 3 Chronic Pancreatitis/ Pain/Narc Seeking	Problem 4 Lacks Insurance Unemployed	Problem 5 R/O Cirrhosis ? Decreased Liver Metab
1/24	R/O thrombophlebitis at IV site due to antibiotic (i.e., erythro)	Review C&S. Repeat blood Cx if temp spikes. Change IV Site/add lido for pain	ETOH binge x 4 days. Cover with thiamine, B vits, and diazepam PO—ETOH W/D protocol	Minimal pain on palpation Pt requests meperidine for HA and ? abd. pain. Try ibuprofen —guaiac neg. stools— amylase & lipase WNL.	Team will contact social worker re coverage for discharge Rx meds	Pt ↑—see if corrects w/SQ Vit K x 3 doses
1/25	Pt c/o constipation needs Rx for laxative—rec. MOM	Cx Kleb pneumon sens. to genta, cefazolin Tmp/Sulfa —but resistant to amp. change to cefazolan from ceftriaxone. Tol. ceph's well despite pcn allergy hx	Pt c/o seeing bugs, BP & temp ↑, tremulous, & confused. Change to IV lorazepam with rapid titration to drowsiness— Mg++ low give MgSO4 1 gm slow IV infusion over 4 hr— check K+	HA OK on ibuprofen - avoid acetaminophen due to liver dis. No new req. for narc's Guaiac neg. and no steatorrhea but ↓ PO intake due to confusion/ withdrawal	Social worker will see once ETOH withdrawal clears	Pt now WNL & albumin 3.0— Expect near normal hep. metabolism Subclinical cirrhosis—small nodular liver— LFT's WNL

(Continued)

FIGURE 13-3: The Clinical Monitoring Note (CMN) Assessment Planning Form. *(Continued)*

Date/ RPH Sig.	Daily Opportunities	Problem 1 Aspiration Pneumonia	Problem 2 ETOH Abuse R/O ETOH Withdrawal	Problem 3 Chronic Pancreatitis/ Pain/Narc Seeking	Problem 4 Lacks Insurance Unemployed	Problem 5 R/O Cirrhosis ? Decreased Liver Metab
1/26		Changed to cefazolin. Legionella DFA negative —DC erythromycin & no beta lactam allergy seen	Sleepy after lorazepam 30mg IV in 12 hr. Cont. with PO now—hold if sleeping	Requests Percocet for abd. pain—limit to 3 doses/24 hr—watch acetaminophen use!	Family hx of ETOH abuse with poor support network via SW	
1/27		No fever and ↓ cough. Tolerating cefazolin well—cont.	Change IV thiamine to PO, cont. B Vits w/FA. Taper lorazepam over 5–8 days to avert seizures	Patient request for Percocet cont. but pt appears OK when team not examining pt	Medicaid coverage OK'd & halfway house may be available on 1/31. SW to arrange & discuss AA	
1/28		Discussed PO AB regimen for discharge. Intern wrote cipro—changed to cephalexin as per guidelines	Rx for lorazepam taper written—pt teaching done	No discharge narc's— will see GI MD in clinic in 2 weeks	As above	

The form for recording the laboratory/disease parameters (see Figure 13–1) is straightforward and typical of many used in various institutions to track laboratory values and detect trends. The uniqueness of this form is its emphasis on tracking only parameters and laboratory data which pertain to active diseases, drugs used to treat those diseases, and drug-related problems (e.g., rising serum levels due to interacting drugs). To assure this narrower focus, the rationale for monitoring is included to the left of the parameter being followed. For example, patients receiving renally eliminated drugs (e.g., allopurinol, digoxin, imipenem/cilastatin, spironolactone), nephrotoxic agents (e.g., amphotericin B, cisplatin, gentamicin), or having a diagnosis of renal insufficiency (e.g., chronic renal disease due to diabetes mellitus or polycystic kidney disease) warrant close monitoring of serum creatinine. Patients with normal kidneys and no risk factors for renal toxicity receive baseline evaluation of serum creatinine, but do not warrant intense monitoring (or documentation) of repetitive serum creatinine values.

It's important to emphasize that parameters *other than* laboratory tests must be monitored routinely to assess the patient's clinical status. Daily weights, ankle swelling (for patients with CHF or ascites), temperatures, energy level (RA, SLE), and stool counts (ulcerative colitis) are examples of non-lab test parameters which may be more indicative of a patient's clinical course than laboratory tests.

The assessment and planning form (see Figure 13–3) demonstrates the use of the clinical monitoring note. The patient in this example has the same clinical problems as used with S-O-A-P format above. The goal of using this form is to focus on documenting the interventions, assessments for efficacy/toxicity, and pharmacist's recommendations, as well as addressing any unresolved drug-related problems. This intensive but highly organized format for clinical monitoring permits any pharmacy practitioner or student who assumes care of the patient to quickly comprehend the patient's current status and historical problems. This combined with the intentional focus of making notes very relevant to the pharmacist's role in providing patient care is an asset of this format.

Intensive Care Unit–Clinical Monitoring Notes (ICU–CMN).

For patients requiring monitoring for medication therapy in an intensive care unit (ICU), the complexity of patient care demands an even more comprehensive monitoring system. Several concomitant diseases, complications of therapy, and multi-organ system failure are common clinical problems which the health care team must carefully monitor and manage. While the S-O-A-P format can be used, the volume of notes quickly becomes too difficult to review and integrate quickly. Further, the CMN grid previously described is too small and unstructured for following complex ICU patients.

To facilitate monitoring of the ICU patient, an adaptation of the CMN was created. The ICU–CMN is subdivided into organ systems (see Figure 13–4). Problems and interventions are noted vertically under the respective organ system. By scanning down the appropriate column, the clinician can quickly review the patient's clinical course by a particular organ system. This approach is critical when the patient's status changes dynamically or when complications begin to occur. A major difference of the ICU–CMN is that organ systems are preprinted on the form and the form is larger (11 x 17 paper) so that each patient's information is contained on one form. Figure 13–4 shows the organization of data and interventions for a confused lung cancer patient with sepsis, neutropenia, supervening renal failure, adult respiratory distress syndrome (ARDS), and a chronic (pre-existing) problem of atrial fibrillation managed with digoxin and verapamil.

As with all monitoring notes, time, date, and initials of the practitioner are a critical step that should not be omitted. This information allows others to contact the appro-

FIGURE 13–4: The Intensive Care Unit—Clinical Monitoring Form (ICU-CMN)

Date/ RPH:	NEURO:	RESP:	ID:	CV:	RENAL/ HEPATIC:	GI/ NUTRITION:	HEME/ ENDO.
	Confusion R/O Brain Mets vs. Meningitis	ARDS Lung CA—OAT Cell	SEPSIS	A Fib Digoxin Verap.	Renal Insuff	Stress Ulcer Proph.	Neutropenic ANC = 5
5/3/89	O x 1 LP results to follow, Gram stain neg and neck supple, head CT neg. Sepsis vs benzo sedation? No sign of mets on CT	On vent with PaO$_2$ = 92 Resisting despite morphine and diazepam Q 1 hr —paralyze with panc and sedate with midazolam drip x 48 hr	Ticar + tobra. Temp to 39.8. Hickman site red, no pus. Blood Cx neg at 48 hr, start vanco 1.5 gm Q 24 hr due to renal insuff — give over 2 hr to avert Redman's syndrome	Continue dig and verap at present dose. If SrCr cont. to rise dec. dig by ¹/2. Repeat Dig Cp in am— last Cp = 2.5 w/good rate control	Serum Cr ↑ to 2.1 from 1.7—daily SrCr. Continue AG for now	Q 2 hr antacids pt has small amt BRB on suction but no ulcer on endoscopy—see heme No diarrhea from AAs, but Dc if Cl$_{Cr}$↓	ANC slowly ↑ ANC = 48. Plt low at 40 K and pt oozing; platelets given 4 U HCT 32

priate individual if a question arises. It also documents input by the pharmacist in providing pharmaceutical care and refocuses their role by making them accountable for optimizing therapy. Finally, if notes are to be included as a permanent part of the patient care chart in the progress notes, the note should be titled "Clinical Pharmacy Note" or "Pharmacy Note," with the appropriate date, time, and practitioner signature. The note must be objective and concise. If written by a student in training, it should be countersigned by a licensed pharmacy practitioner.

SUMMARY

Ongoing, organized, documented clinical monitoring by pharmacists is essential for providing competent and optimal pharmaceutical care. The methods described in this chapter will facilitate the recording of important patient data and identification of drug or compliance problems and enhance the pharmacist's ability to assess therapeutic efficacy while monitoring for potential toxicity. Ultimately, these approaches will increase the practitioner's ability to appropriately intervene and resolve drug-related problems.

Appendix I: Medical Abbreviations, Terms, and Notations

A

ā. Before.

A₂. Aortic second sound.

AA. Amino acid.

AAA. Abdominal aortic aneurysm.

AAO x 3. Awake and oriented to time, place, and person.

Abd. Abdomen abductor.

ABE. Acute bacterial endocarditis.

ABGs. Arterial blood gases.

ABO. Blood group system (A, AB, B, and O).

ABW. Actual body weight.

AC. Before meals.

ACE. Angiotensin-converting enzyme.

ACLS. Advanced cardiac life support.

ACMV. Assist-controlled mechanical ventilation.

ACTH. Corticotropin (adrenocorticotrophic hormone).

ADD. Attention deficit disorder.

ADH. Antidiuretic hormone.

ADL. Activities of daily living.

Ad lib. As desired *or* At liberty.

ADM. Admission.

ADR. Adverse drug reaction.

AF Acid-fast *or* Atrial fibrillation.

AFB. Acid-fast bacilli.

AFEB. Afebrile.

A Fib. Atrial fibrillation.

AFP. Alpha-fetoprotein.

AFVSS. Afebrile, vital signs stable.

AG. Aminoglycoside *or* Anion gap.

A/G. Albumin to globulin ratio.

AGN. Acute glomerulonephritis.

AHF. Antihemophilic factor.

AHFS. American hospital formulary service.

AI. Accidentally incurred *or* Aortic insufficiency.

AICD. Automatic implantable cardioverter/defibrillator.

AIDS. Acquired immunodeficiency syndrome.

AIHA. Autoimmune hemolytic anemia.

AIMS. Abnormal involuntary movement scale *or* arthritis impact measurement scales.

AKA. Above-knee amputation.

Alb. Albumin.

ALG. Antilymphocyte globulin.

ALL. Acute lymphoblastic leukemia *or* Acute lymphocytic leukemia.

Al(OH)³. Aluminum hydroxide.

ALT. Alanine transaminase (SGPT).

AM. Adult male *or* Morning (a.m.).

AMA. Against medical advice *or* American Medical Association.

AMI. Acute myocardial infarction.

AML. Acute myelogenous leukemia.

AMP. Ampicillin *or* Amputation.

ANA. Antinuclear antibody.

ANC. Absolute neutrophil count.

ANF. Atrial natriuretic factor.

ANLL. Acute nonlymphoblastic leukemia.

ANT. Anterior.

Ante. Before.

A & O. Alert and oriented.

A & O x 3. Awake and oriented to person, place, and time.

AOC. Antacid of choice.

AODA. Alcohol and other drug abuse.

AODM. Adult onset diabetes mellitus.

AOM. Acute otitis media.

AP. Alkaline phosphatase *or* Apical pulse.

A & P. Anterior and posterior assessment and plans *or* Auscultation and percussion.

A$_2$>P$_2$. Second aortic sound greater than second pulmonic sound.

APACHE. Acute physiology and chronic health evaluation.

APAP. Acetaminophen.

APC. Aspirin, phenacetin, and caffeine *or* Atrial premature contraction.

Appr. Approximately.

Appt. Appointment.

APPY. Appendectomy.

aPTT. Activated partial thromboplastin time.

ARA-A. Vidarabine.

ARA-C. Cytarabine.

ARC. AIDS related complex.

ARDS. Adult respiratory distress syndrome.

ARF. Acute renal failure *or* Acute respiratory failure *or* Acute rheumatic fever.

AS. Aortic stenosis.

ASA. Aspirin (acetylsalicyclic acid).

AS/AI. Aortic stenosis/aortic insufficiency.

ASAP. As soon as possible.

ASCVD. Arteriosclerotic cardiovascular disease.

ASD. Atrial septal defect.

ASHD. Arteriosclerotic heart disease.

ASO. Antistreptolysin-O titer.

AST. Aspartate transaminase (SGOT)

ATB. Antibiotic.

ATC. Around the clock.

At Fib. Atrial fibrillation.

ATG. Antithymocyte globulin.

ATN. Acute tubular necrosis.

ATPase. Adenosine triphosphatase.

AU. Both ears.

AUC. Area under the curve.

AVF. Arteriovenous fistula.

AVN. Arteriovenous nicking *or* Atrioventricular node *or* Avascular necrosis.

AVR. Aortic valve replacement.

AVSS. All vital signs stable *or* Afebrile, vital signs stable.

AWI. Anterior wall infarct.

AWOL. Absent without leave.

ax. Axillary

AZA. Azathioprine.

AZT. Zidovudine (Azidothymidine).

B

B_1. Thiamine HCl.

B_2. Riboflavin.

B_2M. Beta$_2$ microglobulin.

B_6. Pyridoxine HCl.

B_7. Biotin.

B_8. Adenosine phosphate.

B_{12}. Cyanocobalamin.

BACOP. Bleomycin, adriamycin, cyclophosphamide, vincristine, and prednisone.

BaE. Barium enema.

BAERs. Brain stem auditory evoked response.

BAL. Bronchoalveolar lavage.

BAND. Band neutrophil (stab).

BBB. Bundle branch block.

B Bx. Bone biopsy *or* Breast biopsy.

BC. Birth control *or* Blood culture.

BC/BS. Blue Cross/Blue Shield.

BCC. Basal cell carcinoma.

BCCa. Basal cell carcinoma.

B cell. Large lymphocyte.

BCG. Bacillus Calmette-Guérin vaccine.

BCNU. Carmustine.

BCP. Birth control pills *or* Carmustine, cyclophosphamide, and prednisone.

BE. Barium enema *or* Base excess.

BEP. Bleomycin, etoposide, and cisplatin.

BF. Black female.

B. frag. *Bacillus fragilis.*

Bicarb. Bicarbonate.

BID. Twice daily.

BIL. Bilateral.

Bili. Bilirubin.

BKA. Below-knee amputation.

bld cult. Blood culture.

BLEO. Bleomycin sulfate.

BM. Black male *or* Bone marrow *or* Bowel movement.

BMR. Basal metabolic rate.

BMT. Bone marrow transplant.

BO. Body odor.

B & O. Belladonna and opium (suppositories).

BOM. Bilateral otitis media.

BP. Bathroom privileges *or* Blood pressure.

BPD. Bronchopulmonary dysplasia.

BPH. Benign prostatic hypertrophy.

BPM. Beats per minute *or* Breaths per minute.

BPR. Blood per rectum.

BRBPR. Bright red blood per rectum.

BS. Blood sugar *or* Bowel sounds *or* Breath sounds.

BSA. Body surface area.

BSN. Bachelor of Science in Nursing.

BSO. Bilateral salpingo-oophorectomy.

BUN. Blood urea nitrogen.

Bx. Biopsy.

C

C. Ascorbic acid *or* Celsius *or* Centigrade *or* Hundred.

c̄. With.

C₁...C₇. Cervical nerve 1 through 7 *or* Cervical vertebra 1 through 7.

CII. Controlled substance, class 2.

CIII. Controlled substance, class 3.

CA. Carcinoma *or* Cardiac arrest *or* Carotid artery.

Ca. Calcium.

CAA. Crystalline amino acids.

CABG. Coronary artery bypass graft.

CaCO₃. Calcium carbonate.

CAD. Coronary artery disease.

CAF. Cyclophosphamide, doxorubicin, and fluorouracil.

CAH. Chronic active hepatitis.

CAO. Chronic airway (airflow) obstruction.

CAP. Capsule.

Ca/P. Calcium to phosphorus ratio.

CAPD. Chronic ambulatory peritoneal dialysis.

CAT. Computed axial tomography.

Cath. Catheter *or* Catheterization.

CBC. Complete blood count.

CBD. Common bile duct.

CBI. Continuous bladder irrigation.

CBZ. Carbamazepine.

CC. Chief complaint *or* Cubic centimeter (cc), (mL)

CCE. Clubbing, cyanosis, and edema.

CCNU. Lomustine.

CCPD. Continuous cycling (cyclical) peritoneal dialysis.

C$_{Cr}$. Creatinine clearance.

CCU. Coronary care unit *or* Critical care unit.

CDB. Cough and deep breath.

CDC. Centers for Disease Control.

CEA. Carcinoembryonic antigen *or* Carotid endarterectomy.

CEV. Cyclophosphamide, etoposide, and vincristine.

CF. Cystic fibrosis.

CFNS. Chills, fever, and night sweats.

CHAD. Cyclophosphamide, adriamycin, cisplatin, and hexamethylmelamine.

CHB. Complete heart block.

CHD. Congenital heart disease.

CHF. Congestive heart failure.

CHOP. Cyclophosphamide, doxorubicin, vincristine, and prednisone.

CI. Cardiac index.

CIG. Cigarettes.

Cis-DDP. Cisplatin.

CK. Creatine kinase.

Cl. Chloride.

Cl$_{Cr}$. Creatinine clearence.

CL/CP. Cleft lip and cleft palate.

CLL. Chronic lymphocytic leukemia.

Cl liq. Clear liquid.

CM. Caucasian male *or* Centimeter (cm).

cm³. Cubic centimeter.

CMC. Carpal metacarpal (joint).

CMF. Cyclophosphamide, methotrexate, and fluorouracil.

CMG. Cystometrogram.

CMI. Cell-mediated immunity.

CML. Chronic myelogenous leukemia.

CMML. Chronic myelomonocytic leukemia.

CMV. Cytomegalovirus.

CN. Cranial nerve.

CN II–XII. Cranial nerves 2 through 12.

CNS. Central nervous system *or* Clinical Nurse Specialist.

CO. Carbon monoxide *or* Cardiac output.

C/O. Complained of.

CO$_2$. Carbon dioxide.

COAD. Chronic obstructive airways disease.

COPD. Chronic obstructive pulmonary disease.

CP. Cerebral palsy *or* Chest pain.

CPAP. Continuous positive airway pressure.

CPB. Cardiopulmonary bypass.

CPK. Creatinine phosphokinase (BB, MB, MM are isoenzymes).

CPmax. Peak serum concentration.

CPmin. Trough serum concentration.

CPP. Cerebral perfusion pressure.

CPPB. Continuous positive pressure breathing.

CPR. Cardiopulmonary resuscitation.

CPT. Chest physiotherapy.

CR$_1$. First cranial nerve.

Cr$_{Cl}$. Creatinine clearance.

CREST. Calcinosis, Raynaud's, esophageal dysmotility, sclerodactyl, and telangiectasia.

CRF. Chronic renal failure.

CRIT. Hematocrit.

C & S. Culture and sensitivity.

C/S. Culture and sensitivity.

CsA or CSA. Cyclosporin.

CSF. Cerebrospinal fluid *or* Colony-stimulating factors.

CT. Chest tube *or* Computed tomography.

CTA. Clear to auscultation.

CT & DB. Cough, turn, and deep breath.

CTX. Cyclophosphamide (Cytoxan).

CTZ. Chemoreceptor trigger zone.

Cu. Copper.

CUP. Carcinoma of unknown primary (site).

CV. Cardiovascular.

CVA. Cerebrovascular accident *or* Costovertebral angle.

CVAT. Costovertebral angel tenderness.

CVP. Central venous pressure.

CVS. Cardiovasular surgery.

Cx. Cervix *or* Culture.

CXR. Chest x-ray.

CYSTO. Cystoscopy.

D

D. Day *or* Diarrhea.

D50. 50% dextrose injection.

DA. Dopamine *or* Drug addict.

DAT. Daunorubicin, cytarabine, (ARA-C), and thioguanine.

DAW. Dispense as written.

DB. Date of birth.

DBP. Diastolic blood pressure.

DC, d/c. Decrease *or* Discharge *or* Discontinue.

DDAVP. Desmopressin acetate.

DEA #. Drug Enforcement Administration number.

Decub. Decubitus.

DES. Diethylstilbestrol.

DFO. Deferoxamine.

DHPG. Ganciclovir.

DI. Drug information *or* Diabetes insipidus *or* Drug interactions.

D & I. Dry and intact.

DIC. Disseminated intravascular coagulation.

DIFF. Differential blood count.

DIG. Digoxin.

DIP. Distal interphalangeal (joint).

DJD. Degenerative joint disease.

DKA. Diabetic ketoacidosis.

D_L. Maximal diffusing capacity.

D_5LR. Dextrose 5% in lactated Ringer's solution.

DM. Dermatomyositis *or* Dextromethorphan *or* Diabetes mellitus.

DMARD. Disease modifying antirheumatic drug.

DME. Durable medical equipment.

$D_5^1/_2NS$. Dextrose 5% in 0.45% sodium chloride solution.

DNR. Do not resuscitate.

D_5NSS. 5% dextrose in normal saline solution.

DO. Doctor of Osteopathy.

DOA. Date of admission *or* Dead on arrival.

DOB. Date of birth.

DOC. Drug of choice.

DOE. Dyspnea on exertion.

DOSS. Docusate sodium (dioctyl sodium sulfosuccinate).

DP. Diastolic pressure *or* Dorsalis pedis (pulse).

DPH. Phenytoin (diphenylhydantoin).

DPT. Diphtheria, pertussis, and tetanus (immunization).

DPUD. Duodenal peptic ulcer disease.

Dr. Doctor.

DRG. Diagnosis-related groups.

DS. Double strength.

DSA. Digital subtraction angiography.

DSMIII. Diagnostic & Statistical Manual, 3rd Edition.

DSS. Docusate sodium.

DST. Dexamethasone suppression test.

DT. Delerium tremens *or* Diphtheria tetanus *or* Diphtheria toxoid.

DTIC. Dacarbazine.

DTRs. Deep tendon reflexes.

DTs. Delerium tremens.

DUI. Driving under the influence.

DUR. Drug use review duration.

DVI. Digital vascular imaging *or* Atrioventricular sequential pacing.

DVM. Doctor of Veterinary Medicine.

DVT. Deep vein thrombosis.

D_5W. 5% dextrose in water solution.

DWI. Driving while intoxicated.

Dx. Diagnosis.

E

EC. Enteric coated.

ECG. Electrocardiogram.

ECHO. Echocardiogram.

ECM. Erythema chronicum migrans.

ECMO. Extracorporeal membrane oxygenation (oxygenator).

ECOG. Eastern Cooperative Oncology Group.

ECT. Electroconvulsive therapy.

EDTA. Edetic acid (ethylenedinitrilo tetra-acetic acid).

EEG. Electroencephalogram.

EENT. Eyes, ears, nose, and throat.

EES. Erythromycin ethylsuccinate.

EF. Ejection fraction.

EFAD. Essential fatty acid deficiency.

e.g. For example.

EKG. Electrocardiogram.

ELISA. Enzyme-linked immunosorbent assay.

Elix. Elixir.

EMD. Electromechanical dissociation.

EMG. Electromyogram *or* Electromyograph.

EMIT. Enzyme multiple immunoassay technique.

EMS. Emergency medical services *or* Eosinophilia myalgia syndrome.

EMT. Emergency medical technician.

ENDO. Endoscopy.

ENT. Ear, nose, and throat.

EOC. Enema of choice.

EOM. External otitis media *or* Extraocular movement.

EOMI. Extraocular muscles intact.

EOS. Eosinophil.

EPI. Epinephrine.

EPO. Erythropoietin.

EPS. Electrophysiologic study *or* Extrapyramidal syndrome (symptom)

EPSE. Extrapyramidal side effect.

EPT. Early pregnancy test.

ER. Emergency room.

ER⁺. Estrogen receptor-positive.

ERCP. Endoscopic retrograde cholangio-pancreatography.

ESR. Erythrocyte sedimentation rate.

ESRD. End-stage renal disease.

ET. Endotracheal.

et. And.

et al. And others.

ETC. And so forth *or* Estimated time of conception.

ETCO$_2$. End tidal carbon dioxide.

ETOH. Alcohol.

ETT. Endotracheal tube *or* Exercise tolerance test *or* Exercise thallium test.

Exp Lap. Exploratory laparotomy.

EXT. Extension *or* Extremity.

F

F. Fahrenheit *or* Female.

F II. Factor II (two).

F VIII. Factor VIII (eight).

FA. Folic acid.

FAB. Digoxin immune Fab (Digibind).

FABER. Flexion, abduction, and external rotation.

FAS. Fetal alcohol syndrome.

FB. Fasting blood (sugar) *or* Foreign body.

FBRCM. Fingerbreadth below right costal margin.

FBS. Fasting blood sugar.

5-FC. Flucytosine.

FC. Fever, chills.

F & D. Fixed and dilated.

FDA. Food and Drug Administration.

FDP. Fibrin-degradation products.

FDS. First day surgery *or* For duration of stay.

Fe. Iron.

FEM. Femoral.

Fem-Pop. Femoral popliteal (bypass).

FeSO$_4$. Ferrous sulfate.

FEV$_1$. Forced expiratory volume in one second.

FFP. Fresh frozen plasma.

FH. Family history.

FiCO$_2$. Fraction of inspired carbon dioxide.

FiO$_2$. Fraction of inspired oxygen.

FMH. Family medical history.

FSH. Follicle-stimulating hormone.

FSP. Fibrin split products.

FT. Foot (ft).

FT$_3$. Free triiodothyroxine.

FT$_4$. Free thyroxine.

F/U. Follow-up.

5-FU. Fluorouracil.

FUO. Fever of undetermined (unknown) origin.

FVC. Forced vital capacity.

Fx. Fracture.

FXN. Function.

FYI. For your information.

G

G. Gram (gm) *or* Gravida.

G$^+$. Gram-positive.

G$^-$. Gram-negative.

Ga. Gallium.

GABA. Gamma-aminobutyric acid.

Ga scan. Gallium scan.

GC. *Gonococci* (gonorrhea).

GCSF. Granulocyte colony-stimulating factor.

GE. Gastroesophageal.

GENT. Gentamicin.

GERD. Gastroesophageal reflux disease.

GFR. Glomerular filtration rate.

GGT. Gamma-glutamyl transpeptidase.

GH. Growth hormone.

GI. Gastrointestinal.

GM$^+$. Gram-positive.

GM$^-$. Gram-negative.

gm%. Grams per 100 milliliters.

GMC. General medical clinic.

GM-CSF. Granulocyte macrophage colony-stimulating factor.

GN. Glomerulonephritis.

GNB. Gram-negative bacilli.

GNR. Gram-negative rods.

GP. General practitioner.

G/P. Gravida/para.

G_3P_3. Three pregnancies (gravida), three went to term.

GPC. Gram-positive cocci.

GRD. Gastroesophageal reflux disease.

$Gr_2P_1AB_1$. Two pregnancies, one birth, and one abortion.

GSW. Gunshot wound.

GT. Gastrostomy tube.

GTT. Drop *or* Glucose tolerance test.

GU. Genitourinary.

GVHD. Graft-versus-host disease.

H

H. Heart *or* Hydrogen.

HA. Headache *or* Hemolytic anemia *or* Hyperalimentation.

HAV. Hepatitis A vaccine.

HbA_{1c}. Glycosylated hemoglobin.

HB_eAb. Hepatitis B_e antibody.

HB_cAg. Hepatitis B_c antigen.

HB_eAg. Hepatitis B_e antigen.

HBIG. Hepatitis B immune globulin.

HbS. Sickle cell hemoglobin.

HBsAg. Hepatitis B surface antigen.

HbSC. Sickle cell hemoglobin C.

HBV. Hepatitis B vaccine *or* Hepatitis B virus.

HC. Hydrocortisone.

HCG. Human chorionic gonadotropin.

HCO_3. Bicarbonate.

HCT. Hematocrit.

HCTZ. Hydrochlorothiazide.

HD. Hemodialysis *or* Hodgkin's disease.

HDL. High-density lipoprotein.

HEENT. Head, eyes, ears, nose, and throat.

H flu. *Hemophilus influenzae.*

HG. Hemoglobin.

Hgb. Hemoglobin.

HH. Hiatal hernia.

H & H. Hematocrit and hemoglobin.

HHC. Home health care.

HI. Head injury.

Hi-cal. High caloric.

HIV. Human immunodeficiency virus.

HJR. Hepato-jugular reflex.

HLA(–). Heart, lungs, and abdomen negative.

HLA. Human lymphocyte antigen.

HMO. Health maintenance organization.

H & N. Head and neck.

HO. House officer.

H/O. History of.

H_2O. Water.

H_2O_2. Hydrogen peroxide.

HOB. Head of bed.

H & P. History and physical.

HPI. History of present illness.

HPLC. High-pressure (performance) liquid chromatography.

HR. Heart rate *or* Hour.

HS. Bedtime *or* Herpes simplex.

HSV. Herpes simplex virus.

HSVI. Herpes simplex virus type I.

HSVII. Herpes simplex virus type II.

HT. Height *or* Hypertension.

HTN. Hypertension.

Hx. History.

HZV. Herpes zoster virus.

I

IABP. Intra-aortic balloon pump.

IBD. Inflammatory bowel disease.

IBS. Irritable bowel syndrome.

IBW. Ideal body weight.

ICF. Intermediate care facility.

ICP. Intracranial pressure.

ID. Identification *or* Infectious disease (physician or department).

IDS. Investigational Drug Service.

I & D. Incision and drainage.

IDDM. Insulin-dependent diabetes mellitus.

i.e. That is.

IF. Interferon *or* Internal fixation.

IFN. Interferon.

IFOS. Ifosfamide.

IgA. Immunoglobulin A.

IgD. Immunoglobulin D.

IGDM. Infant of gestational diabetic mother.

IgE. Immunoglobulin E.

IgG. Immunoglobulin G.

IGIV. Immune globulin intravenous.

IgM. Immunoglobulin M.

IHSS. Idiopathic hypertrophic subaortic stenosis.

IJ. Internal jugular.

IL ( ). Interleukin (1, 2, etc.).

IM. Intramuscular.

IMC. Intermediate care *or* Intermediate care unit.

IMI. Inferior myocardial infarction.

IMP. Impression.

In. Inches.

Inc Spir. Incentive spirometer.

IND. Investigational new drug.

ING. Inguinal.

✓ing. Checking.

INH. Isoniazid.

Inj. Injection *or* Injury.

Inpt. Inpatient.

Intol. Intolerance.

Intub. Intubation.

I & O. Intake and output.

IO. Intraocular pressure.

IOF. Intraocular fluid.

IOP. Intraocular pressure.

IP. Intraperitoneal.

IPG. Impedance plethysmography.

IPN. Intern's progress note.

IPP. Inflatable penile prosthesis.

IPPB. Intermittent positive pressure breathing.

IQ. Intelligence quotient.

IRB. Institutional review board.

IRR. Irrigate.

Irreg. Irregular.

IT. Intrathecal.

ITP. Idiopathic thrombocytopenia purpura.

IU. International unit.

IV. Four *or* Intravenous (i.v.) *or* Symbol for class 4 controlled substance.

IVF. Intravenous fluid(s).

IVH. Intraventricular hemorrhage.

IVIG. Intravenous immunoglobulin.

IVP. Intravenous push *or* Intravenous pyelogram.

IVPB. Intravenous piggyback.

J

Jnt. Joint.

JODM. Juvenile onset diabetes mellitus.

JP. Jackson-Pratt (drain).

JRA. Juvenile rheumatoid arthritis.

JT. Jejunostomy tube *or* Joint.

J-Tube. Jejunostomy tube.

Juv. Juvenile.

JVD. Jugular venous distention.

JVP. Jugular venous pressure *or* Jugular venous pulse.

K

K. Potassium *or* Thousand *or* Vitamin K.

K$_1$. Phytonadione.

KA. Ketoacidosis.

kcal. Kilocalorie.

KCl. Potassium chloride.

KD. Kawasaki's disease.

KDA. Known drug allergies.

kg. Kilogram.

KI. Potassium iodide.

kilo. Kilogram.

KISS. Saturated solution of potassium iodide.

Kleb. Klebsiella.

KMnO$_4$. Potassium permanganate.

KO. Keep open.

KOH. Potassium hydroxide.

KTx. Kidney transplant.

KUB. Kidney, ureter, and bladder.

KVO. Keep vein open.

KW. Keith-Wagener (ophthalmoscopic finding, graded I –IV).

L

L. Fifty *or* Left *or* Lente (insulin) *or* Liter.

L$_1$–L$_5$. Lumbar nerve 1–5 *or* Lumbar vertebra 1–5.

LA. Left atrial *or* Left atrium *or* Local anesthesia.

L + A. Light and accommodation.

LAD. Left anterior descending.

LAK. Lymphokine-activated killer.

LAM. Laminectomy.

LAP. Laparoscopy *or* Laparotomy.

L-ASP. Asparaginase.

LAT. Lateral.

LB. Low back *or* Pound.

LBP. Low back pain.

LBW. Lean body weight.

LCD. Coal tar solution *(liquor carbonis detergens)*.

LCFA. Long-chain fatty acid.

LCM. Left costal margin.

LD. Lactic dehydrogenase (formerly LDH) *or* Learning disability *or* Lethal dose *or* Living donor.

LDH. Lactic dehydrogenase (see LD).

LDL. Low-density lipoprotein.

L-dopa. Levodopa.

LE. Left ear *or* Left eye *or* Lower extremities *or* Lupus erythematous.

LES. Lower esophageal sphincter.

LF. Left foot.

LFT(s). Liver function test(s).

LG. Large.

LH. Left hand.

LHF. Left heart failure.

Li. Lithium.

LICM. Left intercostal margin.

Li₂CO₃. Lithium carbonate.

Lido. Lidocaine.

LIG. Ligament.

LIH. Left inguinal hernia.

LIQ. Liquid.

LIS. Left intercostal space *or* Low intermittent suction.

LK. Left kidney.

LKS. Liver, kidneys, and spleen.

LL. Left leg *or* Left lower *or* Left lung *or* Lower lid *or* Lower lobe *or* Lymphocytic leukemia.

LLE. Left lower extremity.

LLL. Left lower lid *or* Left lower lobe (lung).

LLQ. Left lower quadrant (abdomen exam).

LMD. Local medical doctor *or* Low molecular weight dextran.

L/min. Liters per minute.

LMP. Last menstrual period.

LMWD. Low molecular weight dextran.

LOA. Leave of absence.

LOC. Laxative of choice *or* Loss of consciousness.

LOM. Left otitis media *or* Loss of motion.

LOS. Length of stay.

LOZ. Lozenge.

LP. Lumbar puncture.

LPA. Left pulmonary artery.

LPN. Licensed Practical Nurse.

LR. Lactated Ringer's (solution).

L→R. Left to right.

LRD. Living related donor.

LS. Left side *or* Liver spleen *or* Lumbosacral.

L-Spar. Elspar (asparaginase).

LT. Left *or* Light.

LTB. Laryngotracheo-bronchitis.

LTC. Long-term care.

LTCF. Long-term care facility.

LUL. Left upper lobe (lung).

LV. Left ventricle.

LVDP. Left ventricular diastolic pressure.

LVEDP. Left ventricular end diastolic pressure.

LVEDV. Left ventricular end diastolic volume.

LVEF. Left ventricular ejection fraction.

LVF. Left ventricular failure.

LVFP. Left ventricular filling pressure.

LVG. Living.

LVH. Left ventricular hypertrophy.

LVP. Large volume parenteral *or* Left ventricular pressure.

Lymphs. Lymphocytes.

Lytes. Electrolytes (Na, K, Cl, CO_2).

M

M. Male *or* Meter (m) *or* Molar *or* Monday *or* Thousand.

MA. Medical assistance.

MAB. Monoclonal antibody.

MABP. Mean arterial blood pressure.

Mag Cit. Magnesium citrate.

Mag sulf. Magnesium sulfate.

Malig. Malignant.

m-AMSA. Amsacrine.

MAOI. Monoamine oxidase inhibitor.

MAP. Mean airway pressure *or* Mean arterial pressure.

MAR. Medication administration record.

MAST. Mastectomy.

Max. Maximal.

MBC. Minimal bacteriocidal concentration.

MBD. Minimal brain dysfunction.

MCA. Motorcycle accident.

mcg. Microgram (μg).

MCH. Mean corpuscular hemoglobin.

MCHC. Mean corpuscular hemoglobin concentration.

MCT. Medium chain triglyceride.

MD. Manic depression *or* Medical doctor *or* Multi-dose.

MDE. Major depressive episode.

MDI. Metered dose inhaler.

MDR. Minimum daily requirement.

MEC. Meconium.

MED. Medial *or* Medication *or* Medicine *or* Medium.

mEq. Milliequivalent.

mEq/24 hr. Milliequivalents per 24 hours.

mEq/L. Milliequivalents per liter.

MET. Medical emergency treatment *or* Metastasis.

METS. Metastasis.

MG. Milligram (mg).

Mg. Magnesium.

mg%. Milligrams per 100 milliliters.

mg/dL. Milligrams per 100 milliliters.

MGF. Maternal grandfather.

mg/kg. Milligram per kilogram.

mg/kg/hr. Milligram per kilogram per hour.

MGM. Maternal grandmother.

MGN. Membranous glomerulonephritis.

MgO. Magnesium oxide.

MgSO$_4$. Magnesium sulfate (Epsom salt).

MI. Mitral insufficiency *or* Myocardial infarction.

MIC. Minimum inhibitory concentration.

MIN. Minimum *or* Minute (min).

MIP. Metacarpo-interphalangeal (joint).

MISC. Miscellaneous.

mL. Milliliter.

MLC. Mixed lymphocyte culture.

MLNS. Mucocutaneous lymph node syndrome.

MM. Malignant melanoma *or* Millimeter (mm) *or* Mucous membrane.

mM. Millimolar.

M & M. Morbidity and mortality.

mm Hg. Millimeters of mercury.

mmol. Millimole.

MMPI. Minnesota Multiphasic Personality Inventory.

MMR. Measles, mumps, and rubella.

MMWR. Morbidity & Mortality Weekly Report.

MN. Midnight.

Mn. Manganese.

MO. Month (mo) *or* Months old.

MOA. Mechanism of action.

MoAb. Monoclonal antibody.

MOM. Milk of magnesia.

Mono. Infectious mononucleosis.

mOsm. Milliosmole.

mOsmol. Milliosmole.

6-MP. Mercaptopurine.

MPGN. Membranoproliferative glomerulonephritis.

MPSS. Methylprednisolone sodium succinate.

MR. Magnetic resonance *or* May repeat *or* Metal retardation *or* Mitral regurgitation.

MR x 1. May repeat times one (once).

MRI. Magnetic resonance imaging.

MRM. Modified radical mastectomy.

MRSA. Methicillin-resistant *Staphylococcus aureus.*

MRSE. Methicillin-resistant *Staphylococcus epidermitis.*

MS. Mental status *or* Mitral stenosis *or* Morphine sulfate *or* Multiple sclerosis *or* Muscle strength.

MSE. Mental status examination.

MSH. Melanocyte-stimulating hormone.

MSIR. Morphine sulfate immediate-release tablets.

MSL. Midsternal line.

MSPN. Medical student progress note.

MSW. Master of Social Work.

MT. Metatarsal.

MTX. Methotrexate.

MU. Million Units.

mU. Milliunits.

MUGA. Multiple gated acquisition.

MV. Millivolts *or* Mitral valve.

MVA. Motor vehicle accident.

M-VAC. Methotrexate, vinblastine, doxorubicin, and cisplatin.

MVAC. Methotrexate, vinblastine, doxorubicin, and cisplatin.

MVI. Multiple vitamin injection *or* Trade name for parenteral multivitamins.

MVI 12. Trade name for parenteral multivitamins.

MVO$_2$. Myocardial oxygen consumption.

MVR. Mitral valve regurgitation *or* Mitral valve replacement.

Myelo. Myelocytes.

N

N. Negative *or* Negro *or* Nerve *or* Normal *or* NPH insulin *or* Size of sample.

N$_2$. Nitrogen.

Na. Sodium.

NA. Native American *or* Not applicable *or* Not available *or* Nursing Assistant.

NaCl. Sodium chloride (salt).

NAD. No acute distress *or* No apparent distress.

NaF. Nafcillin *or* Sodium fluoride.

NaHCO₃. Sodium bicarbonate.

NaI. Sodium iodide.

NAPA. N-acetyl procainamide.

Na Pent. Pentothal sodium.

NARC. Narcotic(s).

NAS. No added salt.

NB. Note well.

NC. Nasal cannula *or* No change.

NCI. National Cancer Institute.

NDA. New drug application.

NE. Norepinephrine.

NEC. Necrotizing entercolitis.

NEG. Negative.

NF. Negro female.

NG. Nanogram *or* Nasogastric.

NGB. Neurogenic bladder.

NGR. Nasogastric replacement.

NGU. Nongonococcal urethritis.

NGT. Nasogastric tube.

NH. Nursing home.

NH₃. Ammonia.

NH₄Cl. Ammonium chloride.

NHL. Non-Hodgkin's lymphomas.

NICU. Neonatal intensive care unit.

NIDD. Non-insulin-dependent diabetes.

NIDDM. Non-insulin-dependent diabetes mellitus.

NIH. National Institutes of Health.

Nitro. Nitroglycerin.

NJ. Nasojejunal.

NKA. No known allergies.

NKDA. No known drug allergies.

NKMA. No known medication allergies.

NL. Normal.

NLT. Not later than *or* Not less than.

NM. Neuromuscular *or* Negro male.

nmol. Nanomol.

NMP. Normal menstrual period.

NMR. Nuclear magnetic resonance (same as magnetic resonance imaging).

NMS. Neuroleptic malignant syndrome.

NMT. Not more than.

NN. Neonatal.

NO. Nitrous oxide.

N₂O. Nitrous oxide.

N₂O:O₂. Nitrous oxide to oxygen ratio.

Noc. Night.

Noct. Nocturnal.

NOR-EPI. Norepinephrine.

Norm. Normal.

NP. Nasal prongs *or* Nurse Practitioner.

NPH. Isophane insulin.

NPO. Nothing by mouth.

NPR. Normal per rectum.

NPT. Nocturnal penile tumescence.

NR. No refills *or* No response.

NRC. Nuclear Regulatory Commission.

NREM. Nonrapid eye movement.

NREMS. Nonrapid eye movement sleep.

NS. Normal saline solution (0.9% sodium chloride solution) *or* Not significant.

NSA. Normal serum albumin.

NSAIA. Nonsteroidal anti-inflammatory agent.

NSAID. Nonsteroidal anti-inflammatory drug.

NSC. No significant change.

NSG. Nursing.

NSR. Normal sinus rhythm.

1/2 NSS. Sodium chloride 0.45% (or 1/2 normal saline solution).

NSVD. Normal spontaneous vaginal delivery.

NSY. Nursery.

NT. Nasotracheal.

NTI. Nortriptyline.

N & T. Nose and throat.

NTE. Not to exceed.

NTG. Nitroglycerin.

NTP. Nitropaste (nitroglycerin ointment) *or* Sodium nitroprusside.

NTT. Nasotracheal tube.

Nullip. Nullipara.

NV. Nausea and vomiting.

N & V. Nausea and vomiting.

NVD. Nausea, vomiting, and diarrhea *or* Neck vein distention.

NYHA. New York Heart Association (classification for heart disease).

O

O. Eye *or* Objective findings *or* Oral *or* Oxygen *or* Zero.

O₂. Oxygen.

OA. Osteoarthritis.

OB. Obstetrics.

OBG. Obstetrics and gynecology.

Ob-Gyn. Obstetrics and gynecology.

Obj. Objective.

Obl. Oblique.

OC. On call *or* Oral contraceptive.

Occl. Occlusion.

Occup Rx. Occupational therapy.

OCD. Obsessive-compulsive disorder.

OCP. Ova, cysts, and parasites.

OD. Doctor of Optometry *or* Overdose *or* Right eye.

OI. Opportunistic infection.

OJ. Orange juice.

OK. All right.

OLT. Orthotopic liver transplantation.

OM. Otitis media

ON. Ortho-Novum.

ONC. Oncology.

OOB. Out of bed.

OOC. Out of control.

OP. Outpatient.

O & P. Ova and parasites.

op cit. In the work cited.

OPP. Opposite *or* Outpatient pharmacy.

OPS. Operations *or* Outpatient surgery.

OPV. Oral polio vaccine

OR. Operating room *or* Open reduction.

ORCH. Orchiectomy.

ORIF. Open reduction internal fixation.

ORN. Operating room nurse.

OR X 1. Oriented to time.

OR X 2. Oriented to time and place.

OR X 3. Oriented to time, place, and person.

OS. Left eye *or* Ophthalmic suspension *or* Ophthalmic solution.

OSHA. Occupational Safety & Health Administration.

OSN. Off service note.

OSS. Osseous.

OT. Occupational therapy.

OTC. Over the counter.

OTD. Out the door.

OTH. Other.

OTO. Otology.

OT/RT. Occupational therapy/recreational therapy.

OU. Both eyes.

oz. Ounce.

P

P. Para *or* Peripheral *or* Phosphorous *or* Pint *or* Plan *or* Protein.

p̄. After.

PA. Physician's assistant *or* Posterior-anterior *or* Pulmonary artery.

P & A. Percussion and auscultation.

PAB. Premature atrial beat.

PaCO₂. Partial arterial carbon dioxide tension.

PACU. Post-anesthesia care unit.

PAE. Postantibiotic effect.

PAF. Paroxysmal atrial fibrillation.

PAH. Pulmonary arterial hypertension.

PAL. Posterior, anterior, lateral.

Pa Line. Pulmonary artery line.

PALN. Para-aortic lymph node.

PALS. Pediatric advanced life support.

2-PAM. Pralidoxime.

PAN. Polyarteritis nodosa.

PAO₂. Partial arterial oxygen tension.

PAP. Prostatic acid phosphatase *or* Pulmonary artery pressure.

Pap smear. Papanicolaou smear.

PAR. Postanesthetic recovery.

PARA. Number of pregnancies.

para. Paraplegic.

PAS. Pulmonary artery stenosis.

PAT. Paroxysmal atrial tachycardia.

Path. Pathology.

PAWP. Pulmonary artery wedge pressure.

PB. Phenobarbital.

Pb. Lead *or* Phenobarbital.

PBI. Protein-bound iodine.

PBN. Polymyxin B sulfate, bacitricin, and neomycin.

PBS. Phosphate-buffered saline.

PBZ. Phenoxybenzamine *or* Phenylbutazone.

ΦBZ. Phenylbutazone.

PC. After meals *or* Packed cells.

PCA. Patient-controlled analgesia.

PCBs. Polychlorinated biphenyls.

PCE. Erythromycin particles in tablets.

PC & HS. After meals and at

bedtime.

PCKD. Polycystic kidney disease.

PCM. Protein-calorie malnutrition.

PCN. Penicillin.

PCO$_2$. Carbon dioxide pressure (or tension).

PCP. Phencyclidine *or Pneumonocystis carinii* pneumonia.

PCV. Packed cell volume.

PCWP. Pulmonary capillary wedge pressure.

PD. Peritoneal dialysis.

PDA. Patent ductus arteriosus.

PDE. Paroxysmal dyspnea on exertion.

PDN. Prednisone.

PDR. Physician's Desk Reference.

PE. Physical examination *or* Physical exercise *or* Pulmonary edema *or* Pulmonary embolism.

P$_1$E$_1$. Epinephrine 1%, pilocarpine 1% ophthalmic solution.

PEARLA. Pupils equal and retract to light and accommodation.

PEB. Cisplatin, etoposide, and bleomycin.

Peds. Pediatrics.

PEEP. Positive end-expiratory pressure.

PEG. Percutaneous endoscopic gastrostomy *or* Polyethylene glycol.

PEN. Penicillin.

PERC. Percutaneous.

Perf. Perforation.

Peri care. Perineum care.

PERL. Pupils equal, reactive to light.

***Per os*.** By mouth.

PERRLA. Pupils equal, round, reactive to light and accommodation.

PET. Position-emission tomography.

PETN. Pentaerythritol tetranitrate.

PEx. Physical examination.

PF. Preservative free.

PFC. Persistent fetal circulation.

PFT. Pulmonary function test.

PG. Pregnant.

PGE. Posterior gastroenterostomy *or* Prostaglandin E.

PGE$_2$. Prostaglandin E$_2$.

PG-1. Post-graduate year one.

PG-2. Post-graduate year two.

PG-3. Post-graduate year three.

PH. Past history.

PHA. Pharmacist Assistant.

Pharm. Pharmacy.

Pharm. D. Doctor of Pharmacy.

PID. Pelvic inflammatory disease.

Pit. Pitocin.

PIV. Peripheral intravenous.

PKU. Phenylketonuria.

PLS. Plastic surgery.

PLT. Platelet.

PLTs. Platelets.

PM. Afternoon *or* Pacemaker *or* Petit mal *or* Polymyosititis.

PMD. Private medical doctor.

PMH. Past medical history.

PMI. Past medical illness *or* Point of maximal impulse.

PMN. Polymorphonuclear leukocyte.

PMP. Previous menstrual period.

PMS. Premenstrual syndrome.

PNB. Percutaneous needle biopsy.

PNC. Penicillin.

PND. Paroxysmal nocturnal dyspnea.

PNET-MB. Primitive neuroectodermal tumors-medulloblastoma.

PO. By mouth (*per os*).

PO$_2$. Partial pressure of oxygen.

PO$_4$. Phosphate.

POD 1. Postoperative day one.

POMP. Prednisone, vincristine, methotrexate, and mercaptopurine.

Poplit. Popliteal.

POS. Positive.

"Post." Post mortem examination (autopsy).

Post op. Postoperative.

P & P. Policy and procedure.

PPB. Positive pressure breathing.

PPD. Packs per day *or* Purified protein derivative (tuberculin skin test).

PPI. Patient package insert.

PPM. Parts per million.

PPNG. Penicillinase producing *Neisseria gonorrhoeae*.

PPO. Preferred provider organization.

PR. Patient relations *or* Per rectum.

PRBC. Packed red blood cells.

PRC. Packed red cells.

Pred. Prednisone.

Pre-op. Before surgery.

Prep. Prepare for surgery.

PRN. As occasion requires or as needed.

PRO. Protein *or* Prothrombin.

PROM. Passive range of motion.

PSA. Prostate-specific antigen.

PSF. Posterior spinal fusion.

PSGN. Poststreptococcal glomerulonephritis.

PSI. Pounds per square inch.

PSVT. Paroxysmal supraventricular tachycardia.

PT. Paroxysmal tachycardia *or* Patient *or* Pint *or* Prothrombin time.

P & T. Pharmacy and therapeutics *or* Peak and trough.

PTA. Percutaneous transluminal angioplasty *or* Prior to admission.

PTCA. Percutaneous transluminal coronary angioplasty.

PTH. Parathyroid hormone.

PTSD. Post-traumatic stress disorder.

PTT. Partial thromboplastin time.

PTU. Propylthiouracil.

PU. Peptic ulcer.

PUD. Peptic ulcer disease.

PUFA. Polyunsaturated fatty acids.

Pul. Pulmonary.

PUVA. Psoralen-ultraviolet-light (treatment).

PV. Per vagina.

PVB. Premature ventricular beat.

PVC. Polyvinyl chloride *or* Premature ventricular contraction.

PVK. Penicillin V potassium.

PVR. Peripheral vascular resistance *or* Postvoiding residual *or* Pulse-volume recording.

PVT. Private.

PWB. Partial weight bearing.

PWP. Pulmonary wedge pressure.

Px. Physical exam *or* Pneumothorax *or* Prognosis.

PZI. Protamine zinc insulin.

Q

Q. Every.

QA. Quality assurance.

Q AM. Every morning

QC. Quality control.

QD. Every day.

Q 2 hr. Every two hours.

Q hr. Every hour.

Q HS. Every night.

QID. Four times daily.

QOD. Every other day.

Q PM. Every evening.

Qt. Quart.

Q wk. Once a week.

R

R. Rectum *or* Regular *or* Respiration *or* Right.

RA. Rheumatoid arthritis *or* Right atrium *or* Room air.

RAA. Renin-angiotensin-aldosterone.

RAD. Ionizing radiation unit *or* Reactive airway disease.

RAN. Resident's admission notes.

RAS. Renal artery stenosis.

RBBB. Right bundle branch block.

RCA. Right coronary artery.

RCC. Renal cell carcinoma.

RCM. Right costal margin.

R.D. Registered Dietician.

RDA. Recommended daily allowance.

RDS. Respiratory distress syndrome.

RDW. Red (cell) distribution width.

RE. Reticuloendothelial *or* Right ear.

Re ✓. Recheck.

REC. Recommend.

REE. Resting energy expenditure.

Regurg. Regurgitation.

Rehab. Rehabilitation.

REM. Rapid eye movement.

REMS. Rapid eye movement sleep.

REP. Repeat.

RES. Resident *or* Reticuloendothelial system.

Resp. Respirations.

Retic. Reticulocyte.

REV. Review.

RF. Rheumatic fever *or* Rheumatoid factor.

Rh. Rhesus factor in blood.

RHD. Rheumatic heart disease.

rHmEPO. Recombinant human erythropoietin.

RIA. Radioimmunoassay.

R→L. Right to left.

RLD. Related living donor.

RLE. Right lower extremity.

RLL. Right lower lobe.

RLQ. Right lower quadrant.

RM. Room.

RMSF. Rocky Mountain spotted fever.

RN. Registered Nurse.

RO. Routine order.

R/O. Rule out.

ROM. Range of motion *or* Right otitis media *or* Rupture of membranes.

RoRx. Radiation therapy.

ROS. Review of systems.

R. Ph. Registered Pharmacist.

RPT. Registered Physical Therapist.

RQ. Respiratory quotient.

RR. Recovery room.

R/R. Rales-rhonchi.

R & R. Rate and rhythm.

RS. Renal scan.

RSR. Regular sinus rhythm.

RSV. Respiratory syncytial virus.

RT. Respiratory Therapist *or* Right.

RTA. Renal tubular acidosis.

RTC. Return to clinic.

rtPA. Recombinant tissue plasminogen activator.

RTx. Radiation therapy *or* Renal transplant.

RU. Routine urinalysis.

RUA. Routine urine analysis.

RUL. Right upper lobe.

RUQ. Right upper quadrant.

RV. Right ventrical.

RVH. Right ventricular hypertrophy.

S

S. Second(s) *or* Subjective findings *or* Suction *or* Sulfur.

s̄. Without.

S$_1$. First heart sound.

S$_2$. Second heart sound.

S$_3$. Third heart sound (ventricular gallop).

S$_4$. Fourth heart sound (atrial gallop).

S$_1$–S$_5$. Sacral vertebra one through five.

SA. Salicylic acid *or* Sinoatrial *or* Surface area *or* Sustained action.

SAD. Seasonal affective disorder.

SAH. Subarachnoic hemorrhage.

Sang. Sanguinous.

Sat. Saturated *or* Saturation *or* Saturday.

SB. Sinus bradycardia *or* Small bowel *or* Spina bifida.

SBA. Serum bactericidal activity.

SBFT. Small bowel follow through.

SBP. Systolic blood pressure.

SC. Subcutaneous.

SCC. Squamous cell carcinoma.

SCCa. Squamous cell carcinoma.

SCI. Spinal cord injury.

SCID. Severe combined immunodeficiency disorder.

SCr. Serum creatinine.

SD. Septal defect.

SDH. Subdural hematoma.

SE. Side effect.

Se. Selenium.

Sec. Second.

SED. Sedimentation.

SEG. Segment.

SF. Spinal fluid *or* Sugar free.

SG. Serum glucose *or* Specific gravity *or* Swan-Ganz.

SGA. Small for gestational age.

SGOT. Serum glutamic oxaloacetic transaminase (see AST).

SGPT. Serum glutamic pyruvic transaminase (see ALT).

SH. Social history.

SI. International system of units.

SIADH. Syndrome of inappropriate antidiuretic hormone secretion.

SIDS. Sudden infant death syndrome.

Sig. Let it be marked.

SIM. Similac.

SL. Sublingual.

SLE. Systemic lupus erythematosus.

Sl tr. Slight trace.

SLUD. Salivation, lacrimation, urination, and defecation.

SM. Small.

SMA. Sequential multiple analyzer *or* Simultaneous multichannel auto-analyzer.

SNP. Sodium nitroprusside.

SOAP. Subjective, objective, assessment, and plan.

SOB. Shortness of breath.

SOM. Serous otitis media.

S/P. Status post.

SPA. Albumin human (formerly known as salt-poor albumin).

SPF. Split products of fibrin *or* Sun protective factor.

SQ. Subcutaneous.

SR. Sinus rhythm.

SROM. Spontaneous rupture of membrane.

SRT. Sustained-release theophylline.

SS. Half *or* Sliding scale.

S & S. Signs and symptoms.

SSKI. Saturated solution of potassium iodide.

SSS. Sick sinus syndrome.

S/SX. Signs/symptoms.

ST. Sinus tachycardia *or* Skin test.

stab. Polymorphonuclear leukocytes.

Staph. *Staphylococcus aureus*.

STAT. Immediately.

STDs. Sexually transmitted diseases.

STD TF. Standard tube feeding.

STG. Split thickness graft.

STI. Soft tissue injury.

Strep. *Streptococcus*.

STSG. Split thickness skin graft.

SUBL. Sublingual.

Subcu. Subcutaneous.

sub q. Subcutaneous.

SUP. Superior.

Supp. Suppository.

SVPB. Supraventricular premature beat.

SVPC. Supraventricular premature contraction.

SVR. Supraventricular rhythm *or* Systemic vascular resistance.

SVT. Supraventricular tachycardia.

SWOG. Southwest Oncology Group.

Sx. Signs *or* Symptoms.

syr. Syrup.

SYS BP. Systolic blood pressure.

SZ. Seizure.

T

T. Tablespoon (15 mL) or Tender.

t^1/2. Half-life.

T$_3$. Tylenol with codeine 30 mg.

T$_4$. Levothyroxine.

T & A. Tonsillectomy and adenoidectomy.

TAB. Tablet.

TAH. Total abdominal hysterectomy.

TAHBSO. Total abdominal hysterectomy, bilateral salpingo-oophorectomy.

TAO. Troleandomycin.

TB. Tuberculosis.

TBA. To be added or To be admitted or Total body (surface) area.

TBG. Thyroxine-binding globulin.

T bili. Total bilirubin.

tbl. Tablespoon (15 mL).

TBR. Total bed rest.

Tbsp. Tablespoon (15 mL).

TBW. Total body water or Total body weight..

TC. Throat culture or Tissue culture.

T & C. Type and crossmatch.

T & C # 3. Tylenol with 30 mg codeine.

TCA. Tricyclic antidepressant.

T cell. T-lymphocyte.

TCN. Tetracycline.

TD. Tardive dyskinesia or Tetanus-diphtheria toxoid (pediatric use).

Td. Tetanus-diphtheria toxoid (adult type).

TDD. Thoracic duct drainage.

TDM. Therapeutic drug monitoring.

TDNTG. Transdermal nitroglycerin.

TE. Trace elements or Tracheoesophageal.

TEDS. Anti-embolism stockings.

TEE. Transesophageal echocardiography.

TEN. Total enteral nutrition.

TENS. Transcutaneous electrical nerve stimulation (stimulator).

TERB. Terbutaline.

TF. Tube feeding.

TFTs. Thyroid function tests.

TG. Triglycerides.

6-TG. Thioguanine.

TGA. Transposition of the great arteries.

TH. Total hysterectomy.

THAM. Tromethamine.

THC. Tetrahydrocannibinol (dronabinol).

TH CULT. Throat culture.

THR. Total hip replacement.

TI. Tricuspid insufficiency.

TIA. Transient ischemic attack.

TIBC. Total iron-binding capacity.

TID. Three times daily.

TIG. Tetanus immune globulin.

tinct. Tincture.

+tive. Positive.

TIW. Three times per week.

TKA. Total knee arthroplasty.

TKO. To keep open.

TKR. Total knee replacement.

TKVO. To keep vein open.

TLC. Tender loving care *or* Total lung capacity *or* Total lymphocyte count *or* Triple lumen catheter.

TM. Thayer Martin (culture) *or* Tympanic membrane.

TMJ. Temporomandibular joint.

TMP. Trimethoprim.

TMP/SMX. Trimethoprim sulfamethoxazole.

TNA. Total nutrient admixture.

TNF. Tumor necrosis factor.

TNG. Nitroglycerin.

TO. Telephone order.

TOA. Tubo-ovarian abscess.

TOF. Tetralogy of Fallot.

TOGV. Transposition of the great vessels.

Tomo. Tomography.

TOPV. Trivalent oral polio vaccine.

TORCH. Toxoplasmosis, other (syphilis, hepatitis, Zoster), rubella, cytomegalovirus, and herpes simplex (maternal infection).

TOT BILI. Total bilirubin.

TP. Total protein.

TPA. Alteplase, recombinant (tissue plasminogen activator) *or* Total parenteral alimentation.

TPN. Total parenteral nutrition.

TP & P. Time, place, and person.

TPR. Temperature, pulse, and respiration.

T PROT. Total protein.

TR. Trace.

TRA. To run at.

Trach. Tracheal.

TRH. Protirelin (thyrotropin-releasing hormone).

TSF. Tricep skin fold.

TSH. Thyroid-stimulating hormone.

TSP. Total serum protein.

TT. Tetanus toxoid *or* Thrombin time.

TTP. Thrombotic thrombocytopenic purpura.

TU. Tuberculin units.

TUN. Total urinary nitrogen.

TURBT. Transurethral resection bladder tumor.

TURP. Transurethral resection of prostate.

TV. Television *or* Tidal volume.

TVH. Total vaginal hysterectomy.

TW. Tap water.

TWE. Tap water enema.

Tx. Therapy *or* Transfer *or* Transfuse *or* Transplant *or* Treatment.

T & X. Type and crossmatch.

Tyl. Tylenol.

U

U. Ultralente insulin *or* Units.

UA. Umbilical cord *or* Uric acid *or* Urinalysis.

UAC. Umbilical artery catheter.

UC. Ulcerative colitis *or* Urine culture.

UCHD. Usual childhood diseases.

UCX. Urine culture.

UE. Upper extremity.

UES. Upper esophageal sphincter.

UGDP. University Group Diabetes Project.

UGI. Upper gastrointestinal series.

UK. Unknown.

ULQ. Upper left quadrant.

ULYTES. Electrolytes, urine.

umb ven. Umbilical vein.

UNa. Urine sodium.

ung. Ointment.

UNK. Unknown.

UO. Urinary output.

Uosm. Urinary osmolality.

✓up. Checkup.

U/P ratio. Urine to plasma ratio.

UR. Utilization review.

URI. Upper respiratory infection.

Urol. Urology.

URTI. Upper respiratory tract infection.

US. Ultrasonography.

USN. Ultrasonic nebulizer.

USPHS. United States Public Health Service.

ut dict. As directed.

UTI. Urinary tract infection.

UV. Ultraviolet.

UVA. Ultraviolet A light.

UVB. Ultraviolet B light.

V

V. Five.

V̇. Ventilation (L/min).

VA. Valproic acid *or* Veterans Administration.

vag. Vagina.

VAG HYST. Vaginal hysterectomy.

VAH. Veterans Administration Hospital.

VATER. Vertebral, anal, tracheal, esophageal, and renal anomalies.

VBG. Venous blood gases *or* vertical banded gastroplasty.

VBL. Vinblastine.

VC. Vena cava *or* Vital capacity.

VCR. Vincristine sulfate.

VCU. Voiding cystourethrogram.

VD. Venereal disease.

Vd. Volume of distribution.

V & D. Vomiting and diarrhea.

Vdg. Voiding.

VDRL. Venereal Disease Research Laboratory (syphilis test).

VENT. Ventilation *or* Ventilator.

VF. Ventricular fibrillation.

V. Fib. Ventricular fibrillation.

VG. Very good.

VI. Six.

vib. Vibration.

VIP. Etoposide, ifosfamide, and cisplatin *or* Vasoactive intestinal peptide.

VIT. Vitamin.

vit cap. Vital capacity.

VLDL. Very low density lipoprotein.

VM26. Teniposide.

VMA. Vanillylmandelic acid.

VO. Verbal order.

Vocab. Vocabulary.

VOL. Volume *or* VP or etoposide.

VP-16. Etoposide.

VPC. Ventricular premature contractions.

VQ. Ventilation perfusion.

VRI. Viral respiratory infection.

VS. Versus *or* Vital signs.

v. tach. Ventricular tachycardia.

VWD. von Willebrand's disease.

VZ. Varicella zoster virus.

W

w. Week *or* Weight.

WA. While awake.

WB. Weight bearing.

WBC. White blood cell (count).

WBE. Whole blood electrolytes.

W Bld. Whole blood.

WBN. Wellborn nursery.

WC. Ward clerk *or* White count *or* Whooping cough.

WD. Well developed.

W→D. Wet to dry.

WDM. White divorced male.

WDWN-BM. Well-developed, well-nourished black male.

WDWN-WF. Well-developed, well-nourished white female.

WE. Weekend.

WF. White female.

W/. With.

W/I. Within.

wk. Week.

WK. Week.

WM. White male.

WMF. White married female.

WMM. White married male.

WN. Well nourished.

WND. Wound.

W/O. Water in oil *or* Without.

WPW. Wolff-Parkinson-White.

WT. Weight (wt).

W/U. Workup.

W/V. Weight to volume ratio.

X

X. Cross *or* Crossmatch *or* Times.

$\bar{\chi}$. Except.

X3. Orientation as to time, place, and person.

X-ed. Crossed.

XKO. Not knocked out.

XR. x-ray.

XRT. Radiation therapy.

XV. Fifteen.

Z

Z-E. Zollinger-Ellison (syndrome).

ZIG. Zoster serum immune globulin.

ZnO. Zinc oxide.

Other Notations

±	Either positive *or* negative *or* Plus or minus.
>	Greater than.
≥	Greater than or equal to.
<	Caused by *or* Less than.
≤	Less than or equal to.
↑	Elevated *or* Increase.
↓	Decrease *or* Falling.
→	Causes to *or* Results in.
←	Resulted from.
↓↓	Flexor *or* Testes descended.
↑↑	Extensor *or* Positive Babinsky *or* Testes

undescended.

✓	Check.
#	Number *or* pound.
∴	Therefore.
+	Plus *or* Positive *or* Present.
–	Absent *or* Minus *or* Negative.
/	Signifying Per *or* And *or* With.
?	Questionable.
∅	No *or* Not.
@	At.
1°	First degree *or* Primary.
2°	Second degree.
3°	Third degree.
♂	Male.
♀	Female.
■	Deceased male.
●	Deceased female.
□	Living male.
○	Living female *or* Standing *or* Recumbent position *or* Sitting position.
'	Feet *or* Minutes (as in 30').
"	Inches *or* Seconds.
2 × 2	Gauze dressing folded 2" x 2".
4 × 4	Gauze dressing folded 4" x 4".

References

1. Chabner DE. Medical Technology: A Short Course. Philadelphia: WB Saunders Co;1991:156–220.

2. Steves N, Adler J. Introduction to Medical Terminology. Springhouse: Springhouse;1992:252–260.

3. Austrin MG, Austrin HR. Learning Medical Terminology. St. Louis: Mosby Year Book;1991:456–461.

4. Bergman HD. Medical terminology. US Pharm. 1980;1:42–48.

5. Davis NM. Medical Abbreviations: 7000 Conveniences at the Expense of Communication & Safety. Huntington Valley: Davis Associates;1991.

140	100	20
3.8	28	105

Na = 140, Cl = 100, BUN = 20
K = 3.8, CO_2 = 28, glucose = 105

sodium	*chloride*	*BUN*	*glucose*
potassium	*bicarbonate*	*creatines*	

calcium	*protein*	*AST*	*LDH*	*bilirubin*
phosphorous	*albumin*	*ALT*	*Alkalinephos*	

segmented neutrophils	*lymphocytes*	*eosinophils*
banded neutrophils	*monocytes*	*basophils*

hemoglobin	*WBC*
hematocrit	*platlets*

Appendix II: Common Anatomic Terms

Anatomic Planes

Frontal (Coronal Plane). An imaginary line that divides an organ or the body into front and back portions or anterior and posterior portions.

Median (Midsagittal, Midline) Plane. An imaginary plane that passes from the front to the back through the center of the body and divides the body into right and left equal portions.

Sagittal Plane. An imaginary line that divides an organ or the body into a right and left portion.

Transverse Plane. An imaginary line that divides an organ or the body into upper (cranial) and lower (caudal) portions.

Anatomic Positions

Erect. Standing position.

Knee-Chest (Genupectoral). Kneeling with chest resting on same surface.

Lateral Recumbent (Sim's). Lying on left side with thigh and knee drawn up.

Prone. Lying face down.

Reverse Trendelenburg. Lying supine with the *head tilted upward* 45° or less.

Supine (Dorsal). Lying on the back.

Trendelenburg Position. Lying supine with the *head tilted downward* 45° or less.

Regions of the Body
Chest and Abdomen

Axillary. Axillary (armpit) and its borders.

Clavicular. Region on either side of the sternum (breastbone), extending the length of the clavicles (collarbones).

Epigastric. Upper mid area of the abdomen.

Hypochondrium. Right and left areas of the epigastric region.

Hypogastric. Middle region of the lower portion of the abdomen.

Infraclavicular. Region below the clavicles.

Infraspinous. Located below a spinous process.

Infrasternal. Located below the sternum.

Inguinal (Iliac). On either side of the hypogastric region, triangular in shape, also known as the groin area.

Lateral Abdominal. Lying on either side of the umbilical region.

Mammary. Area relating to the breasts.

Pubic. Area near the pubic bone.

Sternal. Region over the front of the sternum.

Subclavian. Region beneath the clavicle.

Subdiaphragmatic (Subphrenic). Located below the diaphragm.

Subingual. Just below the inguinal region.

Supraclavicular. Area above the clavicles.

Suprapubic. Region above the pubic area.

Umbilicus. Umbilical area of the abdomen.

Head

Auricular. Located around the ears.

Buccal. Region pertaining to the cheeks.

Infraorbital. Located immediately beneath or in the floor of the eye.

Mental. Region of the chin.

Occipital. Area relating to the lower back of the head.

Orbital. Region around the orbit or eyes.

Sublingual. Region located beneath the tongue.

Submandibular. Region below the lower jaw.

Submaxillary. Region below the upper jaw.

Submental. Region below the chin.

Supraorbital. Region above the eyebrows.

Posterior Trunk

Coxal. Areas just below the lumbar regions in the back and lateral abdominal regions on either side; they are bordered by gluteal regions (area over the buttocks).

Infrascapular. Area below scapulae (shoulder blades), extending down to the last ribs.

Loin. Part and sides of the body between the ribs and pelvis.

Lumbar. Region immediately below the infrascapular region, extending down to the crest of the ilium.

Medial Region of Back. Central zone of the back, extending from the neck as far down as the base of the sacrum.

Nuchal. Area located at the back of the neck.

Sacroiliac. Area over the sacrum at the base of the median region.

Scapular. Areas on either side covering the scapula.

Suprascapular Region. Region above or in the upper part of the scapula.

Terms for Determining Directions

Abduction. Movement away from the body midline.

Adduction. Movement toward the midline or beyond the body midline.

Anterior. At or near the ventral (front) surface of the body.

Caudal. Toward the lower end of the body (cauda means tail).

Cavity. A hollow part or space in a structure.

Central. Toward the center of the body.

Cranial (Cephalic). Toward the head.

Distal. Away from the point of origin or away from the body.

Eversion. A turning outward.

Extension. The straightening of a limb.

External. Outside.

Flexion. The bending of a limb so that the proximal and distal parts are brought together.

Inferior. Below or beneath some part of a structure.

Internal. Inside.

Inversion. A turning inward.

Lateral. Farther from the midline or to the side of the body.

Medial. Near to or toward the midline.

Palmer. Involving the palm of the hand.

Peripheral. Away from the center of the body.

Posterior. At or near the dorsal (back) surface of the body.

Proximal. Nearest to the point of attachment or to the point of origin.

Superior. Above or over some part of a structure.

Supination. Turning the palmar side upward.

Index

A

Abbreviations A1-1–A1-27

ABGs
See Arterial blood gases

Abdomen
physical examination of 4-14
superficial topography 4-14

Absolute neutrophil count 11-17–11-18

Acetaminophen
pharmacokinetics
See Pharmacokinetics, acetaminophen
poisoning, Matthew-Rumak nomogram for 12-4

Acquired immunodeficiency antibody tests 5-53–5-56
alpha-fetoprotein 5-56
beta$_2$-microglobulin 5-55
ELISA 5-53
erythrocyte sedimentation rate 5-54
lymphocytes 5-54
Western Blot 5-54

Activated partial thromboplastin time
See Coagulation tests, activated partial thromboplastin time

Administration, drugs 7-1–7-7

Admission histories 1-8, 1-10

Adrenal gland diagnostic tests
See specific tests

ACTH stimulation test 5-46, 6-15–6-16

AFP
See Alpha-fetoprotein

AG
See anion gap

Alanine aminotransferase 5-38

Albumin 5-61

Alpha-fetoprotein 5-56

ALT
See Alanine aminotransferase

Alkaline phosphatase 5-38

Alk phos
See Alkaline phosphatase

Aminoglycosides, pharmacokinetics
See Pharmacokinetics, aminoglycosides

Ammonia, laboratory tests 5-40

Amylase, serum 5-37

Anatomic terms A2-1–A2-3

ANC
See Absolute neutrophil count

Anemias, diagnostic tests 5-46–5-49
Also see specific tests

Angiocatheters 7-3

Antithrombin III
See Coagulation tests, antithrombin III

aPTT
See Coagulation tests, activated partial thromboplastin time

Anion gap 5-30

Arterial blood gases 5-27–5-29
oxygen saturation 5-28
partial pressure of carbon dioxide 5-28
partial pressure of oxygen 5-28
pH 5-29

Arteriography 6-62–6-63

Arthrography 6-49

Arthroscopy 6-48–6-49

Aspartate aminotransferase 5-40

AST
See Aspartate aminotransferase

ATIII
See Coagulation tests, antithrombin III

B

C

F

G

H

techniques of 4-1
throat
>See HEENT
vital signs 4-3–4-4
>blood pressure 4-3
>height and weight 4-4
>pulse 4-3
>respiratory rate 4-4
>temperature 4-3

Potassium
>laboratory tests 5-18
>requirements 8-4, 8-7, 8-8
>salt, IV administration guidelines 8-18–8-19
>urine 5-36

Pound to kilogram conversion 11-4–11-5

PPD
>See Tuberculin skin test

PPN
>See Parenteral nutrition

Problem list 13-5–13-6

Procainamide pharmacokinetics
>See Pharmacokinetics, procainamide

Proctoscopy 6-28–6-29

Professional conduct, standards of 2-1–2-9

Prothrombin time
>See Coagulation tests, prothrombin time

Protirelin
>See Thyrotropin releasing hormone test

PT
>See Coagulation tests, prothrombin time

Pulmonary function tests 6-52–6-56

Pulse
>measurement 4-3
>peripheral, recording of 4-16

PVS
>See Peripheral vascular system

Pyelography
>intravenous 6-60–6-61
>retrograde 6-61

Q

Quinidine pharmacokinetics
>See Pharmacokinetics, quinidine

R

RBC count
>See Red blood cell count

Red blood cell count 5-8

Red cell indices 5-9–5-10
>mean corpuscular hemoglobin 5-10
>mean corpuscular hemoglobin concentration 5-10
>mean corpuscular volume 5-9

Rectal exam 4-15–4-16

Renal diagnostic tests 5-35–5-37
>Also see specific tests

Renal scan 6-39–6-40

Respiratory rate, measurement 4-4

Resting energy expenditure calculation 10-2–10-3

Reticulocytes 5-10

Retinal vascular grading systems 6-47

Rheumatologic diagnostic tests 5-53–5-63
>Also see specific tests

S

Salicylates, pharmacokinetics
>See Pharmacokinetics, salicylates

SaO$_2$
>See Oxygen saturation

SBT
>See Serum bactericidal titer

Schlicter's test 5-57

Other Publications from Applied Therapeutics, Inc.:

Drug Interactions & Updates
by Philip D. Hansten and John R. Horn
ISBN 0-8121-1381-0 ISSN 0271-8707

Basic Clinical Pharmacokinetics, 2nd edition.
by Michael E. Winter
ISBN 0-915486-08-3

Bedside Clinical Pharmacokinetics, revised edition.
by Carl C. Peck, Dale P. Conner, and M. Gail Murphy
ISBN 0-915486-10-5

Applied Pharmacokinetics: Principles of Therapeutic Drug Monitoring, 3rd edition.
edited by William E. Evans, Jerome J. Schentag, and William J. Jusko
ISBN 0-915486-15-6

Applied Therapeutics: The Clinical Use of Drugs, 5th edition.
edited by Mary Anne Koda-Kimble and Lloyd Y. Young
ISBN 0-915486-14-8

Handbook of Applied Therapeutics, 2nd edition
by Mary Anne Koda-Kimble, Lloyd Y. Young, Wayne A. Kradjan, and Joseph B. Guglielmo
ISBN 0-915486-16-4

For ordering information contact:
  Applied Therapeutics, Inc.
  P. O. Box 5077
  Vancouver, WA 98668-5077
  (206) 253-7123
  Fax (206) 253-8475